ANESTHESIOLOGY CRITICAL CARE BOARD REVIEW

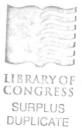

ANESTHESIOLOGY CRITICAL CARE BOARD REVIEW

EDITED BY

George W. Williams, MD, FASA, FCCM, FCCP

ASSOCIATE PROFESSOR OF ANESTHESIOLOGY AND CRITICAL CARE MEDICINE
VICE CHAIR FOR CRITICAL CARE MEDICINE
PROGRAM DIRECTOR, ANESTHESIOLOGY CRITICAL CARE MEDICINE FELLOWSHIP
MEDICAL CO-DIRECTOR, SURGICAL INTENSIVE CARE UNIT
LYNDON B. JOHNSON GENERAL HOSPITAL
HOUSTON, TX, USA

CO-EDITORS

Navneet Kaur Grewal, MD

ASSISTANT PROFESSOR OF ANESTHESIOLOGY AND CRITICAL CARE MEDICINE
ASSISTANT PROGRAM DIRECTOR, ANESTHESIOLOGY CRITICAL CARE
MEDICINE FELLOWSHIP PROGRAM
DIRECTOR OF EDUCATION, MEDICAL/SURGICAL AND
CARDIOVASCULAR INTENSIVE CARE UNITS
MEMORIAL HERMANN SOUTHWEST HOSPITAL
HOUSTON, TX, USA

Marc J. Popovich, MD, FCCM

HELMUT F CASCORBI PROFESSOR AND CHAIR, DEPARTMENT OF ANESTHESIOLOGY
AND PERIOPERATIVE MEDICINE
CASE WESTERN RESERVE UNIVERSITY SCHOOL OF MEDICINE
UNIVERSITY HOSPITALS CLEVELAND MEDICAL CENTER
CLEVELAND, OH, USA

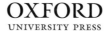

OXFORD
UNIVERSITY PRESS

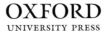

OXFORD
UNIVERSITY PRESS

Oxford University Press is a department of the University of Oxford. It furthers
the University's objective of excellence in research, scholarship, and education
by publishing worldwide. Oxford is a registered trade mark of Oxford University
Press in the UK and certain other countries.

Published in the United States of America by Oxford University Press
198 Madison Avenue, New York, NY 10016, United States of America.

© Oxford University Press 2020

CIP data is on file at the Library of Congress
ISBN 978-0-19-090804-1

This material is not intended to be, and should not be considered, a substitute for medical or other professional advice.
Treatment for the conditions described in this material is highly dependent on the individual circumstances. And, while this
material is designed to offer accurate information with respect to the subject matter covered and to be current as of the time it
was written, research and knowledge about medical and health issues is constantly evolving and dose schedules for medications
are being revised continually, with new side effects recognized and accounted for regularly. Readers must therefore always
check the product information and clinical procedures with the most up-to-date published product information and data
sheets provided by the manufacturers and the most recent codes of conduct and safety regulation. The publisher and the
authors make no representations or warranties to readers, express or implied, as to the accuracy or completeness of this
material. Without limiting the foregoing, the publisher and the authors make no representations or warranties as to the
accuracy or efficacy of the drug dosages mentioned in the material. The authors and the publisher do not accept, and expressly
disclaim, any responsibility for any liability, loss or risk that may be claimed or incurred as a consequence of the use and/or
application of any of the contents of this material.

1 3 5 7 9 8 6 4 2

Printed by Sheridan Books, Inc., United States of America

To God who makes all things possible.

To my beautiful wife and best friend, Erin.

To Eden, Emeri, and Gabriel, who bring immeasurable joy to our lives.

CONTENTS

PREFACE

The *Anesthesiology Critical Care Board Review* was forged as a concept rooted in working to prepare critical care fellow physicians to take and be successful on the American Board of Anesthesiology Critical Care Certification Examination (ABACCCE). This goal is important because it speaks to our purpose as clinicians and educators in preparing the next generation of anesthesiologist intensivists. In my time as a program director (which functionally started in 2011), I found there to be a paucity of materials suited for and tailored to physicians preparing for the examination—in particular, a perioperative and wide-ranging examination such as the ABACCCE. I experienced this myself when I was a recent fellow graduate. As editors of this book, we sought to do everything in our power to prevent others from an anxiety-laden experience resulting from minimal opportunities to practice for a critical care examination with questions written by authors that shared a background in anesthesiology.

It is our hope that, after reading this book, our audience would have learned something new, been able to identify their strengths and weaknesses, and gain a perspective of factual content that is important for a successful clinician and leader in the intensive care unit. The editors and authors put a great deal of effort toward making the questions challenging yet fair, as well as thorough yet straightforward, for the reader. This book was created with the perspective and passion of educators from across the country who hope to make the process of board preparation less stressful and more productive.

Each chapter has been written by an author who actively provides care within the domain of the chapter. Additionally, the editors have endeavored to make the format and style of the questions consistent with an examination's level of difficulty. This book would not have been possible without the hard work of my mentor Dr. Popovich and my partner Dr. Grewal; in this effort, we have generated a lasting partnership focused on education, and they have my thanks. The resulting product is a collective effort of our team, of which I am proud to be a member.

Please allow me to express my gratitude to the physicians and mentors that made this book possible: Dr. Howard Nearman, my chairman during my residency who as an anesthesiologist intensivist inspired me to work as hard as I could to be emulate his example as a compassionate physician and effective leader; my residency program co-directors Dr. Matthew Norcia (another intensivist) and Dr. David Wallace, who strongly encouraged me to pursue a career in critical care; the program director of my fellowship, Dr. Marc Popovich (co-editor), who taught me how to be confident and thorough as an intensivist and provided me with the skills to create and lead a new critical care division at a new institution; my parents, who always insisted that I give 100% effort to everything that I do; my patients, who give me the privilege of caring for them in their darkest hours and who, to this day, teach me something new in my experience of lifelong learning; and finally, my beautiful and incredibly supportive wife and our three children, who sacrificed nights and weekends together to allow this book to come to fruition.

George W. Williams, MD, FASA, FCCM, FCCP

CONTRIBUTORS

Danielle L. Behrens, DO
Assistant Professor of Medicine
Cooper Medical School of Rowan University
Attending Physician
Division of Hematology/Oncology
Department of Medicine
MD Anderson/Cooper Cancer Center
Cooper University Hospital
Camden, NJ, USA

Talia K. Ben-Jacob, MD, MSc
Division Chief of Critical Care Medicine
Department of Anesthesiology
Cooper University Hospital
Assistant Professor of Anesthesiology
Cooper Medical School of Rowan University
Camden, NJ, USA

Robert Brown, MD
Assistant Professor
Department of Neurosurgery
University of Texas Houston Health Science Center
Houston, TX, USA

Jennifer Cortes, PharmD, BCPS, BCCCP
Medical ICU/Respiratory ICU Clinical
    Pharmacy Specialist
Department of Pharmacy Services
Memorial Hermann-Texas Medical Center
Houston, TX, USA

James M. Cross, MD, FACS
Professor of Surgery
McGovern Medical School at UT Health
Medical Director
John S. Dunn Burn Center
Memorial Hermann-Texas Medical Center
Houston, TX, USA

Tonya C. George, PhD, PAC
Physician Assistant
Dallas, TX, USA

Navneet Kaur Grewal, MD
Assistant Professor of Anesthesiology and Critical Care
    Medicine
Assistant Program Director, Anesthesiology Critical Care
    Medicine Fellowship Program
Director of Education, Medical/Surgical and Cardiovascular
    Intensive Care Units
Memorial Hermann Southwest Hospital
Houston, TX, USA

Todd F. Huzar, MD, FACS
Associate Professor
Department of Surgery
McGovern Medical School/UT Health
Houston, TX, USA

Olakunle Idowu, MD
Assistant Professor
Department of Anesthesiology and Perioperative Medicine
Department of Critical Care and Respiratory Care
University of Texas MD Anderson Cancer Center
Houston, TX, USA

Lillian S. Kao, MD, MS
Professor
Department of Surgery
McGovern Medical School at UT Health
Houston, TX, USA

John C. Klick, MD
Associate Professor
Penn State University College of Medicine
Division Chief, Cardiothoracic Anesthesiology
Department of Anesthesiology and Perioperative Medicine
Penn State Milton S. Hershey Medical Center
Hershey, PA, USA

Naveen Kukreja, MD
Assistant Professor
Department of Anesthesiology
University of Colorado
Denver, CO, USA

Ted Lytle, MD
Medical Director
Cardiothoracic Intensive Care University Hospitals
    Cleveland Medical Center
Section Chief Critical Care
Harrington Heart and Vascular Institute University
    Hospitals Cleveland Medical Center
Associate Chief Medical Officer
University Hospitals Cleveland Medical Center
Assistant Professor
Department of Anesthesiology
Case Western Reserve University
Cleveland, OH, USA

Joti Juneja Mucci, MD
Assistant Professor
Case Western Reserve University School of Medicine
Medical Director
Surgical Intensive Care Unit
Program Director
Anesthesiology Critical Care Fellowship
Department of Anesthesiology and Perioperative Medicine
University Hospitals Cleveland Medical Center
Cleveland, OH, USA

Joshua Person, MD
Assistant Professor of Surgery
Division of Acute Care Surgery
Department of Surgery
University of Texas McGovern Medical School at Houston
Houston, TX, USA

Marc J. Popovich, MD, FCCM
Helmut F Cascorbi Professor and Chair
Department of Anesthesiology and Perioperative Medicine
Case Western Reserve University School of Medicine
University Hospitals Cleveland Medical Center
Cleveland, OH, USA

Christopher P. Potestio, MD
Assistant Professor of Anesthesiology
Cooper Medical School of Rowan University
Attending Physician
Division of Critical Care
Department of Anesthesiology
Cooper University Hospital
Camden, NJ, USA

Sophie Samuel, PharmD, BCPS, BCCCP
Critical Care Clinical Specialist, Neurosciences
Department of Pharmacy Services
Memorial Hermann-Texas Medical Center
Houston, TX, USA

George W. Williams, MD, FASA, FCCM, FCCP
Associate Professor of Anesthesiology and Critical
    Care Medicine
Vice Chair for Critical Care Medicine
Program Director, Anesthesiology Critical Care
    Medicine Fellowship
Medical Co-Director, Surgical Intensive Care Unit
Lyndon B. Johnson General Hospital
Houston, TX, USA

Linda W. Young, MD, MS
Critical Care Intensivist
Anesthesiologist
Critical Care Medicine
Halifax Health
Daytona Beach, FL, USA

ANESTHESIOLOGY CRITICAL CARE BOARD REVIEW

1.

CENTRAL NERVOUS SYSTEM

Robert Brown

QUESTIONS

1. A 71-year-old man with a history of heart failure, poorly controlled diabetes, and chronic kidney disease is brought to the emergency department (ED) by his family with altered mental status. He is found to have a serum creatinine of 5.3 mg/dL, blood urea nitrogen (BUN) of 81 mg/dL, glucose of 313 mg/dL, and pH of 7.17. On arrival to the ED, he does not open his eyes but swats your hand away with both arms when you squeeze his trapezius muscles. He moans but does not speak or follow commands. The cranial nerves are intact; however, you notice an irregular breathing pattern of alternating periods of hyperventilation and apnea in a crescendo-decrescendo repeating pattern. Which of the following MOST likely describes this respiratory pattern?

  A. Brainstem injury
  B. Metabolic derangement
  C. Stroke
  D. Seizure

2. An 88-year-old man with a history of heart failure and mild dementia is intubated with a diagnosis of community-acquired pneumonia. He takes donepezil daily. His daughter informs you that he was hospitalized several years ago following a hip fracture and required four-point restraints due to hallucinations, agitation, and injuring a staff member. Which of the following would MOST reduce the risk for a similar issue during this hospitalization?

  A. Avoidance of central alpha agonists
  B. Scheduled haloperidol
  C. Utilization of the ABCDEF bundle
  D. Increased sedation

3. A 67-year-old man is admitted to the intensive care unit (ICU) following a pulseless electrical activity (PEA) arrest with restoration of spontaneous circulation (ROSC) after 17 minutes of cardiopulmonary resuscitation (CPR). Initial examination reveals 3-mm pupils with absent pupillary light reflex bilaterally, absent corneal reflex, and no motor response to pain. He is breathing over the ventilator. He undergoes targeted temperature management with a temperature target of 33° C and is rewarmed slowly after 24 hours. During rewarming, he has diffuse jerking involving spontaneous eye opening and twitching of all four limbs, which are not suppressed with levetiracetam and valproic acid. Which of the following would MOST support a poor prognosis in this patient?

  A. Absent pupillary light reflex before cooling
  B. Bilateral absence of N_2O response with somatosensory evoked potentials (SSEPs)
  C. Early status myoclonus

4. During morning rounds, a 37-year-old patient admitted with severe traumatic brain injury (TBI) now has absent cranial nerve reflexes. On examination, pupils are 5 mm and nonreactive; corneal nerve reflexes, oculocephalic reflex, gag, cough, and motor response to painful stimulation are all absent. The patient's respiratory rate is the same as the prescribed rate on the ventilator. You have reviewed your hospital's brain death policy and confirm that all prerequisites have been met. Which of the following statements is NOT required to declare brain death?

  A. Cerebral blood flow study
  B. Oculovestibular reflex testing (cold calorics)
  C. Normothermia
  D. Lack of vasopressors

5. A 24-year-old female with past medical history significant for polysubstance abuse presents after a witnessed seizure. En route to the hospital, the patient has another seizure and is given 10 mg intramuscular (IM) midazolam. In the ED, she has two more seizures and is given 2 mg intravenous (IV) lorazepam each time, ultimately resulting in intubation with etomidate and rocuronium. What is the next MOST appropriate drug to administer?

A. Propofol
B. Levetiracetam
C. Lacosamide
D. Phenytoin

6. A patient presents with status epilepticus refractory to lorazepam and is intubated in the ED. Convulsive activity stops after treatment with a loading dose of phenytoin and a midazolam infusion. An electroencephalogram (EEG) is obtained and shows frequent epileptiform discharges without seizures. The patient is noted to have a temperature of 38.7° C, and lab results reveal a white blood cell (WBC) count of 18 (80% polymorphonuclear neutrophils [PMNs]). A computed tomography (CT) scan of the head is shown here. What is the next MOST appropriate step?

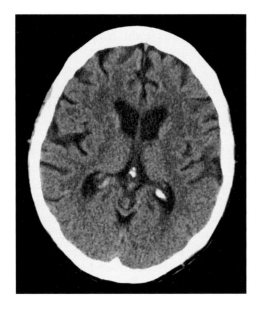

A. Obtain a lumbar puncture
B. Titrate midazolam to obtain a suppression-burst pattern
C. Magnetic resonance imaging (MRI) of the brain with or without contrast
D. Administer vancomycin, ceftriaxone, or acyclovir

7. A 42-year-old male is admitted for sudden onset of severe headache associated with nausea, vomiting, and neck pain. He is otherwise neurologically intact. A CT scan of the brain is completed and shows the following image. What is the next best step in management?

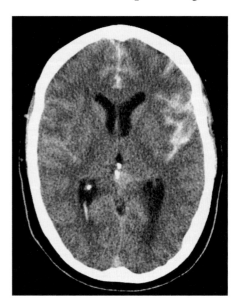

A. Administer levetiracetam
B. Administer nimodipine
C. Ventriculostomy placement
D. CT angiogram of the brain

8. A 62-year-old patient with past medical history of hypertension, hyperlipidemia, type 2 diabetes, and coronary artery disease presents at 5 a.m. with acute onset of confusion. On exam, he has a left gaze preference, has dense right hemiplegia, and is globally aphasic. He was found by his family this morning and was last seen normal at 10 p.m. the previous night. A CT scan of the brain is completed and is remarkable for a dense left middle cerebral artery (MCA) sign with an Alberta Stroke Program Early Computed Tomography (ASPECT) score of 8. What is your next MOST immediate step in management?

A. IV thrombolytics
B. Diffusion-weighted MRI of the brain
C. CT angiogram of the brain with perfusion
D. Aspirin

9. Which of the following is FALSE regarding traumatic intracranial epidural hemorrhage?

A. Good prognosis with early evacuation
B. Biconvex shape
C. Always due to arterial bleeds
D. Most commonly in the temporoparietal region

10. A 53-year-old 70-kg female with a history of myasthenia gravis presents to the ED with dyspnea and worsening dysphagia over the past week. She takes pyridostigmine 90 mg four times daily. On examination, there is weakness of the neck flexors and proximal muscles of the upper extremity, significant dysarthria, and use of accessory muscles of respiration. Forced vital capacity (FVC) is 1 L and negative inspiratory force (NIF) is –17 cm H_2O. Arterial blood gas (ABG) analysis reveals:

pH: 7.42
$PaCO_2$: 37 mm Hg
PaO_2: 90 mm Hg
Hemoglobin saturation: 97% on room air

Which of the following options is the MOST appropriate next step?

A. Close clinical monitoring
B. Endotracheal intubation
C. Prednisone
D. Pyridostigmine

11. A patient with myasthenia gravis on pyridostigmine is admitted with shortness of breath. She is started on biphasic positive airway pressure (BiPAP) with an inspiratory pressure of 12 cm H_2O and expiratory pressure of 5 cm H_2O, with stabilization in her symptoms. She is afebrile and demonstrates no clinical signs of infection. Which of the following is the MOST appropriate next step in this patient's management?

A. High-dose IV methylprednisolone
B. Increased pyridostigmine
C. IV immunoglobulin
D. Levofloxacin

12. A 65-year-old male presents with a 5-day history of progressively worsening mental status and fever. A lumbar puncture is performed, followed by IV vancomycin and ceftriaxone administration. A 20-minute EEG shows periodic lateralized epileptiform discharges (PLEDs). Which diagnostic test would be MOST appropriate to evaluate this patient's condition?

A. CT of the brain with contrast
B. MRI of the brain with contrast
C. Cerebrospinal fluid (CSF) polymerase chain reaction (PCR) testing
D. Continuous EEG

13. A 45-year-old male presents to the ED with progressive lower extremity weakness. The symptoms started 4 days ago with vague tingling in his toes. He denies respiratory symptoms. On exam, his lower extremity strength is 1/5 bilaterally, while his upper extremities are 2/5 distally and 4/5 proximally. Deep tendon reflexes are absent, sensory exam shows partial numbness over all distal extremities without a spinal level, and cranial nerve function is intact. He reports having an upper respiratory illness 1 month ago. He is admitted to the Neurology ICU, where a nerve conduction study/electromyography (NCS/EMG) is performed. What is one of the earliest and MOST sensitive electrophysiological findings in patients with this diagnosis?

A. Absent tibial nerve H reflex
B. Reduced F-wave latency
C. Abnormal sural sensory nerve action potential (SNAP)
D. Absent temporal dispersion of proximal compound muscle action potential (CMAP) responses

14. Which among these are NOT included in the differential diagnosis for a patient presenting with acute flaccid paralysis?

A. Acute poliomyelitis
B. West Nile virus (WNV) meningoencephalitis
C. Critical illness myopathy
D. Charcot-Marie-Tooth syndrome

15. A 37-year-old male suffers a severe asthma attack that results in cardiac arrest. ROSC is achieved in the field, and hypothermia is initiated in the ED. The patient undergoes controlled rewarming on day 2; however, overnight he becomes hypotensive, and norepinephrine is started to maintain mean arterial pressure (MAP) above 60 mm Hg. Over the course of the night, the patient's vasopressor requirement increases significantly, and loss of cranial nerve reflexes is noted. Serum sodium increased from 142 mEq/L the day before to 159 mEq/L currently. Urine output has been 300 to 500mL/hour for the past several hours. Which of the following is the next BEST step?

A. D_5W infusion
B. Isotonic fluid bolus
C. Urine osmolality
D. Brain death testing

16. A 42-year-old female with a history of IV drug abuse presents to the ED complaining of severe back pain. She is reluctant to participate in the neurological examination because of shooting pain with movement; however, she does not seem to have weakness or sensory loss. She denies bowel or bladder dysfunction and is afebrile. Laboratory findings include:

WBC count: 11.2×10^3
Hemoglobin: 12.6 g/dL
Hematocrit: 37%
Platelets: 214×10^9/L

Which of the following is the MOST appropriate next step in management?

A. Urgent MRI of the cervical, thoracic, and lumbar spine
B. No further workup because she is likely drug-seeking
C. Cervical radiograph
D. Lumbar puncture

17. A 57-year-old is involved in a high-speed motor vehicle collision. In the ED, the patient is quadriplegic, breath sounds are shallow, and O_2 saturation is 88% on a non-rebreather mask. The patient undergoes endotracheal intubation, and a CT scan of the spine shows bilateral facet dislocations at C5–6. The patient is taken emergently to the operating room for spinal stabilization and is now admitted to the ICU for further management. On arrival, the patient is awake and alert but has no movement or sensation below the deltoids. Which of the following is FALSE?

A. MAP should be maintained above 85 mm Hg
B. The patient can be safely extubated
C. IV glucocorticoids are not recommended
D. The long-term prognosis for ambulation is poor

18. A 32-year-old male is admitted with severe TBI. Admission Glasgow Coma Scale (GCS) score is 6T; admission CT scan is shown here. A ventriculostomy is in place for intracranial pressure (ICP) monitoring. He is sedated with propofol and fentanyl with an ICP of 15 mm Hg and MAP of 66 mm Hg. He is intubated and mechanically ventilated on assist control mode with a respiratory rate of 20 breaths/minute and tidal volume of 500 mL. The patient's ABG reveals a pH of 7.49, $PaCO_2$ of 29 mm Hg, and PaO_2 of 113 mm Hg. The patient's brain tissue oxygen monitor reads 13 mm Hg; hemoglobin is 7.2 g/dL. Which of the following is LEAST likely to improve the patient's brain tissue oxygenation?

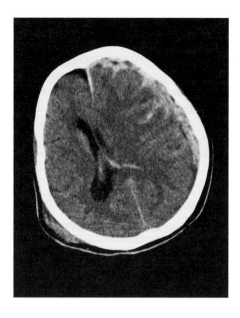

A. Decreasing sedation
B. Reducing the patient's minute ventilation
C. Cerebral perfusion pressure (CPP) augmentation with norepinephrine
D. Red blood cell (RBC) transfusion

19. In a patient with severe TBI undergoing multimodality monitoring, which of the following MOST suggests an increased risk for further neuronal injury?

A. EEG reactivity to painful stimuli
B. Decreased jugular venous bulb O_2 saturation
C. Decreased cerebral lactate-to-pyruvate ratio
D. ICP of 25 mm Hg

20. A 62-year-old female with a history of hypertension, dyslipidemia, and type 2 diabetes mellitus is undergoing a diagnostic cardiac catheterization. She receives 2 mg of IV midazolam before the procedure. Twenty minutes into the procedure, the patient is noted to be unresponsive, although she is breathing well. A closer examination shows that the patient does not open her eyes to stimulation, her pupils are 1.5 mm and reactive, and the left eye is lower than the right eye. The left upper extremity weakly withdraws to noxious stimulation, and there is no motor response on the right. What is the MOST likely cause of the patient's clinical symptoms?

A. Left frontal lobe intracerebral hemorrhage (ICH)
B. Brainstem infarction
C. Left lacunar infarction
D. Oversedation

21. A 50-year-old female admitted with moderate TBI and small bifrontal contusions is found acutely unresponsive by a nurse. Her vital signs are as follows:

Heart rate: 93 bpm
Blood pressure: 162/82 mm Hg
Respiratory rate: 18 breaths/minute (on mechanical ventilation)
Temperature: 99.1° F

The patient localizes bilaterally, opens eyes to sternal rub, has equal and reactive pupils, and has intact gag/cough and corneal reflexes. The patient then has a sudden clinical deterioration manifested by extension in all extremities with a 5-mm nonreactive left pupil. After emergent intubation, what is the next MOST appropriate management?

A. Mannitol
B. Levetiracetam
C. Dexamethasone
D. Hypertonic saline 23.4%

22. A 27-year-old female, G_1P_{1001} at 34 weeks' gestational age, is brought to the ED after she had a witnessed generalized tonic-clonic convulsion at home. She has no prior medical history. Her blood pressure is 163/102 mm Hg. She slowly regains consciousness but has no focal neurological deficits. What would be the MOST appropriate next step in management of this patient?

A. Diazepam
B. Fosphenytoin
C. Magnesium sulfate
D. Levetiracetam

23. A 57-year-old female with no known medical history presents after being found in a confused state by family members. On examination, she is afebrile and appears cachectic and with poor dentition. Neurological examination demonstrates aphasia and a right facial droop. Cardiac examination reveals normal S1 and S2 without murmurs. A CT scan shows an ovoid lesion with surrounding vasogenic edema in the left parietal lobe, which is concerning for cerebral metastasis versus abscess. Which of the following features MOST favor cerebral abscess over metastasis?

A. Rim enhancement
B. Multiple lesions
C. Restricted diffusion on diffusion-weighted imaging (DWI)
D. Vasogenic edema that spares the cortex

24. A 34-year-old woman with a history of a prolactinoma presents to the ED with thunderclap headache. The CT scan of the brain is read as normal. She is drowsy but follows commands and has no focal neurological deficits. Shortly after admission to the ICU, she complains of lightheadedness and is noted to have a blood pressure of 77/40 mm Hg. Serum sodium is 132 mEq/L, and urine output is 80 to 100 mL/hour since admission. Which of the following is the BEST initial treatment?

A. Vasopressin
B. Hydrocortisone
C. Hypertonic saline 3%
D. Norepinephrine infusion

25. A 67-year-old man with a history of hypertension is "found down" by his neighbors. A CT scan of the brain shows ICH in the left basal ganglia (see the following image). His blood pressure is 210/120 mm Hg. On neurological examination, the patient is alert, follows simple commands, and answers simple questions. He extends his right arm and strongly follows with the left arm. The patient's home medications include aspirin and lisinopril. Which of the following is the next BEST step in management?

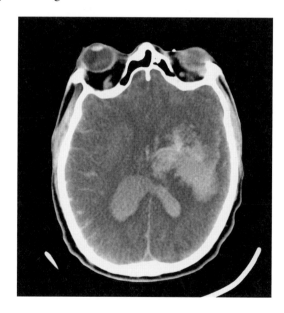

A. Emergent craniotomy and hematoma evacuation
B. Nicardipine infusion
C. Factor VIIa
D. Emergent cerebral angiogram

26. On your rounds, you visit a 49-year-old male who is post-bleed day 6 from an aneurysmal subarachnoid hemorrhage. The patient had an external ventricular drain (EVD) placed on admission for hydrocephalus and then underwent coiling of an anterior communicating artery aneurysm. The clinical course has been unremarkable; however, your resident tells you that the patient's transcranial Doppler ultrasound exams from this morning were abnormal. The results include:

Left MCA velocity: 156 cm/second
Right MCA velocity: 207 cm/second

On examination, you now note a right-sided facial droop and new pronator drift. Which of the following is the MOST appropriate management at this time?

A. Maintenance fluids
B. Vasopressors
C. MRI
D. Brain CT with angiography

27. A 57-year-old female with a history of smoking and hypertension presents with thunderclap headache. On arrival, she does not open her eyes to pain, moans, and localizes bilaterally. A CT scan shows diffuse cisternal subarachnoid hemorrhage with mild hydrocephalus. She is intubated for airway protection, and an external ventriculostomy drain is placed. A CT angiogram is performed that shows a left posterior communicating artery aneurysm. She arrives to the ICU in the evening and is scheduled for a cerebral angiogram in the morning. Which of the following treatments is MOST indicated?

A. Vasopressors
B. Avoidance of antifibrinolytics
C. Phenytoin
D. EVD drainage

ANSWERS

1. ANSWER: B

An often overlooked component of the neurological examination is the patient's respiratory pattern. This is largely because the patient's natural respiratory pattern can be obscured by mechanical ventilation. However, two patterns are commonly seen in the ICU but are often misunderstood. These patterns are post-hyperventilation apnea and Cheyne-Stokes respirations. Cheyne-Stokes respirations can be quite dramatic when observed, and if not familiar with the pattern, healthcare providers usually impute this to a severe structural brain abnormality. However, this is almost never the case. To understand Cheyne-Stokes respiration requires an understanding of post-hyperventilation apnea. While the medullary respiratory center is responsible for controlling the respiratory drive, the frontal lobes have hegemony over the process (this is why one can hold one's breath under water but may hyperventilate when nervous). When a patient is hypocapnic, rather than an apneic period until CO_2 is normalized, the respiratory rate is simple slowed, and tidal volumes are decreased to allow CO_2 to return to normal more gradually. If the frontal lobes are damaged or malfunctioning owing to a systemic process causing encephalopathy (much more common), apnea is commonly seen following periods of hypocapnia. This can be observed by asking an encephalopathic patient to take several deep breaths and observing for apnea; however, in day-to-day practice, apnea is typically encountered in anxious or agitated patients who are causing apnea alarms on a ventilator during spontaneous breathing trials. Instead of returning to an assisted mode of ventilation and delaying extubation, the amount of pressure support can be reduced to avoid large tidal volumes, and the patient can be directed to relax, or other measures to control agitation can be employed. The apnea alarm on the ventilator can also be extended. However, the best way to solve this issue is to extubate the patient. Cheyne-Stokes is a more extreme version of post-hyperventilation apnea and results from a delay between alveolar CO_2 and the partial pressure of CO_2 in the medullary interstitium such that the brain is always trying to "catch up" to the alveolar CO_2. Low-output states can exacerbate this condition because changes in alveolar CO_2 take much longer to reach the medullary respiratory centers. Many clinicians, after observing a patient with this respiratory pattern, assume a severe structural or brainstem injury when in fact the pattern demonstrates intact brainstem reflexes, as is the case with this patient. Respiratory patterns that are reflective of brainstem pathology include apneustic breathing (inspiratory pauses, seen with pontine injuries), ataxic breathing (irregular pattern, seen with rostral medullary lesions), and apnea (seen with caudal medullary lesions). These are typically not observed (with the exception of apnea) owing to early intubation and mechanical ventilation in patients with these brain injuries. This patient's active heart failure with signs of end-organ dysfunction is more likely the cause of this patient's presentation.

Keywords: Central nervous system (CNS) diagnosis; Altered mental status (coma)

REFERENCE

Posner JB, Saper, CB, Schiff ND, Plum F. *Plum and Posner's diagnosis of stupor and coma,* 4th ed. New York: Oxford University Press; 2007, pp. 46–52.

2. ANSWER: C

Delirium is associated with increased mortality, prolonged ICU and hospital length of stay, and post-ICU cognitive impairment. A multifaceted approach should be implemented for its prevention, detection, and treatment. One method is the ABCDEF bundle. This is an acronym for pain **a**ssessment and utilization of **a**nalgesics, daily **a**wakening and spontaneous **b**reathing trials, **c**hoosing an appropriate sedation strategy, employing a delirium **d**etection method, **e**arly mobilization, and **f**amily engagement. Daily awakening periods with interruption of sedatives and spontaneous breathing trials (SBTs) have been shown to decrease delirium incidence and ventilator and ICU lengths of stay. Indeed, a randomized controlled trial of daily sedation interruptions (frequently called "holidays") with SBTs demonstrated reductions in ICU and hospital lengths of stay of 3.8 and 4.3 days, respectively. Benzodiazepines may lead to delirium and prolonged ventilator and ICU lengths of stay, while sedation with dexmedetomidine may have the opposite effect. Depth of sedation should be monitored with an appropriate sedation scale (e.g., Richmond Agitation and Sedation Scale), and sedatives should be regularly titrated to achieve a lighter level of sedation. Additionally, CAM-ICU is a simple assessment tool used to detect delirium and has been shown to have a high sensitivity and specificity. Once delirium has been detected, one can then review potential causes and address them accordingly. Results of trials investigating antipsychotic medication have not been conclusive, although the recent REDUCE trial demonstrated that prophylactic haloperidol (1 or 2 mg) is not effective in preventing delirium. Typical antipsychotics such as haloperidol are not recommended, while atypical antipsychotics should be used only when other measured have failed. Early mobilization has been shown to reduce delirium as well as improve functional status at discharge, likely by reducing the incidence of ICU-acquired weakness. Mobilization and exercise with physical and occupational therapy can be paired with the patient's daily sedation holiday and breathing trial. Restraints, while often necessary to avoid self-extubation or removal of other life-sustaining medical devices (e.g., ventriculostomies), can agitate patients and exacerbate delirium and their use should be minimized.

Keywords: CNS diagnoses; Altered mental status (delirium, hallucinations)

REFERENCES

Barr J, Fraser GL, Puntillo K et al. Clinical practice guidelines for the management of pain, agitation, and delirium in adult patients in the intensive care unit. *Crit Care Med* 2013;41:263–306.
Girard TD, Kress JP, Fuchs, BD et al. Efficacy and safety of a paired sedation and ventilator weaning protocol for mechanically ventilated patients in intensive care (Awakening and Breathing Controlled trial): a randomized controlled trial. *Lancet* 2008;12:126–134.
Morandi A, Brummel NE, Ely EW. Sedation, delirium and mechanical ventilation: the "ABCDE" approach. *Curr Opin Crit Care* 2011;17:43–49.
van den Boogaard M, Slooter AJC, Brüggemann RJM et al. Effect of haloperidol on survival among critically ill adults with a high risk of delirium: The REDUCE Randomized Clinical Trial. *JAMA* 2018;319(7):680–690.

3. ANSWER: B

Prognostication following cardiac arrest is complex and is most accurate when utilizing a multimodal approach. Some features have been consistently associated with a poor prognosis and can thus be used with a high degree of confidence. These include absent pupillary light reflexes at 72 hours and bilateral absence of N_2O response during SSEP testing; loss of N_2O is defined as no negative deflection 20 seconds after stimulation on both sides. Of note, automated methods of assessing pupillary light reflex have been developed and tested and may be expected to be seen more often in the coming years. Other features may be strongly associated but have lower specificity and should therefore not be used as the sole indictor of poor prognosis. These include early (within the first 48 hours) status myoclonus, neuroimaging features (other than frank herniation), and malignant EEG findings. Neuroimaging features associated with poor prognosis include loss of gray-white differentiation and sulcal effacement on CT imaging, and restricted diffusion on MRI. Of note, patchy or regional abnormalities, including isolated basal ganglia abnormalities, do not preclude neurological recovery. Malignant EEG findings that augur poor prognosis include suppression or a suppression-burst pattern, absent reactivity, and low voltage. Hypothermia and sedatives can confound the EEG; thus, the patient should be normothermic and off sedation. Serum biomarkers have also been used, with neuron-specific enolase being the most studied. However, studies have demonstrated a range of

thresholds that predict poor prognosis with high specificity, which has limited their clinical utility.

Keywords: CNS diagnosis; AMS; Other (hypoxic/metabolic encephalopathy); CNS; Diagnostic modalities; Evoked potential; CNS; Diagnostic modalities; EEG

REFERENCES

Oddo M, Rossetti AO. Early multimodal outcome prediction after cardiac arrest in patients treated with hypothermia. *Crit Care Med* 2014;42:1340–1347.
Sandroni C, Cariou A, Cavallaro F et al. Prognostication in comatose survivors of cardiac arrest: an advisory statement from the European Resuscitation Council and the European Society of Intensive Care Medicine. *Resuscitation* 2014;85:1779–1789.
Solari D, Rossetti AO, Carteron L et al. Early prediction of coma recovery after cardiac arrest with blinded pupillometry. *Ann Neurol* 2017;81(6):804–810.

4. ANSWER: D

While guidelines have been published for brain death declaration, some details are left to the discretion of individual hospitals. In general, however, the first step in declaring brain death is confirming that all prerequisites have been met and that there are no confounding factors. This involves knowing the cause of injury and having that be compatible with causing brain death. For example, severe Guillain-Barré syndrome (GBS) has mimicked brain death, including absent cranial nerve reflexes, absent motor response, and failed apnea testing. A brain death examination would incorrectly diagnose brain death, yet cerebral function might be normal. A patient who is "found down" with an unknown cause of injury should be approached cautiously. Severe metabolic derangements should be excluded because these may confound the examination, although what defines a severe derangement is mostly left to the provider. The patient should be adequately resuscitated, normothermic, and normotensive (although vasopressors to achieve normotension do not preclude the ability to declare brain death). Brain imaging compatible with brain death is not mandatory but is performed almost universally. For example, in a patient with anoxic brain injury, imaging demonstrating herniation and diffuse loss of gray-white differentiation is not required and often not present because CT imaging may be performed before the development of cerebral edema; however, a CT scan obtained on day 4 without evidence of anoxic injury would not be consistent with brain death. Medications that may confound the examination, including benzodiazepines, barbiturates, and opiates, should be held, and testing should be delayed until these medications have been fully metabolized. The brain death examination should demonstrate lack of response to simulation, absent pupillary light reflex, corneal reflex, oculocephalic reflex, oculovestibular reflex, gag reflex, cough reflex, and motor response. Finally, a formal apnea test should be performed to demonstrate no respiratory effort despite an arterial $PaCO_2$ higher than 60 mm Hg (or 20 mm Hg above baseline in patients with chronic CO_2 retention). This is typically performed by disconnecting the patient from the ventilator and providing continuous oxygen through a catheter inserted into the endotracheal tube (passive oxygenation). Patients may become hypotensive during apnea testing as acidosis develops; however, this can be managed with vasopressor titration and does not usually prevent one from completing the test. Because brain death is a clinical diagnosis, ancillary tests are not required unless part of the clinical examination cannot be performed. It is also for this reason that one should use the term "ancillary test" rather than "confirmatory test" to avoid the misconception that the brain death examination requires confirmation. Acceptable ancillary tests include EEG, transcranial Doppler ultrasound, catheter angiography, and cerebral blood flow testing using single photon emission computed tomography (SPECT). The latter is typically the most commonly used test because of its availability and ease of performance. Importantly, while brain death is considered "whole brain death," certain features such as absence of diabetes insipidus and blood pressure variability do not preclude the diagnosis.

Keywords: CNS; Diagnoses; Brain death; Basic physiology; CNS; Brain death; CNS; Diagnostic modalities; Nuclear medicine studies

REFERENCES

Bonetti MG, Ciritella P, Valle G, Perrone E. 99mTc HM-PAO brain perfusion SPECT in brain death. *Neuroradiology* 1995;37(5):365.
Wijdicks EF, Varelas PN, Gronseth GS et al. Evidence-based guideline update: determining brain death in adults. A report of the Quality Standards Subcommittee of the American Academy of Neurology. *Neurology* 2010;74:1911–1918.

5. ANSWER: D

Status epilepticus is defined as a seizure duration of greater than 5 minutes or recurrent seizures without return to baseline. Benzodiazepines, including midazolam (IV or IM) and lorazepam (IV), have the highest efficacy and are thus first-line agents to arrest a seizure. Phenytoin is an appropriate second-line agent. Phenytoin can cause hypotension if infused too quickly and also has the risk for skin necrosis if the infusion infiltrates, a condition known as purpleglove syndrome. For these reasons, a recent guideline has recommended fosphenytoin, a prodrug of phenytoin, if available because it can be infused rapidly. Fosphenytoin is

hydrolyzed to phenytoin by serum phosphatases with a conversion half-time of 15 minutes; the loading dose is 20 mg/kg (considered phenytoin equivalents) and is infused at a rate of 100 to 150 mg/minute. It should be noted that while hypotension is less likely to be seen with phosphenytoin, it may still be occur, and hemodynamic monitoring remains indicated.

Levetiracetam can be considered in this case, but evidence for its efficacy in aborting status epilepticus is unclear. An appropriate dose per guidelines is 20 to 60 mg/kg, up to a maximum of 4500 mg. The mechanism of action for levetiracetam is not known, although it is hypothesized to modulate GABA receptors indirectly and bind to protein SV2A (which has been linked to seizures in animal models). Since levetiracetam does not induce CYP, it has minimal interactions with other drugs such as immunosuppressants, and IV to oral dosing and bioequivalence are identical.

Lacosamide works by helping inactivate sodium channels, thereby preventing repetitive firing of neurons, and it can be used to treat focal-onset seizures; unfortunately, lacosamide has no role in treating generalized status epilepticus. If the patient does not respond to phenytoin, while second-line alternatives or third-line agents such as valproic acid and phenobarbital are acceptable, an infusion of midazolam or propofol has a higher likelihood of aborting the status epilepticus.

Keywords: CNS; Diagnoses; Seizures and status epilepticus; CNS; Management strategies; Anticonvulsants

REFERENCES

Chokshi R, Openshaw J, Mehta N, Mohler E. Purple glove syndrome following intravenous phenytoin administration. *Vasc Med* 2007;12:29–31.
Glauser T, Shinnar S, Gloss D et al. Evidence-based guideline: treatment of convulsive status epilepticus in children and adults: a report of the guideline committee of the American epilepsy society. *Epilepsy Currents* 2016;16:48–61.

6. ANSWER: D

Antibiotics to cover both bacterial meningitis and herpes encephalitis are indicated. Ceftriaxone would cover the most likely bacterial agents (*Streptococcus pneumoniae*, *Haemophilus influenzae*, and *Neisseria meningitidis*), while vancomycin would cover beta-lactam-resistant pneumococcus. Acyclovir would cover herpes encephalitis. Ampicillin would be added in immunocompromised or elderly patients or to cover *Listeria monocytogenes*. Additionally, it is appropriate to include dexamethasone until pneumococcal meningitis is ruled out because this may improve mortality and reduce neurological sequalae.

Glucocorticoids should be administered shortly before (or at the same time as) antibiotics because this approach has been shown to reduce unfavorable outcomes. It is hypothesized that glucocorticoid administration (usually dexamethasone) reduces cerebral edema as well as cytokine levels in the CSF. A lumbar puncture should be performed ideally within 6 hours of starting treatment in order to improve yield from cultures. A diagnosis on the basis of the CSF profile can still be made if the lumbar puncture is delayed more than 6 hours but may yield less useful information, especially in cases of meningococcal meningitis. While a CT scan was appropriate in this patient, it is not necessary in most patients and if performed often leads to an unnecessary delay in treatment, as would waiting for results of the lumbar puncture. Continuous EEG monitoring should be applied because the patient could be having subclinical events; however, starting treatment for the likely infection is of utmost importance. The advantage of titrating sedation to a suppression-burst pattern if the patient is no longer seizing is unclear and thus would not be the most appropriate next step in this patient. The head CT shown is normal, and while an MRI would likely assist with diagnosis and prognosis, it would be the last step in the management of this patient.

Keywords: CNS; Diagnoses; Infectious; Encephalitis/meningitis; CNS; Diagnostic modalities; EEG; CNS; Diagnostic modalities; Lumbar puncture; CNS; Management strategies; Antimicrobials

REFERENCE

Hasbun R, Abrahams J, Jekel J, Quagliarelllo VJ. Computed tomography of the head before lumbar puncture in adults with suspected meningitis. *N Engl J Med* 2001;345:1727.

7. ANSWER: B

The patient has spontaneous subarachnoid hemorrhage (SAH), which is most commonly caused by a ruptured aneurysm. SAH affects nearly 30,000 patients in the United States each year and has a mortality rate of around 45%. CT angiography of the brain will assist both in accurate diagnosis and surgical planning if an aneurysm is found. The yield of CT angiography in aneurysmal detection is approximately 95% when compared with digital subtraction angiography. This makes it a quick and important step in the workup before surgical interventions. Although seizure prophylaxis is commonly used for patients with SAH, there are no studies suggesting that it improves outcomes. Furthermore, there is evidence demonstrating that long-term treatment with

anticonvulsants may lead to worse cognitive outcomes, although these studies were performed with phenytoin. It should be noted that generalized status epilepticus has an incidence of 0.2%, but *nonconvulsive* status epilepticus occurs 31% of the time when SAH patients have stupor or coma; such seizures are associated with poor neurological outcome. Nimodipine may improve neurological outcomes and reduce the incidence of cerebral infarctions in patients with aneurysmal SAH but does not reduce the actual rate of vasospasm. Nimodipine is normally administered in doses of 60 mg every 4 hours and can be given less frequently in smaller doses when hypotension is seen after administration. The most important first step in a patient with SAH is to prevent aneurysmal rebleeding. This is done by surgical clipping or endovascular coiling. There is no clear evidence that dexamethasone is beneficial.

Keywords: CNS; Diagnoses; Stroke; Hemorrhagic (SAH); Diagnostic modalities; Other imaging (e.g., CTA)

REFERENCES

Diringer MN, Bleck TP, Claude Hemphill J 3rd et al. Critical care management of patients following aneurysmal subarachnoid hemorrhage: recommendations from the Neurocritical Care Society's Multidisciplinary Consensus Conference. *Neurocrit Care* 2011;15:211–240.

Dorhout Mees S, Rinkel GJE, Feigin VL et al. Calcium antagonists for aneurysmal subarachnoid haemorrhage. *Cochrane Database Syst Rev* 2007;(3):CD000277.

Feigin VL, Anderson N, Rinkel GJE et al. Corticosteroids for aneurysmal subarachnoid haemorrhage and primary intracerebral haemorrhage. *Cochrane Database Syst Rev* 2005;(3):CD004583.

Kelliny M, Maeder P, Binaghi S et al. Cerebral aneurysm exclusion by CT angiography based on subarachnoid hemorrhage pattern: a retrospective study. *BMC Neurol* 2018;11: 8.

8. ANSWER: C

The ASPECTS score was used to predict outcome with thrombolytic use and demonstrated improved outcomes in patients with scores of 8 or higher. Patients with "wake-up stroke" such as this one often present outside of the acceptable window for administration of IV thrombolytics (up to 4.5 hours from last seen normal). This does not, however, exclude them from receiving treatment for their stroke by endovascular modalities, and the ASPECT score is one modality that has been used in selecting patients who may have favorable outcome with mechanical thrombectomy. A recent study known as the DAWN trial demonstrated that mechanical thrombectomy improves outcome in patients presenting 6 to 24 hours from when they were last seen normal who still have a mismatch between clinical deficits and infarct volume. In this case, the patient's neurological symptoms and dense MCA sign (hyperdensity of the MCA) suggest a proximal occlusion of the MCA. CT angiography of the brain would confirm this, while a CT perfusion study would assess for a "mismatch" between infarcted, and hence unsalvageable tissue (the core) and ischemic but not yet infarcted tissue (penumbra). While MRI of the brain is indicated to diagnose the location and size of the infarct, revascularization strategies are paramount and can usually be accomplished faster with the CT perfusion route over an MRI. Although aspirin is indicated for patients not receiving IV tissue plasminogen activator, revascularization has primacy in the management of acute ischemic stroke.

Keywords: CNS; Diagnoses; Stroke; Embolic/thrombotic and ischemic

REFERENCES

Aviv RI, Mandelcorn J, Chakraborty S et al. Alberta Stroke Program Early CT scoring of CT perfusion in early stroke visualization and assessment. *Am J Neuroradiol* 2007;28:1975–1980.
Hill MD, Rowley HA, Adler F et al. ASPECTS score to select patients for endovascular treatment: the IMS-III trial. *Stroke* 2014;45(2):444–449.
Nogueira RG, Jadhav AP, Haussen DC et al. Thrombectomy 6 to 24 hours after stroke with a mismatch between deficit and infarct. *N Engl J Med* 2018;378:11–21.
Ryu CW, Shin HS, Park S et al. Alberta Stroke Program Early CT score in the prognostication after endovascular treatment for ischemic stroke: a meta-analysis. *Neurointervention* 2017;12.1:20–30.

9. ANSWER: C

Although epidural hemorrhages are commonly arterial in nature and secondary to shearing of meningeal arteries, occasionally an epidural hemorrhage can form as a result venous bleeding such as a torn venous sinus with an associated skull fracture. About 15% of the time, an injury to one of the dural sinuses is the source be of the hemorrhage. More than 95% of epidural hemorrhages are supratentorial, and about 85% are associated with the presence of a skull fracture. The temporoparietal region is the most common location, and most result from tearing of the middle meningeal artery. Although patients can decompensate rapidly, prognosis is good if surgical evacuation is carried out promptly, and most patients make full neurological recovery with no residual deficits. In contrast to subdural hematomas, epidural hematomas typically do not cross suture lines owing to the tight adherence of the dura to the skull at these points. Additionally, from a test-taking strategy perspective, the word "always" *may* be a warning that the answer is a trap.

Keywords: CNS; Diagnoses; Epidural hemorrhage

REFERENCE

Bullock MR, Chesnut R, Ghajar J et al. Surgical management of acute epidural hematomas. Surgical Management of Traumatic Brain Injury Author Group. *Neurosurgery* 2006;58(3 Suppl):S7.

10. ANSWER: B

Patients in myasthenic crisis should be admitted urgently to an ICU because they can decompensate rapidly. Frequent respiratory assessments with FVC and NIF are essential. Indications for intubation in patients with myasthenic crisis include FVC ≤15 mL/kg (normal, ≥60 mL/kg), NIF ≤20 cm H_2O (normal, ≥70 cm H_2O), and peak expiratory flow (PEF) 40 cm H_2O (normal, ≥100 cm H_2O). ABG is not a reliable guide to determine need for intubation because this can remain normal just before respiratory collapse. Endotracheal intubation is best performed electively before this. Several studies have shown BiPAP to be effective in patients with myasthenic crises because it can reduce rates of intubation and decrease lengths of stay. However, BiPAP should be used on a case-by-case basis. Hypercapnia predicts BiPAP failure and should warrant immediate intubation. Severe bulbar dysfunction and difficulty managing secretions are a contraindication to BiPAP.

Pyridostigmine has a rapid onset of action with peak action at 2 hours, but because of the bulbar signs of weakness exhibited by this patient, this would not be the immediate optimal management strategy given information presented in this vignette. High-dose glucocorticoids can be helpful in management of myasthenia gravis in general; however, the clinical effect can take 2 to 3 weeks to become optimal, and nearly 50% of patients can experience deterioration about a week after glucocorticoids are initiated. Therefore, steroids do not have an immediate role when respiratory insufficiency is being urgently addressed.

Keywords: CNS; Management strategies; Plasmapheresis; CNS; Diagnoses; Neuromuscular disease; Myasthenia gravis

REFERENCES

Jani-Acsadi A, Lisak RP. Myasthenic crisis: guidelines for prevention and treatment. *J Neurol Sci* 2007;261(1–2):127–133.
Seneviratne J, Mandrekar J, Wijdicks EF, Rabinstein AA. Noninvasive ventilation in myasthenic crisis. *Arch Neurol* 2008;65(1):54–58.

11. ANSWER: C

About 20% of patient with a diagnosis of myasthenia gravis present at some point with myasthenic crisis.

Myasthenic crisis can be associated with acute respiratory failure from fatigue of the diaphragm. Clinical examination of face for eyelid weakness, bulbar weakness (i.e., difficulty swallowing, fatigue with chewing), tachypnea with a paradoxical respiratory pattern, and limb weakness are clinical signs consistent with myasthenic crisis. Monitoring of vital capacity and negative inspiratory force can help establish a threshold for preemptive intubation. The threshold for intubation in myasthenic crisis is generally agreed to be an FVC of <15 mL/kg or an NIF of <20 cm H_2O.

IV immunoglobulin and plasmapheresis are both treatments of choice in patients with myasthenic crisis because studies have not demonstrated clear superiority of one over the other. Plasmapheresis is likely to work more quickly, whereas IV immunoglobulin may have a lower incidence of serious side effects. In addition to myasthenic crisis, plasma exchange also has a role before and after thymectomy and at the start of immunosuppressive drug therapy. The volume and number of plasma exchanges indicated for the treatment of myasthenic crisis are not rigid, but treatment is generally planned for several exchanges each of 2 to 3.5 L, with a goal amount of around 125 mL/kg; these exchanges are commonly performed over a week. In general, a 2-L exchange will remove 80% of circulating antibodies, although there is not a tight correlation between a reduction in antibodies and the degree of clinical improvement. Because the sensitivity to anticholinesterase drugs may be increased after plasma exchange, they should be held and their dosage adjusted as the patient recovers respiratory function.

Steroids, if used by themselves in myasthenic crisis, can cause transient worsening of symptoms. If the patient is already intubated and on mechanical ventilation, there is little downside to starting steroids; however, in patients who are not intubated, steroids should be started at a low dose and titrated slowly as needed. Pyridostigmine has little role in the management of myasthenic crisis and can increase airway secretions and are thus often held initially.

Keywords: CNS; Diagnoses; Neuromuscular disease; Myasthenia gravis; CNS; Management strategies; Steroids

REFERENCES

Barth D, Nabavi Nouri M, Ng E et al. Comparison of IVIg and PLEX in patients with myasthenia gravis. *Neurology* 2011;76(23):2017–2023.
Bershad EM, Feen ES, Suarez JI. Myasthenia gravis crisis. *South Med J* 2008;101(1):63–69.
Jani-Acsadi A, Lisak RP. Myasthenic crisis: guidelines for prevention and treatment. *J Neurol Sci* 2007;261(1-2):127–133.
Ropper AH, Samuels MA, Klein JP. Myasthenia gravis and related disorders of the neuromuscular junction. In: Ropper AH, Samuels MA, Klein JP, eds. *Adams and Victor's principles of neurology*, 10th ed. New York: McGraw-Hill; 2014.

12. ANSWER: C

This patient likely has herpes simplex virus encephalitis (HSE) secondary to herpes simplex virus type 1 (HSV 1). Morbidity and mortality are high especially if untreated or if treatment is delayed. EEG is usually abnormal, with focal slowing being the most frequent finding, but epileptiform discharges, including PLEDs, are commonly encountered. CSF PCR study is the diagnostic test of choice for HSV and has a sensitivity and specificity of 98% and 94%, respectively. CT and MRI are commonly abnormal, with asymmetrical involvement of the temporal lobes being the most common. Treatment of HSE requires early initiation of acyclovir to reduce the risk for severe neurological sequelae.

Keywords: CNS; Management strategies; Antimicrobials; CNS; Diagnostic modalities; EEG; CNS; Diagnosis; Infectious; Encephalitis

REFERENCES

Boivin G. Diagnosis of herpesvirus infections of the central nervous system. *Herpes* 2004;11(Suppl 2):48A.
Whitley RJ. Herpes simplex encephalitis: adolescents and adults. *Antiviral Res* 2006;71(2–3):141–148.

13. ANSWER: A

This patient likely has GBS or acute inflammatory demyelinating polyneuropathy (AIDP). While NCS/EMG studies very early in the course of AIDP can be normal, absent H reflex is one of the earliest and most common findings, which clinically is essentially a confirmation of loss of ankle reflexes. F-wave latencies are often prolonged and are another early neurophysiological marker for AIDP. Increased temporal dispersion is often seen in distal (early) as well as proximal (late) CMAPs during the course of the disease. Sural SNAPs are often normal.

Electrodynamic studies, as well as CSF examination, are accepted parts of the diagnostic paradigm for AIDP. CSF is usually under normal pressure and acellular, although occasionally some lymphocytes are seen. In the acute setting where the patient clinically appears consistent with AIDP and NCS/EMG studies are available, a CSF analysis is not needed.

Paresthesias in the toes and fingers are the earliest symptoms of AIDP. The major clinical manifestation of AIDP is weakness in a symmetrical pattern evolving over several days to 1 to 2 weeks. The proximal and distal muscles of the limbs are involved; usually the lower extremities are symptomatic before the upper extremities. Ten percent of patients will have dysautonomia resulting in hypotension requiring volume administration and vasopressors, although usually briefly. Five percent of AIDP patients will progress to have complete neuromuscular failure, with extreme cases involving the oculomotor nerve; even the pupils may become unreactive.

Keywords: CNS; Diagnoses; Neuromuscular disorders; GBS; CNS; Diagnoses; Neuromuscular disorders; Critical illness polyneuropathy, myopathy, other; CNS; Diagnostic studies; NCS/EMG

14. ANSWER: D

With the exception of Charcot-Marie-Tooth syndrome, all of the options presented can cause an acute flaccid paralysis and can mimic GBS/AIDP. Polio, although extremely rare in developed countries, is resurfacing owing to resistance to vaccination in many societies. WNV is an important pathogen to be aware of; fever and rash are commonly present, and concurrent symptoms of meningoencephalitis may be noted. GBS/AIDP can be distinguished from both WNV and poliomyelitis by the absence of CSF pleocytosis. This "albuminocytologic dissociation" is seen in more than 75% of patients, although CSF pleocytosis can be seen in GBS patients with human immunodeficiency virus (HIV). Neuromuscular weakness is common in patients with critical illness, and critical illness myopathy (CIM) is the most common form. CSF studies are negative, and EMG typically shows coexisting myopathic changes. Serum creatine kinase is frequently elevated but may be normal in patients receiving steroids. Critical illness polyneuropathy (CIP) can be clinically indistinguishable from CIM. NCS/EMG shows decreased sensory and motor nerve amplitudes, normal F-waves, and fibrillation potentials. Both CIM and CIP can cause failure to wean from mechanical ventilation. Treatment is supportive and often requires months to reverse.

Charcot-Marie-Tooth syndrome is an inherited disorder that most commonly presents with athletic imprecision in youth and a gradual decline in neuromuscular function in the distal extremities (i.e., foot drop, hand weakness).

Keywords: CNS; Diagnoses; Infectious; Encephalitis

REFERENCES

Wijdicks EF, Klein CJ. Guillain-Barré syndrome. *Mayo Clin Proc* 2017;92:467–479.
Zhou C, Wu L, Ni F et al. Critical illness polyneuropathy and myopathy: a systematic review. *Neural Regen Res* 2014;9:101–110.

15. ANSWER: B

The patient has likely progressed to brain death given the lack of cranial nerve findings. Hypotension is common after brain death owing to the loss in sympathetic tone. However, brain death per se rarely results in profound hypotension requiring high doses of vasopressors. If a brain-dead patient requires high vasopressor support, a concomitant etiology should be looked for. This is often due to underresuscitation following trauma, diuresis following mannitol administration, cardiac dysfunction, or in this case, diabetes insipidus (DI). Arterial waveform pulse contour analysis is of particular value in this clinical situation.

After DI is diagnosed, a common tendency is to focus on correcting the abnormal serum sodium (especially if markedly elevated). However, the most important first step is volume resuscitation using isotonic fluids. Correction of the patient's water deficit can occur after the patient is euvolemic. Hormonal replacement should occur concomitantly with volume resuscitation and can be accomplished using arginine vasopressin (AVP) or desmopressin (DDAVP).

Of note, in brain-dead donors, the use of AVP has been associated with an increased rate of successful organ procurement and is an excellent option in patients with both hypotension and DI. It is also reasonable in hypotensive patients without DI. If the patient already has DI, a bolus of 5 to 10 units is necessary before starting the infusion. Alternatively, especially in patients without hypotension, desmopressin can be administered. We typically administer 4 mcg IV for DI in the setting of brain death. The tendency to underbolus AVP or DDAVP should be avoided given the detrimental effects of ongoing DI on organ procurement success. Oliguria following DDAVP administration is NOT secondary to overdosing the medication, but rather to inadequate replacement of fluids lost before treatment of the DI. It is important to note that the DDAVP dose administered for platelet dysfunction is much higher (0.3–0.4 mcg/kg).

While DI is diagnosed by the triad of polyuria, hypernatremia, and low urine osmolality, in this case, it would be incorrect to delay fluid resuscitation in order to confirm the diagnosis because the likelihood of DI is nearly certain. It would also be incorrect to proceed to formal brain death testing without first treating the patient for reasons discussed previously.

Keywords: CNS; Management strategies; Vasoactive drugs; CNS; Basic pathophysiology; Brain death

REFERENCES

Callahan DS, Neville A, Bricker S et al. The effect of arginine vasopressin on organ donor procurement and lung function. *J Surg Res* 2014;186:452.
Plurad DS, Bricker S, Neville A et al. Arginine vasopressin significantly increases the rate of successful organ procurement in potential donors. *Am J Surg* 2012;204:856–860.

16. ANSWER: A

While the classic triad for spinal epidural abscess (SEA) is fever, neurological deficits, and back pain, all three are rarely present. While back pain is essentially universal, neurological deficits are unlikely early in the course, and fever may be present in less than 50% of patients. For these reasons, the diagnosis is commonly delayed, and most patients have had prior visits with similar complaints. This can have severe consequences because neurological deficits may not be reversible. While SEA should be strongly considered in patients with more than one feature of the classic triad, the diagnosis should also be considered in patients with spinal pain who have risk factors for SEA. These include IV drug use, hemodialysis, recent bacteremia, diabetes mellitus, alcoholism, and HIV. About two thirds of cases are caused by *Staphylococcus aureus*. MRI is the diagnostic test of choice; and given the potential for more than one lesion, an MRI of the entire spine is preferred.

Keywords: Diagnoses; Infectious; Abscess; Diagnoses; Spinal cord injury

REFERENCES

Chen WC, Wang JL, Want JT et al. Spinal epidural abscess due to *Staphylococcus aureus*: clinical manifestations and outcomes. *J Microbiol Immunol Infect* 2008;41:215.

Darouiche RO. Spinal epidural abscess. *N Engl J Med* 2006;355:2012.

17. ANSWER: B

Proper management of patients with acute traumatic spinal cord injury requires a multidisciplinary approach. Despite the lack of strong evidence, current guidelines recommend maintaining MAP of at least 85 mg Hg to optimize spinal cord perfusion. In patients with cervical cord injury, impaired sympathetic tone (sympathetic nerves arise from cells in the intermediolateral nuclei in the thoracolumbar region) may result in both arterial hypotension and bradycardia such that this goal often requires vasopressors and volume administration to achieve. Despite their promise from animal studies, current guidelines do not recommend glucocorticoids. The efficacy of IV glucocorticoids was evaluated in the National Acute Spinal Cord Injury Studies 1–3. NASCIS 1 compared a low dose (100 mg) to a higher dose (1000 mg) of methylprednisolone and did not show a difference in neurological outcome at 1 year. NASCIS 2 compared a 30-mg/kg methylprednisolone bolus followed by 5.4 mg/kg per hour over 23 hours to placebo and also did not show a difference in neurological outcome. However, patients treated with steroids within 8 hours of injury were noted to have a slight improvement in motor scores at 1 year, which prompted the NASCIS 3 study in which all patients received a steroid bolus within 8 hours of injury. Following this bolus, patients were randomized into three groups: a 24-hour infusion, a 48-hour infusion, or the lipid peroxidation inhibitor tirilazad mesylate. Again, there were no differences overall; however, in the subgroup of patients treated between 3 and 8 hours, the longer steroid infusion led to a greater motor recovery compared with the other treatments. While the controversy surrounding these studies is beyond the scope of this discussion, since the studies were overall negative and because sepsis and pneumonia were more common in patients receiving the 48-hour steroid infusion, steroids are no longer recommended.

The need for mechanical intubation is common in patients with cervical spinal cord injury. While the diaphragm receives its innervation from the C3–5 segments, it is important to remember that accessory muscles receive innervation from C2–7 (scalenes) as well as T1–6 (intercostals) and that the cough reflex involves these segments as well as T5–L1 (rectus abdominus). The implications are that patients with lower cervical cord injury and even thoracic injury are not without risk for respiratory failure in settings requiring accessory muscle use (pulmonary edema, pneumonia) or a strong cough (thick secretions, mucous plugging). These should all be considered before attempting extubation.

Of note, the American Spinal Cord Injury Association (ASIA) Impairment Scale is a common method used to grade spinal cord injury. This patient is likely an ASIA A, in which rates of ambulation at 1 year are typically poor.

Keywords: CNS; Basic pathophysiology; CNS; Spinal cord injury; CNS; Management strategies; Steroids; CNS; Management strategies; Neuroprotectants

REFERENCES

Bracken MB, Shepard JM, Collins WF et al. Methylprednisolone or naloxone treatment after acute spinal cord injury: 1 year follow up data. Results of the second National Acute Spinal Cord Injury Study. *J Neurosurg* 1992;76:23.

Bracken MB, Shepard JM, Holford TR et al. Methylprednisolone or tirilazad mesylate administration after acute spinal cord injury: 1 year follow up data. Results of the third National Acute Spinal Cord Injury Study. *J Neurosurg* 1998;89:699.

Ryken TC, Hurlbert RJ, Hadley MN et al. The acute cardiopulmonary management of patients with cervical spinal cord injuries. *Neurosurgery* 2013;72:84–92.

18. Answer: A

Part of a multimodality monitoring strategy in the management of severe brain injury includes monitoring brain tissues oxygen. One strategy is to directly measure brain tissue oxygen tension with a probe inserted into the patient's white matter. Normal levels are typically 25–50 mm Hg with critical brain hypoxia defined as <15mm Hg. While low brain oxygen measured in this manner has been associated with worse outcome after TBI, the threshold at which treatment should be initiated is not well-established but is typically done between 15–20 mm Hg. Therapies that improve cerebral oxygenation either increase cerebral oxygen delivery (e.g. augmenting cerebral blood flow or increasing arterial oxygen content) or decrease oxygen utilization (e.g. sedation). Therefore, decreasing the patient's sedation may increase cerebral metabolic activity and increase oxygen requirements, which might exacerbate the imbalance between delivery and demand. RBC transfusion may increase oxygen delivery by increasing blood oxygen content. CPP can be increased by blood pressure augmentation or ICP reduction, which could improve cerebral blood flow. While hyperventilation is effective at lowering ICP, it may decrease CBF by vasoconstriction. In this case, the patient is mildly hyperventilated. Assuming ICP is maintained, reducing this patient's minute ventilation to a CO_2 of 35 to 40 mm Hg may have a salutary effect on cerebral oxygenation.

Keywords: CNS; Basic pathophysiology; Cerebral blood flow; CNS; Diagnoses; Head injury

REFERENCE

De Georgia MA. Brain tissue oxygen monitoring in neurocritical care. *J Intensive Care Med* 2015;30:473–483.

19. ANSWER: B

Patients with severe brain injury are at significant risk for secondary neuronal injury. While ICP monitoring is considered the sine qua non of TBI management, a number of devices are currently being used that may provide more specific information regarding cellular function. These include jugular venous O_2 saturation monitoring, brain tissue oxygen tension monitoring, cerebral microdialysis, intraparenchymal blood flow monitors, near infrared spectroscopy, and electroencephalography. A full review of these devices is beyond the scope of this chapter. In brief, various ICP thresholds ranging typically between 20 and 25 mm Hg have been associated with worse outcomes after TBI. While potentially a surrogate for a more severe initial brain injury, elevations in ICP can decrease cerebral blood flow, strain axonal tracts, or precipitate herniation. Measuring O_2 saturation from a catheter inserted into the jugular vein with its tip at the skull base provides information synonymous to central and mixed venous O_2 saturation. That is, a reduction in jugular venous saturation from increased cerebral oxygen extraction suggests inadequate oxygen delivery and may precede ischemia. One step closer to actual cellular function is the cerebral microdialysis catheter, in which elevations in the lactate-to-pyruvate ratio occur during ischemia. Additionally, increased velocity on transcranial Doppler may be a harbinger of ischemia. While less common than in patients with aneurysmal subarachnoid hemorrhage, post-traumatic vasospasm does occur. Based on the formula that flow is equal to velocity times area, assuming cerebral blood flow is unchanged, an increase in blood flow velocity implies a reduction in area (cerebral vasospasm). Finally, EEG reactivity to stimuli is a normal finding and, in the setting of severe brain injury, suggests a favorable prognosis.

Keywords: CNS; Diagnostic modalities; ICP measurement; CNS; Diagnostic modalities; Jugular venous saturation; CNS; Diagnostic modalities; Transcranial Doppler; CNS; Diagnostic modalities; Microdialysis

REFERENCES

Kirkman MA, Smith M. Multimodality neuromonitoring. *Anesthesiol Clin* 2016;34:511–523.
Le Roux PD, Levine J, Kofke A. *Monitoring in neurocritical care*. Philadelphia: Elsevier; 2013.

20. ANSWER: B

Stroke after cardiac catheterization has been reported in up to 0.6% of patients. ICH may occur given the use of anticoagulants and antiplatelet medications, although most cases are related to ischemic strokes from the procedure itself. This typically occurs from the catheter dislodging an atheromatous plaque in the aortic arch or proximal cervical vessels, although de novo thrombus may form on the catheter and subsequently embolize. Although this patient received midazolam, it is unlikely to account for her severe depression in arousal and focal findings on examination. The decreased arousal and weakness of both extremities are very concerning for a posterior circulation event involving the brainstem. This is essentially confirmed by the presence of a skew deviation. A skew deviation is a vertical strabismus of the eyes that most commonly occurs after injury to the brainstem. In the setting of stroke, vertebral or basilar thrombosis should be assumed.

Keywords: Basic pathophysiology; CNS; Stroke; Embolic/thrombotic; Basic pathophysiology; CNS; Stroke; Ischemic

REFERENCE

Keane JR. Ocular skew deviation: analysis of 100 cases. *Arch Neurol* 1975;32:185–190.

21. ANSWER: A

The Monro-Kellie doctrine states that because of the fixed volume of the intracranial vault, the ICP is a result of the volumes of the individual components within it. If the volume of one component increases, the volume of another must decrease, or the pressure will rise. For example, in the setting of increasing cerebral edema, CSF can be shunted out of the ventricles and subarachnoid space into the lumbar cistern, and blood can be shunted out of the dural sinuses and cerebral veins. Eventually, this compensatory reserve is exhausted, and pressure rises. A related concept is that of cerebral compliance. Compliance represents the change in ICP to a given change in volume. When compensatory mechanisms are limited, small changes in volume can have dramatic effects on pressure (poor compliance).

This patient's acute decline is presumably related to increased ICP, which can be secondary to either worsening hemorrhage or worsening edema. Mannitol is a safe and efficient option for lowering ICP in an emergent situation such as this one and has its clinical effect by (1) osmotic diuresis, (2) increasing CSF reabsorption, (3) inducing blood dilution to decrease viscosity, and (4) cerebral vasoconstriction.

Hypertonic saline is an alternative to mannitol; however, concentrations of 3% and greater require administration through a central venous catheter, which would delay treatment. Bolus doses using higher concentrations are effective at reducing ICP when severe ICP elevation is noted or the patient is refractory to other therapies. Hypertonic saline may be particularly helpful when low-volume resuscitation is needed after brain injury. Other mainstays of treatment for an ICP crisis would be elevation of the head of bed to 30 degrees with the head in neutral position, loosening of cervical collar if present, hyperventilation to a PCO_2 of 30 to 35 mm Hg, sedation, analgesia, and neuromuscular paralysis. While a seizure may explain the initial change, the decline into coma with partial loss of brainstem reflexes cannot be explained by seizure alone. High-dose dexamethasone is indicated in patients with herniation from vasogenic edema related to a malignancy; however, it has been associated with worse outcome in patients with TBI.

Keywords: Basic pathophysiology; CNS; Intracranial compliance; CNS; Management strategies; ICP controlling medications

REFERENCE

Alnemari AM, Krafcik BM, Mansour TR, Gaudin D. A comparison of pharmacologic therapeutic agents used for the reduction of intracranial pressure after traumatic brain injury. *World Neurosurg.* 2017;106:509–528.

22. ANSWER: C

Given the lack of prior seizure history and hypertension, this patient has eclampsia. The treatment of choice is IV magnesium sulfate. Magnesium sulfate was found to be superior to benzodiazepines and phenytoin in reducing recurrent seizures in patients with eclamptic seizures. If seizures continue despite magnesium therapy, a benzodiazepine may be added. There is no role for starting antiepileptic drugs (AEDs) like phenytoin or levetiracetam for eclampsia without a previous history of seizure disorder.

While the pathogenesis of eclampsia is not completely understood, hypertension is considered the sine quo non. Neuroimaging may show changes consistent with reversible posterior leukoencephalopathy syndrome, including T2/fluid attenuated inversion recovery (FLAIR) hyperintensities, typically in the parietal and occipital white matter.

Keywords: Basic pathophysiology; CNS; Seizures and status epilepticus; CNS; Management strategies; Anticonvulsants

REFERENCE

Which anticonvulsant for women with eclampsia? Evidence from the Collaborative Eclampsia trial. *Lancet* 1995;345:1455–1463.

23. ANSWER: C

The differential diagnosis of rim-enhancing lesions can be remembered by the mnemonic MAGIC DR: metastasis, abscess, glioma, infarct, contusion, demyelinating disease, and radiation necrosis. While the clinical history often narrows this differential substantially, certain radiographic features can suggest some diagnoses over others. For example, ring enhancement that is open toward the cortex suggests demyelination, while thick, nodular enhancement suggests malignancy. Cerebral edema may be seen in all diagnoses, although extensive edema relative to the lesion size favors abscess. Vasogenic edema can often be distinguished from cytotoxic edema on CT imaging (seen with infarction) by the relative sparing of the cortex. This has to do with the fact that cell bodies are located in the cortex, which increases the resistance to entry of fluid into the cortex. Edema may distribute extensively through the less densely packed white matter before entering the cortex to a significant degree.

While multiple ring-enhancing lesions favor both metastases and abscesses over the other diagnoses, solitary metastases and abscesses are not uncommon (45% of metastases and 25% of abscesses were solitary lesions in one study). The major distinguishing feature of abscess over metastasis is the presence of restricted diffusion on MRI, which is a result of densely packed white blood cells and microbial debris (puss).

Keywords: CNS; Diagnoses; Abscess

REFERENCE

Brouwer MC, Tunkel AR, McKhann GM et al. Brain abscess. *N Engl J Med* 2014;371:447–456.

24. ANSWER: B

This patient has pituitary apoplexy, which occurs after hemorrhage or infarction of the pituitary gland. This most commonly occurs in patients with pituitary adenomas, but may occur as a result of enlargement of the anterior pituitary during pregnancy (Sheehan syndrome). The most frequent presentation is with a headache, which is usually sudden in onset and severe (i.e., thunderclap headache). Like aneurysmal rupture, pituitary apoplexy is in the differential diagnosis for thunderclap headache and should be considered when the evaluation is negative for SAH. While frank hemorrhage can extend into the cavernous sinus, and hyperdensities in the region of the sella turcica can be seen on CT, CT imaging is often unremarkable. MRI, in particular with a specific pituitary gland protocol, is more sensitive.

While deficiencies of all anterior pituitary hormones are common, the most immediate life-threatening risk is adrenal insufficiency. Patients with signs or symptoms of adrenal insufficiency (hemodynamic instability, nausea, hyponatremia, altered mental status) should be treated with 100 to 200 mg of IV hydrocortisone. DI may occur but is rare because involvement of the posterior pituitary is uncommon. This patient does not show signs of diabetes insipidus (e.g., hypernatremia, polyuria).

Keywords: CNS; Diagnoses; Pituitary disorders

REFERENCE

Ranabir S, Baruah M. Pituitary apoplexy. *Indian J Endocrinol Metab* 2011;15:S188–S196.

25. ANSWER: B

Significant hematoma expansion (>33% increase in volume) occurs in about 38% of patients with spontaneous ICH and is an independent predictor of poor outcome. Risk factors include coagulopathy, larger hematoma size, and hypertension. While reversal of coagulation factor deficiencies and anticoagulants such as warfarin, factor Xa inhibitors, and direct thrombin inhibitors is crucial, reversal of antiplatelet agents is controversial. Factor VIIa has been shown to reduce hematoma growth by statistically significant amounts; however, this did not translate into improved clinical outcomes in a randomized trial. Given the potential for increased thromboembolic and arterial thrombotic events, recombinant factor VIIa is currently not recommended in this clinical circumstance.

Blood pressure management following ICH has been an important area of research. Hypertension can increase the risk for hematoma expansion and is associated with worse outcome; however, there is some concern about the need for slightly elevated blood pressures to maintain cerebral perfusion, in particular in the perihematomal region. The INTERACT2 trial randomized patients to systolic blood pressure <140 versus <180 mm Hg and did not find a difference in mortality or severe disability, suggesting that aggressive blood pressure reduction to 140 mm Hg is safe. Furthermore, modified Rankin scores, a measure of disability after stroke, were improved in patients with the 140-mm Hg target. A more recent trial, ATACH 2, also randomized patients to 140 versus 180 mm Hg and did not find a difference in death or disability but did find an increased incidence of acute kidney injury in the more intensive treatment group. While the exact treatment threshold is unclear, control of extreme blood pressure elevation is indicated.

Because this patient is following commands and does not have hydrocephalus, insertion of an EVD is not indicated. A deep bleed (basal ganglia, thalamus, pons, cerebellum) in a hypertensive patient is likely hypertensive in etiology; thus, vascular imaging has a low clinical yield. While an urgent CT angiogram is reasonable, treatment of blood pressure is paramount. The benefit of craniotomy and hematoma evacuation in patients with ICH has been studied in a randomized controlled trial (STICH), which did not show a statistically significant improvement in neurological outcomes. A subgroup analysis of patients whose hemorrhage was 1cm or less from the cortical surface showed a potential benefit, prompting a follow-up study in these patients (STICH 2), which was also negative. Of note, cerebellar hemorrhages and patients with active or impending herniation were not included in these trials. Because the outcome of isolated cerebellar hemorrhage is excellent and posterior fossa hemorrhages have a high risk for herniation, there should be a low threshold for surgical evacuation in these patients. The benefit of minimally invasive hematoma evacuation remains under investigation.

Keywords: Basic pathophysiology; CNS; Stroke; Hemorrhagic; CNS; Management strategies; Surgical interventions

REFERENCES

Anderson CS, Heeley E, Huang Y et al. Rapid blood-pressure lowering in patients with acute intracerebral hemorrhage. *N Engl J Med* 2013;368:2355–2365.

Hemphill JC, Greenberg SM, Anderson CS et al. Guidelines for the management of spontaneous intracerebral hemorrhage. *Stroke* 2015;46:2032–2060.

Mayer SA, Brun NC, Begtrup D et al. Efficacy and safety of recombinant activated factor VII for acute intracerebral hemorrhage. *N Engl J Med* 2008;358:2127–2137.

Qureshi AI, Palesch YY, Barsan WG et al. Intensive blood-pressure lowering in patients with acute cerebral hemorrhage. *N Engl J Med* 2016;375:1033–1043.

26. ANSWER: B

The patient has vasospasm on transcranial Doppler ultrasound as demonstrated by the increased mean velocity in the MCAs. Cerebral vasospasm peaks around day 7 after hemorrhage and occurs in up to two thirds of patients. Half of these patients will develop symptoms or complications (i.e., infarction) from this. The development of ischemic symptoms with or without vasospasm, is known as delayed cerebral ischemia (DCI). DCI is managed by restoring adequate cerebral blood flow. Hypovolemia is a significant risk factor for DCI and should be corrected. Fluid administration may also benefit by lowering serum viscosity and improving blood flow through the cerebral microcirculation; therefore, maintenance fluids alone would usually be inadequate. In general, the patient's volume status should always be positive in aneurysmal subarachnoid hemorrhage. Augmentation of MAP by vasopressors has been shown to reverse neurological deficits and is best done by augmenting MAP in a stepwise fashion (e.g., 10–15%) until deficits are reversed. Institutional protocols general dictate actual blood pressure goals, being mindful of the paradigm just mentioned. Cerebral angiography and administration of vasodilators or angioplasty is another effective means for reversing DCI. Whether all patients with DCI undergo angiography or only cases refractory to medical therapy is dependent on the institution and providers. CT angiography would not be useful because of relatively limited resolution compared with formal angiography and lack of ability to immediately treat any diagnosed vasospasm.

Keywords: CNS; Management strategies; Interventional radiology; CNS; Diagnostic modalities; Angiography

REFERENCE

Francoeur CL, Mayer SA. Management of delayed cerebral ischemia after subarachnoid hemorrhage. *Crit Care* 2016;20:277.

27. ANSWER: A

Rebleeding of ruptured cerebral aneurysm is the leading cause of early morbidity and mortality in survivors of aneurysmal SAH. Excluding an aneurysm from the circulation, either with surgical clipping or endovascular coiling, is the only proven method to prevent this complication. Given that rebleeding risk is highest early after aneurysmal rupture (up to 13.6% on day 1 and gradually falling to 1–2% per day over 2 weeks) and because management of cerebral vasospasm and ischemia may require blood pressure augmentation, the aneurysm should be secured as soon as possible. Patients presenting overnight will typically await definitive treatment until the following day. While blood pressure lowering has not been shown to reduce the risk for rebleeding, the theoretical risks of elevated blood pressure warrant that "extreme" hypertension should be avoided. The exact threshold at which blood pressure should be treated is unknown. Antifibrinolytic agents have been shown to reduce the risk for rebleeding; although when used over an extended period, this benefit is offset by an increase in thromboembolic complications. In this patient, who will wait several hours overnight for her angiogram, a short course of fibrinolytics is reasonable. Finally, as the transluminal pressure across an aneurysm is the pressure within the aneurysm minus the pressure outside of the aneurysm (ICP), sudden and dramatic drops in ICP should be avoided. Therefore, EVDs are managed conservative and generally kept at 20 cm H_2O height and open. This prevents a buildup of elevated pressure while minimizing drainage. As phenytoin "burden" has been associated with worsened cognitive outcomes after aneurysmal SAH, levetiracetam has become the preferred AED, although the use of AEDs for seizure prophylaxis in general is uncertain.

Keywords: Basic pathophysiology; CNS; Vascular malformations; CNS; management strategies; CSF drainage

ACKNOWLEDGMENT

Special thanks to Dr. Rahul Shah and Dr. Niral Patel for their contributions to this chapter.

REFERENCES

Brown RJ, Dhar R. Aneurysmal subarachnoid hemorrhage: case study and commentary. *JCOM* 2011;18:223–237.

Diringer MN, Bleck TP, Hemphill C et al. Critical care management of patients following aneurysmal subarachnoid hemorrhage: recommendations from the Neurocritical Care Society's multidisciplinary consensus conference. *Neurocrit Care* 2011;15: 211–240.

2.

OBSTETRIC CRITICAL CARE

Marc J. Popovich

QUESTIONS

The following case applies to questions 1 to 3:

A 24-year-old, 90-kg G3P2 female with estimated 37 weeks' gestation presents to the emergency department (ED) with obtundation and the following vital signs:

Temperature: 39.3° C
Heart rate (HR): 130 bpm
Blood pressure (BP): 80/50 mm Hg

A fetal monitor is placed, demonstrating a fetal HR of 170 bpm. On physical exam, the uterus is tender to palpation, and vaginal exam indicates dilation and effacement with copious vaginal discharge. The patient is taken to labor and delivery, where she undergoes an urgent delivery. Periprocedurally, the patient has extensive uterine hemorrhage. She receives intravenous (IV) oxytocin and multiple units of red blood cells and fresh frozen plasma (FFP) but continues to hemorrhage. She is admitted to the intensive care unit (ICU), where a central venous catheter is placed and a norepinephrine infusion is started. In the ICU, the following laboratory values are available:

Hemoglobin (Hgb): 7.1 mg/dL
White blood cell (WBC) count: 21,000
Platelets (PLT): 103,000
International normalized ratio (INR): 1.8
Fibrinogen: 100 mg/dL

1. Which of the following would be the MOST effective next line of treatment?

A. Double the dose of oxytocin
B. Transfuse 2 units of FFP
C. Transfuse one 5-unit pack of platelets
D. Transfuse 2 units of cryoprecipitate

2. The patient in question 1 continues to show evidence of postpartum hemorrhage. In addition to supportive care, which of the following represents the BEST next line of management?

A. Urgent hysterectomy
B. Thromboelastography (TEG)
C. Recombinant activated factor VIIa
D. Tranexamic acid

3. Immediately before undergoing urgent delivery, the patient in questions 1 and 2 received hydrocortisone 100 mg IV plus ampicillin 2 g IV (with orders to receive every 6 hours × two doses) and gentamicin 450 mg IV (with orders to receive one additional dose the next day). On postdelivery day 3 in the ICU, norepinephrine has been weaned off, but the patient remains febrile with pelvic and back pain, uterine tenderness, and a persistent vaginal discharge. Antibiotics should be tailored for which of the following MOST likely etiologies?

A. Group A streptococci
B. *Chlamydia trachomatis*
C. *Ureaplasma urealyticum*
D. Polymicrobial (aerobic and anaerobic)

The following case applies to questions 4 and 5:

A 41-year-old, 90-kg female, pregnant with 37 weeks' gestation and with known pre-eclampsia, presents to the ED with mid-epigastric and back pain, right upper quadrant (RUQ) pain and tenderness, nausea, vomiting, and malaise. Her HR is 100 bpm and BP is 140/90 mm Hg. The emergency medicine physician requests an ICU bed for BP management in order to complete an evaluation for presumed acute cholecystitis.

4. In addition to a complete blood count (CBC), comprehensive metabolic panel, and IV fluids, which of the following is the MOST indicated step?

    A. Urine for proteins
    B. Peripheral blood smear
    C. Hepatitis screen
    D. RUQ ultrasound

5. The decision is made to deliver the patient. In the recovery room after delivery, the patient develops a generalized tonic-clonic seizure. After positioning the patient in a left lateral position and maintaining a patent airway, which of the following initial treatments is MOST indicated?

    A. Magnesium sulfate
    B. Mannitol
    C. Diazepam
    D. Fosphenytoin

6. A 32-year-old female status post instrumented vaginal delivery develops sudden onset of profound hypotension, bradycardia, oxygen desaturation, and obtundation. The patient is intubated, a central venous catheter is placed, and fluids are administered. The patient is placed on 100% forced inspiratory oxygen (FiO$_2$) and positive end-expiratory pressure (PEEP) of 5 cm H$_2$O and yet remains hypoxemic and hypotensive. A transthoracic echocardiogram demonstrates an ejection fraction of 45%. Which of the following is the MOST appropriate next step in management?

    A. Insert a pulmonary artery catheter
    B. Increase PEEP and start dobutamine
    C. Place an Impella
    D. Start venovenous extracorporeal membrane oxygenation (ECMO)

The following case applies to questions 7 and 8:

An obese 28-year-old heroin-addicted parturient was admitted to the ED. Continuous epidural analgesia was attempted, but the patient became agitated and a catheter was unable to be placed. She was admitted to the ICU for withdrawal symptoms.

7. The patient is now demanding pain relief. Which of the following is LEAST likely to be of benefit?

    A. Lumbar sympathetic block
    B. Nitrous oxide inhaled by handheld face mask
    C. Tramadol
    D. Butorphanol

8. The patient develops worsening hyperactive delirium. Which of the following management strategies is MOST accurate?

    A. Midazolam can prolong labor
    B. Dexmedetomidine does not cross the placenta
    C. Ketamine may decrease uteroplacental perfusion
    D. Butorphanol does not cause respiratory depression

The following case applies to questions 9 and 10:

A 31-year-old, 70-kg female with 35 weeks' gestation is admitted to the ICU with an acute exacerbation of asthma complicating a viral upper respiratory infection. The patient has a known history of asthma, which is well controlled with bronchodilators. On arrival, the patient's HR is 130 bpm, her respiratory rate is 36 breaths/minute, and she demonstrates intercostal retractions with accessory muscle use and is struggling to talk. Auscultation of the chest demonstrates very faint breath sounds bilaterally.

9. Which of the following is the most appropriate initial management?

    A. Aerosolized albuterol
    B. IV isoproterenol
    C. Inhaled and IV methylprednisolone
    D. Endotracheal intubation

10. After intubation of the patient described in question 9, a blood gas analysis is obtained that demonstrates:

pH: 7.25
Partial pressure of carbon dioxide (PCO$_2$): 56 mm Hg
Partial pressure of oxygen (PO$_2$): 62 mm Hg
Bicarbonate (HCO$_3$): 22 mEq/L
Oxygen saturation by pulse oximetry (SpO$_2$): 92%

The patient is placed on the following ventilator settings:

Volume control ventilation: rate 16
FiO$_2$: 100%
Tidal volume: 800 mL
PEEP: 5 cm H$_2$O

After a few minutes, the patient becomes extremely hypotensive. Which of the following is the most appropriate?

    A. Reduce respiratory rate to 12 breaths/minute
    B. Reduce the tidal volume to 400 mL
    C. Reduce PEEP to 0 cm H$_2$O
    D. Start norepinephrine infusion

ANSWERS

1. ANSWER: D

The patient has postpartum hemorrhage with evidence of consumption of fibrinogen. Pregnant patients trend to have fibrinogen levels of 400 to 600 mg/dL; patients with fibrinogen levels in excess of 400 mg/dL typically do not develop postpartum hemorrhage. Although FFP contains fibrinogen, cryoprecipitate provides a higher concentration. Transfusion of FFP (or red blood cells) is less likely to treat the underlying pathology.

Keywords: Complications of pregnancy; Coagulopathy, bleeding disorders

REFERENCE

James AH, McClintock C, Lockhart E. Postpartum hemorrhage: when uterotonics and sutures fail. *Am J Hematol* 2012;87:S16–S22.

2. ANSWER: C

Recombinant activated factor VIIa is an acceptable treatment in recalcitrant postpartum hemorrhage; recent studies have demonstrated a benefit in avoiding hysterectomy. Tranexamic acid is less effective and is fraught with more side effects, such as nausea and vomiting, and risk for thrombotic events. Repeating lab values may not reflect qualitative coagulation. While a thromboelastogram may be more representative of coagulation function, obtaining useful results will take at least 30 to 60 minutes and thus may not be reasonably timely in this situation.

Keywords: Diagnoses; Coagulopathy, bleeding disorders

REFERENCE

James AH, McClintock C, Lockhart E. Postpartum hemorrhage: when uterotonics and sutures fail. *Am J Hematol* 2012;87:S16–S22.

3. ANSWER: D

The patient presented in early labor with premature rupture of membranes, which likely led to septic shock as a result of chorioamnionitis. Typically, this resolves after a short course of antibiotics, as was ordered. Persistent fever, signs, and symptoms days after delivery are concerning for uterine endometritis, which is more commonly a polymicrobial (aerobic and anaerobic) infection. A lone organism isolated and causing infection is typically group B streptococcus; group A streptococci (and *Staphylococcus* species) are associated with a more virulent, toxic shock–like syndrome (not consistent with this patient's status). Isolated sexually transmitted and urinary mycoplasma infections are much rarer causes but may require further diagnostic (e.g., culture) efforts if the patient does not respond.

Keywords: Diagnoses; Peripartum infection

REFERENCE

Watts DH, Eschenbach DA, Kenny GE. Early postpartum endometritis: the role of bacteria, genital mycoplasmas, and *Chlamydia trachomatis. Obstet Gynecol* 1989;73:52–60.

4. ANSWER: B

A patient with known pre-eclampsia and the constellation of symptoms mentioned in the question, particularly RUQ pain, is at high risk for HELLP (hemolysis, elevated liver enzymes, and low platelet count) syndrome. While the comprehensive metabolic panel and CBC will identify elevated liver enzymes and low platelets, respectively, a peripheral blood smear demonstrating a microangiopathic hemolytic anemia with schistocytes is diagnostic. Because the patient is known to have pre-eclampsia, checking urine for proteins would not provide additional diagnostic information. An imaging investigation should be undertaken only if HELLP syndrome is ruled out.

Keywords: Diagnoses; Liver function abnormalities (e.g., acute fatty liver, HELLP syndrome)

REFERENCE

Stone JH. HELLP syndrome: hemolysis, elevated liver enzymes, and low platelets. *JAMA* 1998;280:559–562.

5. ANSWER: A

Magnesium sulfate is considered grade 1A and remains the standard for management of postpartum seizures (eclampsia) even after delivery. Mannitol is generally considered to be contraindicated in eclampsia management. The other treatments are second line for seizures refractory to magnesium.

Keywords: Diagnoses; Pre-eclampsia, eclampsia; Management strategies; Anticonvulsants

REFERENCE

Sibai BM. Diagnosis, prevention, and management of eclampsia. *Obstet Gynecol* 2005;105:402–410.

6. ANSWER: B

This patient's presentation of abrupt shock after an instrumented delivery is likely a result of an amniotic fluid embolus. The transthoracic echo finding of an ejection fraction of 45% is abnormal but not catastrophic; hypoxemia is likely noncardiogenic. Thus, the hypoxemia, bradycardia, and shock could initially be managed with increased PEEP and the beta-1 inotropic support of dobutamine. A pulmonary artery catheter is unlikely to provide additional useful information. An afterload-increasing agent such as vasopressin would help raise BP, but vasoconstriction in the presence of left ventricular dysfunction may reduce overall organ perfusion. Extracorporeal devices may be second- or third-line management strategies, particularly if left ventricular function worsens.

Keywords: Diagnoses; Emboli (e.g., amniotic fluid, thromboemboli)

REFERENCE

Gist RS, Stafford IP, Leibowitz AB, Beilin Y. Amniotic fluid embolism. *Anesth Analg* 2009;108:1599–1602.

7. ANSWER: D

Butorphanol, as an agonist-antagonist, may exacerbate withdrawal symptoms. Nitrous oxide has been described for usage in laboring parturients and generally results in satisfaction by patients who have received it, while objective analgesic benefit remains variable. Laboring nitrous oxide is most commonly used in Europe. Tramadol is a weak opioid agonist Some literature suggests a reduction in the duration of labor with tramadol; benefits of tramadol include clinical effect within 10 minutes when administered IM and reduced maternal lethargy. Neonatal depression is less common because neonates posses the hepatic capacity to metabolize tramadol. Lumbar sympathetic block was a previously relatively common method of providing labor analgesia which has clinically become seldomly used over the past 20–30 years. It is effective in providing pain relief during the first stage of labor, but not after; parturients tend to have faster cervical dilatation, shorter second stage of labor and lower risk of fetal bradycardia than a paracervical block. It is more technically challenging than an epidural but may be performed when previous back surgery prevents placement of an epidural.

Keywords: Management strategies; Delivery

REFERENCES

Jones L, Othman M, Dowswell T et al. Pain management for women in labour: an overview of systematic reviews. *Cochrane Database Syst Rev* 2012;(3):CD009234.

Likis FE, Andrews JC, Collins MR et al. Nitrous oxide for the management of labor pain: a systematic review. *Anesth Analg* 2014;118:153–167.

8. ANSWER: C

Ketamine acts as a sedative and can be used to treat delirium but has an adverse effect on uteroplacental blood flow. Dexmedetomidine crosses the placenta, but its effects in pregnancy are otherwise unknown.

Keywords: Management strategies; Delivery

REFERENCE

Jones L, Othman M, Dowswell T et al. Pain management for women in labour: an overview of systematic reviews. *Cochrane Database Syst Rev* 2012;(3):CD009234.

9. ANSWER: D

Acute asthma exacerbation is a life-threatening situation, regardless of pregnancy status. Accessory muscle use, inability to talk, and quiet auscultation indicate impending respiratory collapse. The other treatments are all indicated after intubation.

While IV isoproterenol infusions are well described, it is important to remember that isoproterenol (like epinephrine) is not beta-2 selective. Magnesium sulfate infusions may be helpful as an adjunct to nebulized broncodilator and steroid therapy in adults as it augments the relaxation of the upper airways and is given as 25–50 mg/kg IV over 20 minutes (max 2gm); this therapeutic choice could be clinically useful if magnesium is required to manage a parturient.

REFERENCE

Bain E, Pierides BE, Clifton VL et al. Interventions for managing asthma in pregnancy. *Cochrane Database Syst Rev* 2014;(10):CD010660.

10. ANSWER: B

Given the severity of the patient's obstructive disease, it is likely that the tidal volumes of more than 10 mL/kg are exacerbating dynamic hyperinflation and auto-PEEP, which is affecting venous return. The first step would be to reduce the tidal volume so that the patient can exhale more effectively, allowing expiratory flow to reach baseline before the next breath ensues. Reducing the respiratory rate won't help if the patient's own rate remains high. Because the patient's hemodynamics are being affected by intrathoracic pressure, administering vasopressors will not effectively treat or resolve this patient's presentation.

REFERENCE

Bain E, Pierides BE, Clifton VL et al. Interventions for managing asthma in pregnancy. *Cochrane Database Syst Rev* 2014;(10):CD010660.

3.

HEMATOLOGY AND ONCOLOGY

Talia K. Ben-Jacob, Danielle L. Behrens, and Christopher P. Potestio

QUESTIONS

1. A 70-year-old male with a past medical history of alcoholic cirrhosis, chronic renal insufficiency, hypertension, and coronary artery disease (CAD) is admitted to the intensive care unit (ICU) after an open abdominal aortic aneurysm (AAA) repair for ruptured AAA. The patient was resuscitated in the operating room with a ratio of 1:1:1 packed red blood cells (PRBCs), thawed plasma, and platelets for a total of 25 units of PRBCs, 24 units of thawed plasma, and five packs of platelets by rapid transfuser. He arrives to the ICU intubated and sedated with the following vitals: blood pressure (BP) 70/40 mm Hg, heart rate (HR) 134 bpm, sinus tachycardia with prolonged QT and new T-wave inversion in all leads, respiratory rate (RR) of 28 breaths/minute, temperature of 35.5° C, and O_2 saturation of 92% on forced inspiratory oxygen (FiO_2) of 100%. His BP did not respond to aggressive volume replacement. The most likely cause of his instability is:

A. Disseminated intravascular coagulation (DIC)
B. Dilutional thrombocytopenia
C. Citrate toxicity
D. Hypothermia

2. A 51-year-old female with a history of acquired immunodeficiency syndrome (AIDS), with a CD4 count of 80, was recently started on highly active antiretroviral therapy (HAART). She has a recent diagnosis of deep vein thrombosis (DVT) while on anticoagulation. She presented to the hospital with complaints of fatigue and was found to have a gastrointestinal (GI) bleed, which was determined to be caused by diffuse large B-cell lymphoma, germinal center type in her stomach. She suffered worsening respiratory distress and required intubation and mechanical ventilation. She also developed circulatory shock requiring vasopressors, acute renal failure requiring continuous dialysis, and

worsening electrolyte derangement consisting of a phosphorus level of 5.1, potassium level of 6.5, lactate dehydrogenase (LDH) of 1700, uric acid of 12.4, and lactate of 8 because of her large tumor burden. The next step in management of this patient is administration of:

A. Rasburicase 3 g
B. Allopurinol 100 mg
C. Etoposide 125 mg
D. Cyclophosphamide 480 mg

3. An 82-year-old female presented to the emergency department (ED) with left-sided facial droop, expressive aphasia, and slurred speech. Her BP was 162/93 mm Hg. Head computed tomography (CT) showed early ischemic change without evidence of hemorrhage. Tissue plasminogen activator (tPA) was administered 45 minutes after the onset of her symptoms. Initially, the patient's symptoms began to improve, but 30 minutes into the administration of alteplase, the patient became more aphasic, with headache, and developed a large, unreactive pupil. The tPA was stopped immediately. Follow-up CT revealed significant subdural hematoma with midline shift. The best method to reverse the effects of tPA in this situation is:

A. Four-factor prothrombin complex concentrate (PCC)
B. Fresh frozen plasma (FFP)
C. Hemodialysis
D. Cryoprecipitate

4. A 77-year-old 95-kg African American male with a history of poorly controlled hypertension, coronary artery disease, paroxysmal atrial fibrillation, and chronic obstructive pulmonary disease (COPD) is admitted to the ICU after undergoing an aortic-bifemoral bypass. The patient arrives to the ICU intubated and with fenoldopam and nitroglycerin (0.75 µg/kg per minute)

infusing for BP control. He is extubated uneventfully later that evening. On the first postoperative day, the patient's pulse oximetry value falls to 90% despite being on 50% oxygen by aerosol face mask. On physical examination, he has labored breathing, with a RR of more than 20 breaths/minute and diminished air entry bilaterally. Despite two albuterol and ipratropium nebulizer treatments, dyspnea and O_2 saturation do not improve, and the patient is intubated. After intubation, despite an O_2 saturation of 95%, the patient developed cyanosis. When arterial blood gas (ABG) samples were obtained, it was noted that the blood was chocolate brown in color. ABG results were 7.15/58/250. The best treatment option for this patient is:

A. Hyperbaric chamber
B. Methylene blue
C. Insulin
D. Glucagon

5. A 59-year-old female patient with a past medical history of hypertension, diabetes mellitus, coronary artery disease, and receiving warfarin for atrial fibrillation presents to the hospital with severe abdominal pain and respiratory distress. She was found to be febrile with a temperature of 39.4° C, HR 140 bpm, BP 100/50 mm Hg, and pulse oximetry 89% on room air. An electrocardiogram (ECG) shows atrial fibrillation at a rate of 145 bpm. Blood tests revealed anemia with hemoglobin of 9.4 g/day and leukocytosis of 20,600 G/L. Blood cultures were sent, and CT scan of the chest/abdomen and pelvis was performed showing a 10- × 8- × 12-cm tubo-ovarian abscess. After the CT scan, the patient continues to deteriorate, requiring intubation for respiratory failure, and she develops septic shock requiring vasopressors. Gynecology is consulted, and the patient is scheduled for the operating room for source control. Given her long-term oral anticoagulation with warfarin, an international normalized ratio (INR) was ordered and found to be 10. The best method to correct this coagulopathy before the operating room is:

A. FFP
B. Protamine
C. PCC
D. Vitamin K

6. A 17-year-old female was brought to the ED after being found unconscious and covered in emesis while camping. Her propane heater was found to be defective. Her ECG was significant for tachycardia. She was intubated for airway protection. Her O_2 saturation was found to be 100% by pulse oximetry on FiO_2 of 40%. She was afebrile with HR 120 bpm and BP 80/42 mm Hg.

After intubation, she was noted to be hypotonic. The best confirmatory test to make an accurate diagnosis is:

A. Carboxyhemoglobin level
B. Methemoglobin level
C. ABG
D. Folic acid level

7. A 22-year-old female presents to a community hospital after being found unresponsive by friends. Initial head CT demonstrates an acute right-sided subdural hematoma, and she is immediately taken to the operating room for craniectomy. She remains intubated and unresponsive after surgery. Her temperature is 39.3° C, BP is 87/45 mm Hg, HR is 140 bpm and regular, RR is 14 breaths/minute, and O_2 saturation is 100% on FiO_2 of 40%. Laboratory examination reveals a white blood cell (WBC) count of 2.62×10^9/L with an absolute neutrophil count of 0.9×10^9/L, hemoglobin of 10.2 g/dL, platelet count of 17×10^9/L, creatinine of 1.65 mg/dL, total bilirubin of 2.6 mg/dL, LDH of 1521 U/L, and haptoglobin of 137 mg/dL. Coagulation studies show a prothrombin time (PT) of 21.6 seconds, partial thromboplastin time (PTT) of 39.8 seconds, INR of 1.9, fibrinogen of 73 mg/dL, and D-dimer greater than 21.60 μg/mL. Her peripheral smear shows numerous schistocytes, diminished platelet count without clumping, and scattered mature lymphocytes. Numerous promyelocytes are also noted (see the following image).

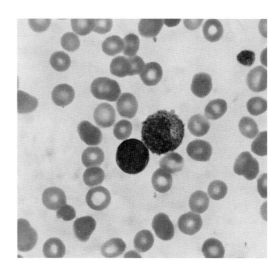

What is the next appropriate step in the management of this patient?

A. Initiate plasmapheresis with FFP replacement
B. Initiate all-*trans*retinoic acid (ATRA); transfuse cryoprecipitate, FFP, and platelets

C. Initiate 30 mL/kg of normal saline and broad-spectrum antibiotics.
D. Administer high-dose corticosteroids and intravenous immunoglobulin (IVIG).

8. A 57-year-old female is brought to the ED by her daughter for altered mental status, blurry vision, and headache. The blurry vision began 3 days ago and has progressively worsened. Her mental status change began approximately 9 hours ago. On exam, she is awake but is not following commands. She is agitated at times. Her medical history is significant for hepatitis C, hypertension, and diabetes mellitus. Her current medications include losartan and metformin. Her vital signs are temperature of 37.8° C, BP of 157/84 mm Hg, HR of 112 bpm, RR of 16 breaths/minute, and an O_2 saturation of 100% on room air. Laboratory analysis results include a WBC count of $20.65 \times 10^9/L$, hemoglobin of 8.4 g/dL, platelet count of $32 \times 10^9/L$, creatinine of 1.78 mg/dL, LDH of 1821, and haptoglobin of less than 10 mg/dL. Coagulation studies are performed and show a prothrombin time (PT) of 12.6 seconds, partial thromboplastin time (PTT) of 28.8 seconds, INR of 1.2, fibrinogen of 643 mg/dL, and D-dimer of 6.56 μg FEU/mL. Direct antiglobulin test (Coombs) is negative. Her peripheral smear shows numerous schistocytes with a diminished platelet count (see the following image). CT of the head without intravenous (IV) contrast is performed and demonstrates multiple acute/subacute nonhemorrhagic infarcts at the cerebral hemispheres in multiple vascular territories.

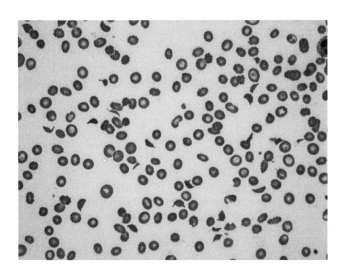

Which of the following is the most appropriate treatment for this patient's condition?

A. Plasmapheresis with FFP replacement
B. Platelet transfusion and administration of IV heparin
C. Plasmapheresis with albumin replacement
D. Transfusion of cryoprecipitate, FFP, and platelets

9. A 19-year-old male presents to the ED with a 3-week history of bruising and mucosal bleeding. He had a prodromal influenza-like illness before the development of spontaneous ecchymoses and epistaxis as well as mild hematuria. On entering the parking lot of the hospital, he developed a frontal headache. He now has left hand numbness as well as photophobia. Physical exam is notable for numerous ecchymoses on his arms, legs, flank, and abdomen. Abdominal exam does not demonstrate splenomegaly or hepatomegaly. Laboratory analysis shows a WBC count of $7.85 \times 10^9/L$ with an absolute neutrophil count (ANC) of $5.34 \times 10^9/L$, a hemoglobin of 15.5 g/dL, and a platelet count of $2 \times 10^9/L$ Coagulation studies are performed and reveal a PT of 11.6 seconds, PTT of 25.1 seconds, and INR of 1.1. Stat CT of the head is performed and shows an acute left-sided subdural hematoma with a 0.4-cm midline shift. Peripheral smear shows normocytic, normochromic red blood cells, a diminished platelet count, and scattered large platelets (see the following image).

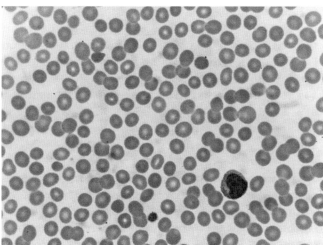

Which of the following is the most appropriate next step in the management of this patient?

A. Administration of PCC
B. Administration of recombinant factor VIIa and platelet transfusions
C. Initiation of high-dose corticosteroids, IVIG, and platelet transfusions
D. Platelet transfusions and neurosurgical consultation followed by evacuation of the subdural hematoma

10. A 68-year-old female presents to the ED with dyspnea and chest discomfort that started 45 minutes ago. The pain is substernal, nonradiating,

and associated with nausea and epigastric discomfort. Her medical history is significant for hypertension, for which she takes a thiazide diuretic. Her vital signs show a temperature of 38.8° C, BP of 102/65 mm Hg, HR of 137 bpm and regular, RR of 20 breaths/minute, and O_2 saturation of 92% on room air. ECG shows sinus tachycardia. Ten minutes after arrival, she develops hypotension with a BP of 72/38 mm Hg. Peripheral IV access cannot be obtained, and a right internal jugular vein triple lumen catheter is placed. Immediately after the procedure, she develops a rapidly expanding hematoma on the right side of her neck with tracheal deviation and airway compromise. She is intubated for airway protection. Imaging shows the triple-lumen catheter in proper position, without arterial injury. Laboratory analysis shows a WBC count of 12.5×10^9/L, hemoglobin of 9.3 g/dL, platelet count of 245×10^9/L, creatinine of 0.9, bilirubin of 1.1, PT of 10.8 seconds, INR of 1.2, and PTT of 78 seconds. Mixing study is performed and shows an initial value of 68 seconds and a 2-hour postincubation value of 76 seconds. Chest radiography is performed and shows a left lower lobe infiltrate consistent with pneumonia. Which of the following is the most appropriate treatment for this patient's coagulopathy?

A. Administration of recombinant factor IX
B. Administration of cryoprecipitate and FFP
C. Administration of recombinant factor VIII
D. Administration of activated PCC (aPCC), steroids, and cyclophosphamide

11. A 61-year-old male presents with fatigue and dyspnea. His symptoms began 2 weeks ago and have been progressively worsening. He is unable to given a full history because of tachypnea with accessory muscle use. O_2 saturation is 78% on room air. He is placed on a non-rebreather mask and transitioned to high-flow noninvasive ventilation. His RR decreases, and he appears more comfortable. His medical history is significant for diabetes mellitus, COPD, hypertension, and hyperlipidemia. Vital signs show a temperature of 37.4° C, BP of 147/68 mm Hg, RR of 18 breaths/minute, and O_2 saturation of 98% on 70% FiO_2. Laboratory analysis is performed and shows a WBC count of 215×10^9/L with 85% blasts, hemoglobin of 6.8 g/dL, and platelet count of 8×10^9/L. Peripheral smear is shown in the following image. Chest radiograph shows hyperinflation with diaphragmatic flattering and diffuse bilateral interstitial infiltrates. Which of the following is the most appropriate treatment for this patient's dyspnea?

A. Bilevel positive airway pressure
B. PRBC transfusions

C. Intubation and mechanical ventilation
D. Leukapheresis

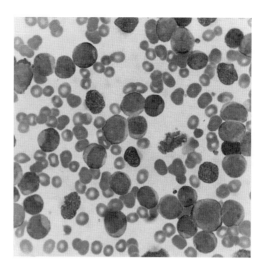

12. A 28-year-old female presents with a 2-month history of progressive dyspnea as well as a 25-lb weight loss. She has also noted a right anterior chest wall mass, which has been rapidly expanding over the past 7 days. On presentation, her vital signs show a temperature of 38.3° C, BP of 86/48 mm Hg, HR of 128 bpm, RR of 22 breaths/minute, and an O_2 saturation of 100% on 2 L by nasal cannula. Laboratory analysis is performed and shows a WBC count of 6.57×10^9/L, hemoglobin of 6 g/dL, platelet count of 429×10^9/L, LDH of 752 U/L, creatinine of 0.59, and total bilirubin of 0.4 mg/dL. CT of the chest is performed and shows a large mediastinal mass (measuring $9.8 \times 9.3 \times 11.9$ cm) with mass effect on the right side of the heart and mediastinum, mildly displacing it to the left of the midline; chronic occlusion of the superior vena cava with collateral vessels; severe encasement of the right pulmonary artery extending into the lower lobe branch; severe narrowing of the upper lobe branch; and a moderate to large pericardial effusion (see the following image). Echocardiography is performed and shows a large circumferential pericardial effusion with respiratory variation suggestive of tamponade. A pericardial drain is placed. Right chest wall biopsy is performed. Core biopsy shows large cells with scattered mitoses (positive for CD20, MUM1, BCL2 [subset], BCL6, and CD23 and a Ki67 of >95%). Which of the following is the most appropriate next step in the treatment of this patient?

A. External-beam radiation
B. Administration of cytotoxic chemotherapy and corticosteroids
C. Surgical resection of the mass
D. Referral to hospice

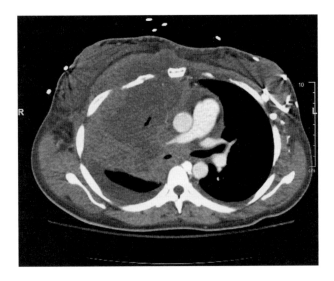

C. Hemophilia B is four times more common than hemophilia A

D. Approximately 70% of patients with hemophilia A will develop factor inhibitors

14. A 63-year-old male with a history of hypertension, prostate cancer, recurrent DVT, and CAD is now postoperative day (POD) 7 from three-vessel coronary artery bypass graft. His postoperative course was complicated by hypoxemic respiratory failure and acute kidney injury. His acute postoperative issues seem to be resolved, but his platelet count decreases from 116×10^9 to 52×10^9 (see the trend in the following table). He has received warfarin for the past 3 days in an attempt to transition to outpatient anticoagulation from an unfractionated heparin infusion. He has no evidence of thrombosis.

PREOP	POD 1	POD 2	POD 3	POD 4	POD 5	POD 6	POD 7
Platelet count ($\times 10^6$)	158	142	141	136	133	116	52
INR	1.2	1.1	1.1	1.0	1.0	1.0	1.4

The best option for management of this patient's anticoagulation status is:

A. Resume warfarin at home dose

B. Stop warfarin; start enoxaparin; send heparin-induced thrombocytopenia (HIT) antibody assay

C. Stop warfarin; start argatroban; send HIT antibody assay

D. Stop warfarin; start argatroban; send HIT antibody assay; give vitamin K

13. A 45-year-old male presents to the ED after a motor vehicle collision. He is visibly intoxicated and accompanied by police. He denies pain but is a poor historian. His medical history is significant for hemophilia A with a baseline factor level of less than 1%, human immunodeficiency virus (HIV), and hepatitis C. He is unable to provide a history regarding prior hemophilia treatments or recent factor dosing. Vital signs show a temperature of 37.2° C, BP of 110/68 mm Hg, HR of 107 bpm, RR of 18 breaths/minute, and O_2 saturation of 96% on room air. On exam, he has superficial abrasions on his arms, legs, and face. He has no cervical spine, chest wall, or abdominal tenderness. Laboratory analysis shows a WBC count of 5.8×10^9/L, hemoglobin of 11.6 g/dL, platelet count of 106×10^9/L, PT of 12.4 seconds, INR of 1.1, and PTT of 44.4 seconds. CT scans of the head, neck, chest, abdomen, and pelvis are performed. Imaging reveals a small acute subdural hematoma along the posterior aspect of the interhemispheric falx, right renal laceration with active bleeding and perinephric hematoma, laceration with partial transection of the pancreatic head with active hemorrhage, and right nondisplaced posterolateral rib fractures 6 to 9. He is taken emergently to the operating room. Arterial embolization of the right lower pole of the kidney is performed. Exploratory laparoscopy, lysis of adhesions, and drain placement are also performed. After surgery, he is admitted to the ICU. Which of the following statements regarding patients with hereditary hemophilia is true?

A. Recombinant factor VIIa is a first-line treatment option for hereditary hemophilia patients with active hemorrhage and no acquired inhibitors

B. The leading cause of death in patients with hemophilia is intracranial hemorrhage (ICH)

15. A 67-year-old female with COPD presented to the ED for COPD exacerbation requiring intubation. She is maintained on mechanical ventilation for several days, and she is started on inhaled albuterol, inhaled budesonide, IV methylprednisolone, and IV famotidine. On hospital day 4, the patient develops fever, leukocytosis, and thick sputum. She is started on vancomycin and cefepime for empiric therapy for ventilator-associated pneumonia. She remains hemodynamically stable and is extubated 8 days after presentation. During the course of her hospitalization, she develops thrombocytopenia, with a nadir platelet count of 50×10^9 on hospital day 7. All other lab values are within normal limits, including fibrinogen, WBC count, hemoglobin, hematocrit, and INR. The most likely cause of the patient's thrombocytopenia is:

A. Sepsis-induced thrombocytopenia

B. Drug-induced thrombocytopenia

C. Disseminated intravascular coagulopathy

D. Bone marrow suppression

16. A 27-year-old female with no significant past medical history presents to the ED with the following vital signs: sinus tachycardia of 155 bpm, BP of 88/62 mm Hg, and SaO$_2$ of 87% on 10 L of supplemental oxygen by face mask, afebrile. She is emergently intubated, and CT reveals pulmonary embolism. Laboratory values reveal WBC count of 10.1×10^9, hemoglobin of 19.4, hematocrit of 56%, and platelets 224×10^6. Red blood cell count is elevated, and erythropoietin (EPO) level is normal. What is the most likely cause of thromboembolic disease?

A. Polycythemia vera (PCV)
B. Undiagnosed malignancy
C. Pregnancy
D. Secondary erythrocytosis from smoking

17. An 82-year-old man presents to the ED after three episodes of emesis in the past hour. He has a past medical history significant for atrial fibrillation, for which he takes metoprolol and dabigatran. On presentation, his vital signs are stable, but after another episode of hematemesis, his HR increases to 132 bpm and is irregularly irregular. His BP drops to 82/39 mm Hg. In addition to synchronized cardioversion and blood transfusion, what is the best next step toward stabilizing this patient?

A. Administer vitamin K
B. Initiate emergent dialysis
C. Administer PCC
D. Administer idarucizumab

18. An obese 55-year-old male (height 5'8", weight 110 kg, body mass index 37) with hypertension and gastroesophageal reflux underwent pancreatoduodenectomy for pancreatic head mass and is admitted to the ICU after his procedure. On postoperative day 2, he develops acute hypoxic respiratory failure and is diagnosed with pulmonary embolism. He is started on heparin infusion but is switched to enoxaparin 4 days after the event. On postoperative day 9, he is extubated and doing well. His vital signs are stable—HR of 107 bpm, BP of 147/82 mm Hg, SaO$_2$ of 97, and temperature of 97.3° F. Laboratory values are as follows: sodium 137 mmol/L, potassium 3.9 mmol/L, chloride 97 mmol/L, serum bicarbonate 24 mmol/L, blood urea nitrogen 22 mg/dL, creatinine 1.1 mg/dL, glucose 107 mg/dL, WBC count 10.1×10^3 μL, hemoglobin 12.3 g/dL, hematocrit 37.2 g/dL, platelets 186×10^3 μL, and INR 1.1. His medications include hydromorphone, acetaminophen, amlodipine, pantoprazole, and enoxaparin 1.5 mg/kg total body weight daily dosing for therapeutic

anticoagulation. At this time, the patient has an acute worsening of mental status. Head CT reveals hemorrhagic stroke. Of the following options, which is the most likely cause of this spontaneous intracranial bleed?

A. Malignancy
B. Enoxaparin overdose
C. Hypertensive emergency
D. Acute liver failure

19. An 82-year-old unidentified man presents to the ED after being found unconscious in his home. Emergency medical services cannot provide any additional information. You notice that the patient has a well-healed sternotomy scar. He has a head laceration and no other notable injuries. CT scan reveals large thalamic bleed with midline shift. Labs are as follows: sodium 142 mg/dL, potassium 4.1 mg/dL, chloride 102 mg/dL, serum bicarbonate 23 mg/dL, blood urea nitrogen 22 mg/dL, creatinine 0.9 mg/dL, glucose 97 mg/dL, WBC count 10.2×10^9, hemoglobin 12.5 mg/dL, hematocrit 37.9%, platelets 222 $\times 10^6$, and INR 1.1. The thromboelastogram (TEG) is pictured in the Figure Q19.1. A normal TEG is provided in the Figure Q19.2.

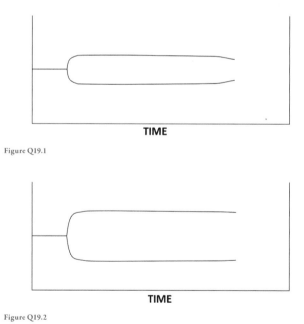

Figure Q19.1

Figure Q19.2

What is the most likely cause of this patient's head bleed?

A. Disseminated intravascular coagulopathy
B. Warfarin-induced coagulopathy
C. Clotting factor deficiency
D. Platelet dysfunction

20. A 67-year-old female with alcoholic cirrhosis is admitted to the ICU for upper GI bleeding from esophageal varices. She is appropriately resuscitated, receiving several units of PRBCs, thawed plasma, and platelets. Now her labs are as follows: INR 2.2, and platelets 39. These appear to be her baseline values. During her recovery, she developed a lower extremity thromboembolism in the left femoral vein. She continues to have a platelet count less than 30 and an INR greater than 2 without any anticoagulation. What is the best next step in the management of this patient?

A. Place permanent inferior vena cava (IVC) filter
B. Initiate heparin infusion with plan to convert to warfarin for 6 months
C. Initiate heparin infusion with plan to convert to dabigatran for 6 months
D. Initiate low-molecular-weight heparin for 6 months

ANSWERS

1. ANSWER: C

Citrate toxicity results when the citrate in the transfused blood binds to calcium in the patient's body and administration of IV calcium is not adequately performed to replenish the bound calcium. Hypotension not responding to volume resuscitation should alert the treatment team to this complication in patients undergoing massive transfusion protocol. Citrate is used to prevent clotting of stored blood products, and 90% of the citrate in blood products is found in platelets and FFP. A side effect of this preservative is that it chelates calcium and magnesium. Symptoms do not usually occur unless the rate of transfusion exceeds 1 unit every 5 minutes (about 6 units/hour or 35 mL/minute). Treatment is administration of IV calcium. Signs and symptoms of citrate toxicity include but are not limited to hypotension, decreased pulse pressure, arrhythmias, mental status changes, tetany, and laryngospasm. It can also lead to myocardial depression and vasoplegia. Circumstances that increase the likelihood of developing citrate intoxication may include hypothermia, hyperventilation, alkalosis, and liver disease/transplantation because citrate metabolism is primarily hepatic.

DIC is characterized by consumption of platelets and clotting factors in conjunction with fibrin formation and activation of fibrinolysis leading to pathologic clotting. It may be precipitated by tissue injury, obstetric complications, malignancies, and infections. Patients present with spontaneous bruising or excessive bleeding from minor wounds such as venipuncture sites. They may also have serious complications such as renal failure, acute respiratory distress syndrome, microangiopathic hemolytic anemia, and even death. DIC is associated with a combination of depleted clotting factors (i.e., prolonged PT and activated PTT), a low platelet count, schistocytes, increased D-dimer levels, and decreased fibrinogen levels. Management of DIC includes treating the underlying cause and correcting the hemostatic abnormalities with blood products. This answer choice is not correct because arrhythmias are not usually present in DIC, and characteristic signs such as bleeding around IV catheters are absent.

Dilutional thrombocytopenia is incorrect because the patient was transfused in a 1:1:1 ratio. There are studies that discuss the inability of transfusion to maintain normal concentrations of RBCs, platelets, and coagulation factors during massive transfusion protocol. The process used to create blood components out of whole blood results often requires dilution of all components with preservative leading to a reduction in the amount of platelets. Therefore, recombining the components (1 unit each of PRBCs, platelets, and FFP) does not result in a product equivalent to whole blood. However, this answer is incorrect in the previously mentioned case because dilutional thrombocytopenia in and of itself would not lead to the ECG changes noted.

The risk for hypothermia during massive blood transfusion and its subsequent complications is an absolute indication for the warming of all blood products administered. The coagulation cascade is significantly affected by hypothermia. There is a 10% reduction in coagulation factor activity for each 1° C drop in temperature below 33° C. Hypothermia can lead to other complications, such as peripheral vasoconstriction, metabolic acidosis, coagulopathy, and infection as well as exacerbate citrate toxicity. However, in this case, a temperature of 35.5° C is not low enough to cause coagulopathy, and cardiac morbidities seen in the patient described in the question.

Keywords: Management strategies: Transfusion and factor replacement

REFERENCES

Elmer J, Wilcox SR, Raja AS. Massive transfusion in traumatic shock. *J Emerg Med* 2013;44(4):829–838.

Patil V, Shetmahajan M. Massive transfusion and massive transfusion protocol. *Indian J Anaesth* 2014;58(5): 590–595.

Sihler KC, Napolitano LM. Complications of massive transfusion. *Chest* 2010;137(1):209–220.

2. ANSWER: A

Tumor lysis syndrome occurs in malignancies that are highly proliferative and have high tumor burdens, such as lymphomas and leukemias. Hyperuricemia as defined by a uric acid level ≥8 mg/dL is a diagnostic finding of tumor lysis syndrome. The other metabolic abnormalities found in tumor lysis syndrome include hyperphosphatemia, hyperkalemia, and hypocalcemia. The standard therapy for preventing tumor lysis syndrome is hydration, alkalinization of the urine with sodium bicarbonate, and allopurinol. However, allopurinol only prevents the formation of uric acid from purine catabolism and does not affect the uric acid developed before treatment. On the other hand, rasburicase affects already developed uric acid by converting uric acid to allantoin. Clinical trials have demonstrated that rasburicase is effective in lowering plasma uric acid levels in pediatric and adult patients in both prophylactic and treatment settings and is therefore the first-line treatment for tumor lysis syndrome. Etoposide and cyclophosphamide are incorrect answer choices because although they are appropriate to treat large B-cell lymphoma, starting chemotherapy in a patient with spontaneous tumor lysis syndrome from large tumor burden would exacerbate the condition.

Keywords: Diagnoses; Tumor lysis syndrome

REFERENCES

Alakel A, Middeke JM, Schetelig J, Bornhäuser M. Prevention and treatment of tumor lysis syndrome, and the efficacy and role of rasburicase. *Onco Targets Ther* 2017;10:597–605.

Bose P, Qubaiah O. VA review of tumour lysis syndrome with targeted therapies and the role of rasburicase. *J Clin Pharm* 2011;36:299–326.

3. Answer: D

The tPA mechanism of action involves the conversion of plasminogen to plasmin. Plasmin then degrades fibrinogen to fibrin, which causes thrombolysis. Plasminogen activators are categorized as fibrin selective and fibrin nonselective. Fibrin-nonselective plasminogen activators cleave both fibrinogen and fibrin, producing an anticoagulant state that can promote hemorrhage. About 2 to 7% of patients with ischemic stroke who receive IV alteplase develop intraparenchymal hemorrhage with mass effect. Thrombolytic infusions should be stopped immediately in any patient with acute clinical changes suggestive of ICH. Emergent noncontrast head CT should be performed for confirmation of hemorrhage. If fibrinogen levels are still very low 24 hours after administration of tPA and only slowly correct over days, it is reasonable to replace fibrinogen immediately. Cryoprecipitate contains fibrinogen (200 mg/unit), von Willebrand factor, fibronectin, factor VIII, and factor XIII. Ten units of cryoprecipitate will raise fibrinogen levels by roughly 70 mg/dL in a 70-kg patient. Current guidelines recommend a fibrinogen level of 150 mg/dL for adequate reversal.

FFP also contains fibrinogen, but in a lower concentration than cryoprecipitate. A larger volume of FFP must be transfused because of lower concentrations of fibrinogen. Therefore, cryoprecipitate is suggested over FFP.

Four-factor PCC does not contain fibrinogen. The factors in PCC include II, IX, and X, and some versions also contain factor VII. It is not indicated in this case. Alteplase, which was used in the aforementioned case, is metabolized by the liver. Reteplase is the only thrombolytic agent that is metabolized by the kidney. There are no reported cases of reteplase-associated symptomatic ICH managed with dialysis. Given its short plasma half-life (13–16 minutes), there appears to be no role for dialysis in the reversal of reteplase.

Keywords: Management strategies, anticoagulants, thrombolytics

REFERENCES

Frontera JA, Lewin JJ, Rabinstein AA et al. Guideline for reversal of antithrombotic in intracranial hemorrhage. *Neurocrit Care* 2016;24:6–46.

Yaghi S, Boehme AK, Dibu J et al. Treatment and outcome of thrombolysis-related hemorrhage: a multicenter retrospective study. *JAMA Neurol* 2015;72(12):1451–1457.

4. ANSWER: B

While methemoglobinemia can be congenital, the most common etiology in adults is ingestion or skin exposure to oxidizing agents. There is a large list of common medications that have been found to produce methemoglobinemia (Table 3.1). It appears likely that our patient formed methemoglobin in response to his continuous IV nitroglycerine infusion. Nitroglycerine accelerates oxidation of oxyhemoglobin to methemoglobin through the NADPH reductase system when metabolized in the liver by glutathione reductase. Large doses and increased rates of infusion of nitroglycerin are risk factors for the development of methemoglobinemia. Because multiple factors contribute to the risk for developing methemoglobinemia (i.e., patient age, weight, renal and hepatic function, arterial oxygen, anemia, pulmonary and cardiac disease, peripheral vascular disease, shock, sepsis, acidosis, and genetics), the exact dose and rate of nitroglycerin necessary to cause methemoglobinemia remain unknown. Signs and symptoms of methemoglobinemia include but are not limited to shortness of breath, cyanosis, headache, fatigue, dizziness, seizures, coma, and death.

Pulse oximetry is a poor indicator of the actual percentage of methemoglobin in the blood and of tissue oxygenation in patients with methemoglobinemia and can often lead to misdiagnosis. This is because a pulse oximeter gauges light absorbance at two wavelengths: 660 and 940 nm, and methemoglobin absorbs light almost equally at both 660 and 940 nm. Therefore, at 100% methemoglobin in the blood, the absorbance ratio is

Table 3.1 **COMMON DRUGS OR TOXINS THAT CAN CAUSE METHEMOGLOBINEMIA**

CLASSES OF DRUGS	SPECIFIC DRUG
Antibiotics	Trimethoprim, dapsone, sulfonamides
Local anesthetics	Benzocaine, prilocaine, articaine, Cetacaine, lidocaine
Environmental toxins	Aniline dyes, exhaust fumes, pesticides, industrial chemicals
Nitrates/nitrites	Nitroglycerine, sodium nitroprusside, bismuth nitrate, nitric oxide, nitrous oxide, silver nitrate, sodium nitrite
Other drugs	Metoclopramide, rasburicase, phenazopyridine

approximately 1, which corresponds to an 85% O_2 saturation reading by pulse oximetry. ABG values can also be misleading. The arterial PO_2 is a measure of dissolved oxygen and does not directly correlate with oxygen molecules bound to hemoglobin. This explains why patients with life-threatening methemoglobinemia may have normal PO_2 values. In addition, an ABG analyzer calculates the O_2 saturation from the pH and PCO_2 values, using the Henderson-Hasselbach equation for serum bicarbonate under the assumption of presence of normal hemoglobin. The presence of methemoglobin shifts the oxygen–hemoglobin dissociation curve to the left, resulting in false elevations of the O_2 saturation levels. Co-oximetry using spectrophotometry is the most accurate way of measuring methemoglobin levels because it measures the absorbance of light at four different wavelengths. When methemoglobinemia is in the differential, it is important to specifically request a methemoglobin level so that the blood may be processed in a co-oximeter because methemoglobin levels are not routinely performed on ABG analyzers.

Two simple tests can be used to diagnose methemoglobinemia at the bedside. Blood that is saturated with methemoglobin appears chocolate brown. The first test involves placing one to two drops of the patient's blood on a piece of white filter paper. When exposed to oxygen, deoxyhemoglobin will brighten in color, whereas methemoglobin will remain chocolate brown. The second test distinguishes between sulfhemoglobin and methemoglobin. The addition of potassium cyanide (Drabkin's reagent) turns methemoglobin bright red but does not alter sulfhemoglobin.

Methylene blue and removal of the causative agent are the first lines of therapy when the diagnosis of symptomatic methemoglobinemia is made. Methylene blue works by returning methemoglobin to an unoxidized state at a dose of 1 to 2 mg/kg over a 3- to 5-minute interval. An additional dose of 1 mg/kg may be repeated after 30 minutes if the methemoglobinemia does not resolve. An infusion of dextrose should be administered in conjunction with methylene blue because it upregulates the glycolytic cycle. Dextrose is necessary to form NADPH through the pentose phosphate pathway. Vitamin C can occasionally reduce cyanosis associated with chronic methemoglobinemia but has no role in treatment of acute acquired methemoglobinemia.

A hyperbaric chamber is used to treat carboxyhemoglobin from carbon monoxide poisoning and is not first-line treatment for methemoglobinemia. Insulin and glucagon are not indicated in the treatment of methemoglobinemia.

Keywords: Diagnoses- Hemoglobin Abnormalities- Methemoglobin

REFERENCE

Cortazzo JA, Lichtman AD. Methemoglobinemia: a review and recommendations for management. *J Cardiothorac Vasc Anesth* 2014;28(4):1043–1047.

5. ANSWER: C

PCC, also known as four-factor or factor IX complex, is a medication made up of blood clotting factors II, IX, and X, and some versions also contain factor VII. These products do not require ABO matching and can be reconstituted and administered quickly. PCCs have an extremely low infection risk because they are purified and contain no living cells. In a prospective, randomized controlled trial of vitamin K antagonist reversal in hemorrhaging patients, three-factor PCCs reliably reversed vitamin K antagonist anticoagulation within 30 minutes, and the effect persisted for up to 24 hours. The magnitude of correction and hemostasis was greater in the PCC group than the FFP group, and hemostasis was better in the PCC group. These results led the American College of Chest Physicians to recommend PCC as the first-line treatment for hemorrhaging patients who have been taking vitamin K antagonists. Table 3.2 describes the management of reversal of vitamin K antagonists at varying INR levels in patients who require surgery. Side effects of PCC include allergic reactions, headache, vomiting, and blood clots, which may result in a heart attack, stroke, pulmonary embolism, or DVT.

FFP is the most commonly used treatment to replace the deficiency of clotting factors caused by vitamin K antagonists because it is inexpensive and widely available. However, it is not first line in this case for various reasons. Our patient required rapid correction for the operating room, and PCC has a quicker onset of action. In addition, to reverse an INR of 10, high volumes of FFP are required. The operating room could be delayed because FFP requires type-specific units and thawing of frozen units. The large volume can put the patient at increased risk for congestive heart failure exacerbation or transfusion-related lung injury. There is also an increased infection risk with FFP compared with PCC.

Protamine is used for reversal of heparin and low-molecular-weight heparins such as enoxaparin. While vitamin K does reverse the effects of warfarin and can even sustain the effects and duration of PCC, it is not first-line treatment. Vitamin K, regardless of route of administration, corrects the INR to below 3 within 24 hours, and this patient requires emergency surgery with need for rapid correction.

Keywords: Coagulopathies, acquired; Vitamin K coagulopathy

INR VALUE	URGENT SURGERY OR PROCEDURE	SURGERY OR PROCEDURE SCHEDULED IN 24–48 HOURS
INR >1.5 but <1.9	No dose reduction may be required Monitor INR again before lowering the dose Treatment with FFP if needed	No dose reduction may be required Monitor INR again before lowering the dose Vitamin K 1 mg PO if needed
INR >1.9 but <5 in patients who require reversal for a procedure No significant bleeding currently	For rapid (<12 hr) reversal: FFP + vitamin K 1–3 mg slow IV	Vitamin K 1–2.5 mg PO If INR still elevated in 24 hr, repeat
INR >5 but <9 in patients who require surgery No significant bleeding currently	For rapid (<12 hr) reversal: FFP + vitamin K 2–5mg slow IV	Vitamin K 2.5–5 mg PO If INR still elevated in 24 hr, give vitamin K 1–2 mg PO
INR ≥9.0 No significant bleeding currently	Hold vitamin K antagonist therapy and give prothrombin concentrate complex supplemented with vitamin K_1 (10 mg by slow IV infusion) Monitor from the fourth hour after prothrombin complex concentrate	Hold vitamin K antagonist therapy Give oral vitamin K_1 at higher dose (5–10 mg) with the expectation that the INR will be reduced substantially in 24 to 48 hr Monitor daily and give additional vitamin K_1 if necessary Resume at lower dose when INR is in therapeutic range
Major bleeding at any elevation of INR	Hold vitamin K antagonist therapy and give prothrombin concentrate complex supplemented with vitamin K_1 (10 mg by slow IV infusion) Monitor from the fourth hour after prothrombin complex concentrate	

IV = intravenous (administration); FFP = fresh frozen plasma; INR = international normalized ratio; PO = oral (administration).

REFERENCES

Ageno W, Gallus AS, Wittkowsky A et al. Oral anticoagulant therapy: antithrombotic therapy and prevention of thrombosis, 9th ed. American College of Chest Physicians evidence-based clinical practice guidelines. *Chest* 2012;141:e44S–e88S.

Ghadimi K, Levy JH, Welsby IJ. Prothrombin complex concentrates for bleeding in the perioperative setting. *Anesth Analg* 2016;122(5):1287–1300.

Holbrook A, Schulman S, Witt DM et al. Evidence-based management of anticoagulant therapy: antithrombotic therapy and prevention of thrombosis, 9th ed. American College of Chest Physicians evidence-based clinical practice guidelines. *Chest* 2012;141(2 Suppl):e152S-e184S.

Meltzer J, Guenzer JR. Anticoagulant reversal and anesthetic considerations. *Anesthesiol Clin* 2017;35(2):191–205.

6. ANSWER: A

The diagnosis of carbon monoxide poisoning is made by a history of exposure. Possible methods of exposure include inhalation of internal combustion engine exhaust, smoke inhalation, improperly adjusted gas or oil heating, charcoal or gas grills, or exposure to paint stripper containing methylene chloride. Confirmation of the diagnosis is made by finding elevated carboxyhemoglobin in either arterial or venous blood. ABG tests are the most reliable source for samples. Of note, smokers can have a carboxyhemoglobin level of up to 9% as baseline. Patients generally do not have symptoms if levels are less than 10%, with overt signs developing at about 15%. Of note, carboxyhemoglobin measurement is an insufficient marker for assessing the severity of disease. In case of suspected carbon monoxide intoxication, the investigation should also include a complete blood count, a liver function test, and determination of electrolyte, urea, and glucose levels. A co-oximeter may be used to measure the carrying state of hemoglobin in a blood specimen from the patient. It is able to measure the carbon monoxide bound to hemoglobin, as distinguished from simple oximetry, which measures hemoglobin bound to molecular oxygen. The use of a regular pulse oximeter is not effective in the diagnosis of carbon monoxide poisoning because people with carbon monoxide poisoning may have a normal O_2 saturation level on a pulse oximeter. This is because the carboxyhemoglobin can be misrepresented as oxyhemoglobin and therefore absorbs light similarly at the two wavelengths measured.

Clinical presentation of carboxyhemoglobinemia is unspecific. Symptoms include nausea, dizziness, confusion, headache, dyspnea, and tachycardia. Specific cardiovascular manifestations include electrocardiographic

QT prolongation, myocardial ischemia, low BP, cardiac dysfunction (systolic and diastolic), and ventricular arrhythmia. Neurological effects associated with carboxyhemoglobin include status epilepticus, polyneuropathy, and hypotonia.

Treatment involves immediate oxygen through a 100% non-rebreather face mask. The increased oxygen promotes cellular respiration and reduces the elimination half-life of carboxyhemoglobin from 4 to 5 hours to 1 to 2 hours. Glucose should be closely monitored because extremes of blood sugars have the potential to exacerbate neuronal cell death. In case of severe toxicity or unremitting symptoms, treatment with hyperbaric oxygen (HBO) should commence. HBO is enhances elimination of carboxyhemoglobin, with a half-life average of 20 minutes at 3 atmospheres. A secondary benefit of HBO may be in regeneration of cytochrome oxidase and inhibition of leukocyte adherence to the microvascular endothelium.

Methemoglobin level is useful in diagnosis of methemoglobinemia, which is usually identified as a continuous pulse oximeter saturation of 85%, despite intervention.

ABG is the primary source from which the carboxyhemoglobin levels are measured but in of itself cannot make a diagnosis of carbon monoxide poisoning.

Folic acid level is used to determine diagnosis of megaloblastic anemia.

Keywords: Diagnoses; Hemoglobin abnormalities, carboxyhemoglobin

burns, placental abruption, amniotic fluid embolism, and vascular malformations. Consumption of platelets, anticoagulant proteins, and fibrinogen, as well as increased fibrinolysis, lead to formation of microvascular thrombi and hemorrhage. Cytokines play an active role in the procoagulant process. The incidence of DIC at presentation or during initial treatment is greater than 90% in patients with acute promyelocytic leukemia. Treatment of DIC consists of supportive care, transfusions (plasma, cryoprecipitate, and platelets), and management of the underlying systemic process.

TTP is characterized by fever, altered mental status, microangiopathic hemolytic anemia, thrombocytopenia, and renal insufficiency. All five symptoms are not necessary to make the diagnosis. Treatment of TTP consists of plasmapheresis with FFP replacement. The coagulation studies should be normal in TTP.

Although sepsis can cause DIC, this patient has evidence of acute promyelocytic leukemia. ATRA should be initiated immediately, while awaiting confirmation of the 15:17 translocation.

IVIG and corticosteroids are the primary treatment for immune thrombocytopenia. In immune thrombocytopenia, patients have an isolated low platelet count, with large platelets and a normal-sized spleen. Coagulation studies should also be normal in immune thrombocytopenia.

Keywords: DIC; Leukemia; Thrombocytopenia; Coagulopathies, acquired; Coagulation studies

REFERENCES

Bleecker ML. Carbon monoxide intoxication. *Handb Clin Neurol* 2015;131:191–203.

Reumuth G, Alharbi Z, Houschyar KS et al. Carbon monoxide intoxication: what we know. *Burns* 2018 Aug 14. doi: 10.1016/j.burns.2018.07.006 [Epub ahead of print].

REFERENCES

Kayser S, Schlenk R, Platzbecker U. Management of patients with acute promyelocytic leukemia. *Leukemia* 2018;32(6):1277–1294.

Levi M, Scully M. How I treat disseminated intravascular coagulation. *Blood* 2018;131:845–854.

Levi M, Seligsohn U. Disseminated intravascular coagulation. In: Kaushansky K, Lichtman MA, Prchal JT et al, eds. *Williams hematology,* 9th ed. New York: McGraw-Hill; 2016.

7. Answer: B

This patient presented with ICH in the setting of pancytopenia. Her peripheral smear demonstrates schistocytes, which are seen in DIC as well as other microangiopathic hemolytic processes, such as thrombotic thrombocytopenic purpura (TTP) and hemolytic uremic syndrome (HUS). Additionally, promyelocytes with Auer rods are present. The coagulation parameters show prolonged PT, PTT, and INR. Additionally, the fibrinogen is low, and the D-dimer is incalculable. These laboratory abnormalities are most consistent with DIC. DIC is not a primary hematologic condition, but rather is a hematologic manifestation of a systemic process. Causes of DIC include infection, malignancies (both solid tumors and hematologic malignancies), trauma,

8. ANSWER: A

This patient presented with altered mental status in the setting of microangiopathic hemolytic anemia and thrombocytopenia. Additionally, she has renal insufficiency and normal coagulation studies. These findings are consistent with a diagnosis of TTP. TTP is caused by antibodies against ADAMTS13 (a disintegrin and metalloprotease with a thrombospondin type 1 motif member 13). ADAMTS13 is responsible for cleaving von Willebrand multimers and is found in plasma. Treatment of TTP consists of emergent plasmapheresis with FFP replacement to remove antibodies and replace ADAMTS13. If plasmapheresis is not available or is delayed, simple transfusion of FFP should be performed. The mortality rate for untreated TTP is greater than 90%.

As stated previously, ADAMTS13 is found in plasma. Plasmapheresis with albumin replacement would remove ADAMTS13 antibodies but would fail to replete levels of functional ADAMTS13.

Transfusion of cryoprecipitate, FFP, and platelets would be recommended if this patient presented with DIC. In DIC, the coagulation studies would be elevated, and the fibrinogen would be low. This patient has normal coagulation studies, which are consistent with TTP.

Keywords: Thrombocytopenia; Anemia; Thrombotic thrombocytopenic purpura; Plasmapheresis; Plasma exchange; Platelet abnormalities

REFERENCES

Joly B., Coppo C, Veyradier A. Thrombotic thrombocytopenic purpura. *Blood* 2017;129:2836–2846.

Levi M, Scully M. How I treat disseminated intravascular coagulation. *Blood* 2018;131:845–854.

Sadler J. Thrombotic microangiopathies. In: Kaushansky K, Lichtman MA, Prchal JT et al., eds. *Williams hematology*, 9th ed. New York: McGraw-Hill; 2016.

9. ANSWER: C

This clinical presentation is most consistent with immune thrombocytopenia. The patient presented with ICH in the setting of severe thrombocytopenia. On exam, he has mucosal bleeding and ecchymoses, which are characteristic of a platelet abnormality, also referred to as "platelet-type bleeding." His spleen is not palpable. His complete blood count reveals a normal leukocyte count and normal hemoglobin. Peripheral smear is notable for a significantly diminished platelet count with scattered large platelets. In immune thrombocytopenia, the risk for life-threatening hemorrhage increases when the platelet count is less than 10 × 10^9/L. The reported frequency of ICH in adults with immune thrombocytopenia is approximately 1.5%. Treatment of severe or life-threatening hemorrhage in patients with immune thrombocytopenia consists of combined treatment with corticosteroids, IVIG, and platelet transfusions.

PCC is a three- or four-factor product containing inactive vitamin K–dependent factors, protein C, protein S, and heparin (to prevent activation of factors). Three-factor concentrates contain factors II, IX, and X. Four-factor concentrates contain factors II, VII, IX, and X. KCentra (four-factor concentrate) was approved for use in the United States in 2013. The main indication for PCC is reversal of vitamin K antagonists (warfarin) in severe or life-threatening hemorrhage. It is also approved for patients taking vitamin K antagonists who require emergent surgery or procedures. PCC is not the treatment of choice in this patient because his hemorrhagic complication is due to severe thrombocytopenia and not factor deficiency or vitamin K antagonists.

Recombinant factor VIIa is approved for bleeding events and periprocedural management in patients with hemophilia A or B who have acquired inhibitors. It is also indicated in the management of patients with Glanzmann thrombocythemia, who are refractory to platelet transfusions, as well as patients with congenital factor VII deficiency and adults with acquired hemophilia. This patient has ICH associated with immune thrombocytopenia; therefore, recombinant factor VIIa is not the treatment of choice.

Neurosurgical consultation is appropriate in the setting of ICH; however, evacuation should not be performed at this time. Corticosteroids, IVIG, and platelets should be administered with frequent neurological monitoring and repeat imaging.

Keywords: Thrombocytopenia; Immune thrombocytopenia; Routine blood studies; Platelet abnormalities

REFERENCES

Arnold D. Bleeding complications in immune thrombocytopenia. *ASH Education Book* December 5, 2015;2015(1):237–242.

Diz-Küçükkaya R, López JA. Thrombocytopenia. In: Kaushansky K, Lichtman MA, Prchal JT et al., eds. *Williams hematology,* 9th ed. New York: McGraw-Hill; 2016.

Franchini M, Lippi G. Prothrombin complex concentrates: an update. *Blood Transfus* 2010;8(3):149–154.

Kcentra (prothrombin complex concentrate) prescribing information. Kankakee, IL: CSL Behring LLC; 2017.

NovoSeven RT prescribing information. Bagsvaerd, Denmark: Novo Nordisk A/S; 2016.

Roberts HR, Monroe DM, White GC. The use of recombinant factor VIIa in the treatment of bleeding disorders. *Blood* 2005;104(13):3858–3864.

Sin J, Berger K, Lesch C. Four-factor prothrombin complex concentrate for life-threatening bleeds or emergent surgery: a retrospective evaluation. *J Crit Care* 2016;36:166–172.

10. ANSWER: D

This patient developed a rapidly expanding hematoma after central line placement. Coagulation studies revealed a prolonged PTT. The differential diagnosis includes a factor deficiency, such as hemophilia, versus a factor inhibitor (also known as acquired hemophilia). A mixing study was performed and failed to correct both initially and 2 hours after incubation. In patients with hereditary hemophilia, the mixing study should normalize the PTT. This patient, therefore, has a factor inhibitor.

Acquired hemophilia A is a condition that results from antibodies against factor VIII. Factor VIII antibodies, although rare, are the most common antibodies against the coagulation cascade. Approximately 50% of cases are idiopathic. Additional causes include malignancy, autoimmune conditions, and medications. Treatment consists of controlling bleeding and suppressing autoantibody formation or treating the underlying cause, if present.

aPCC (also known as factor VIII inhibitor bypassing activity, or FEIBA) and recombinant factor VIIa are first-line treatment options for bleeding in patients with acquired hemophilia. Additionally, immunosuppression is necessary to eliminate autoantibodies to factor VIII. This can be achieved with steroids and cyclophosphamide.

This patient has a factor VIII inhibitor; therefore, administration of recombinant factor IX alone will be insufficient to treat both the bleeding complication and the factor inhibition.

Recombinant factor VIII may be used to replete factor VIII levels if antibody titers are low; however, this patient developed a life-threatening hemorrhage and requires both management of the hemorrhage and suppression of the immune system.

Keywords: Coagulopathies; Factor replacement; Coagulation studies

REFERENCES

Franchini M, Lippi G. Acquired factor VIII inhibitors. *Blood* 2008;112(2):250–255.
Stowell SR, Lollar J, Meeks SL. Antibody-mediated coagulation factor deficiencies. In: Kaushansky K, Lichtman MA, Prchal JT et al., eds. *Williams hematology*, 9th ed. New York: McGraw-Hill; 2016.

11. ANSWER: D

The patient presents with hypoxic respiratory failure due to acute leukemia. He has hyperleukocytosis, with a WBC count of 215×10^9/L. The calculated absolute blast count is 182.75×10^9/L. Hyperleukocytosis is defined as a leukocyte count greater than 100×10^9/L. Leukostasis refers to the clinical symptoms that are due to increased viscosity and organ infiltration from hyperleukocytosis. The lungs, liver, and kidney are the most commonly involved organs. Leukapheresis is considered for symptomatic patients with hyperleukocytosis. IV hydration should be administered, and hydroxyurea should also be started for cytoreduction.

Although he is anemic, this patient should receive leukapheresis before PBRC transfusion. Red cell transfusions may increase viscosity and worsen symptoms of leukostasis.

This patient is hemodynamically stable on high-flow noninvasive ventilation (Vapotherm); therefore, he does not need to be transitioned to bilevel positive airway pressure (BiPAP) or intubated.

Keywords: Leukemia; Leukocytosis; Leukapheresis; WBC disorder

REFERENCES

Liesveld JL, Lichtman MA. Acute myelogenous leukemia. In: Kaushansky K, Lichtman MA, Prchal JT et al., eds. *Williams hematology*, 9th ed. New York: McGraw-Hill; 2016.
Röllig C, Ehninger G. How I treat hyperleukocytosis in acute myeloid leukemia. *Blood* 2016;125(21):3246–3252.

12. ANSWER: B

This patient presented with a large mediastinal mass, superior vena cava occlusion, a large pericardial effusion, and biopsy results consistent with primary mediastinal B-cell lymphoma. The differential diagnosis for an anterior mediastinal mass includes thymoma or thymic carcinoma, teratoma, thyroid mass, germ cell tumor, and lymphoma. Current treatment recommendations include rituximab and anthracycline chemotherapy, with or without radiation therapy.

B-cell lymphoma is sensitive to both chemotherapy and radiation therapy. This patient is newly diagnosed and has not seen prior systemic therapy. While she may require radiation for residual disease after treatment, radiation should not be initiated before chemotherapy.

Surgical resection is not appropriate because lymphoma is a chemosensitive and radiosensitive malignancy.

The patient has a curable malignancy; therefore, referral to hospice is not the appropriate recommendation.

Keywords: Lymphoma

REFERENCES

Giulino-Roth L. How I treat primary mediastinal B-cell lymphoma. *Blood* 2018;132(8):782–790.
Juanpere S, Cañete N, Ortuño P et al. A diagnostic approach to the mediastinal masses. *Insights Imaging* 2013;4(1):29–52.
Smith SD, Press OW, Smith SD et al. Diffuse large b-cell lymphoma and related diseases. In: Kaushansky K, Lichtman MA, Prchal JT et al., eds. *Williams hematology*, 9th ed. New York: McGraw-Hill; 2016.

13: ANSWER: B

The leading cause of death in hemophilia is due to ICH. In patients with severe factor deficiency (defined as less than

1% activity), significant bleeding may occur with even mild trauma.

Hemophilia A and B are the only two sex-linked hereditary factor deficiencies. Their genes are located on the long arm of chromosome X. Hemophilia A is approximately five times more common than hemophilia B. The higher incidence of hemophilia A is attributed to its larger size, which contains 26 exons.

Recombinant factor VIIa is indicated for treatment of hemorrhagic complications in patients with hereditary hemophilia who have acquired inhibitors, factor VII deficiency, or Glanzmann thrombocythemia that is refractory to platelet transfusions, and for bleeding complications and perioperative management of adult patients with acquired hemophilia.

Approximately 30% of patients with hemophilia A will develop inhibitors to factor replacement; therefore answer D is incorrect.

Keywords: Hemophilia, congenital; Coagulation studies; Factor replacement; Coagulopathies

REFERENCES

Escobar MA, Key NS. Hemophilia A and hemophilia B. In: Kaushansky K, Lichtman MA, Prchal JT et al., eds. *Williams hematology*, 9th ed. New York: McGraw-Hill; 2016.

Meeks SL, Batsuli G. Hemophilia and inhibitors: current treatment options and potential new therapeutic approaches. *Hematology* 2016;2016(1):657–662.

NovoSeven RT prescribing information. Bagsvaerd, Denmark: Novo Nordisk A/S; 2016.

14. ANSWER: D

This patient's thrombocytopenia is concerning for Heparin Induced Thrombocytopenia (HIT) and anticoagulation should be maintained only with nonheparinoid drugs. In addition, warfarin should be reversed because vitamin K antagonists cause decreased level of protein C and increase the patient's risk for developing venous limb gangrene.

HIT is an important complication of heparin exposure. There are two types of HIT. Type 1 is a nonimmune disorder that results from a direct effect of heparin on platelet activation. Type 2 is drug-induced, immune-mediated thrombocytopenia that typically occurs 4 to 10 days after exposure to heparin with the development of HIT type 2 antibodies (immunoglobulin G) and creates an increased risk for thrombosis. When we refer to HIT, we typically mean type 2 HIT.

The risk for HIT is independent of age, sex, heparin dose, and route of administration. Unfractionated heparin portends higher risk than low-molecular-weight heparin, although any heparin-containing product can be implicated, and all should be stopped if diagnosis of HIT is suspected. Heparin exposure related to surgery, especially cardiac surgery, also increases

risk. The incidence of HIT has been cited as high as 1.2% of all patients who receive heparin for 4 days.

The mortality rate is approximately 20%, and approximately 10% of patients suffer from major morbidity like amputation. Complications of HIT include DVT, arterial thrombosis, pulmonary embolism, stroke, myocardial infarction, limb ischemia, and warfarin-induced venous limb gangrene.

The probability of any individual patient having HIT can be quantified by using the 4Ts scoring system. The 4T score is calculated by assigning a value of 0 to 2 in four categories, all of which begin with the letter T (sort of): Thrombocytopenia, Timing, Thrombosis, and oTher causes. For Thrombocytopenia, a score of 0 indicates a drop of less than 30% in platelet count or a nadir less than 10×10^6; a score of 1 indicates a drop of 30 to 50% in platelet count, or a nadir between 10 to 19×10^6. For Timing, a score of 0 indicates platelet drop less than 4 days from heparin exposure; a score of 1 indicates platelet drop more than 10 days from heparin exposure; and a score of 2 indicates platelet drop between 4 and 10 days of heparin exposure. For Thrombosis, a score of 0 indicates no thrombosis; a score of 1 indicates suspected thrombosis; and a score of 2 indicates proven thrombosis or skin necrosis after exposure to heparin. For oTher causes, a score of 0 indicates that other causes of thrombocytopenia are likely; a score of 1 indicates that other causes of thrombocytopenia are possible; and a score of 2 indicates that no other causes of thrombocytopenia can explain the patient's condition.

A 4Ts score of 0 to 3 means there is low probability that the patient has HIT antibodies (<5%); score of 4 or 5 means intermediate probability (14%) that the patient has HIT antibodies; and a score greater than 5 means there is a high probability (64%) of HIT. Intermediate scores are particularly challenging because conditions like sepsis or simply post–cardiac bypass syndrome can yield an intermediate score in the absence of HIT antibodies. Of note, the nadir of platelets in HIT is typically greater than $20 \times 10^9/L$, so a nadir lower than that indicates lower risk for HIT compared with a nadir greater than or equal to $20 \times 10^9/L$. Because of the high morbidity and mortality associated with HIT, it is advisable to treat intermediate-risk patients conservatively by discontinuing heparin exposure and sending HIT antibody assay.

This patient has a 4T score of 5 points (2 points for Thrombocytopenia, 2 points for Timing, 0 points for Thrombosis, 1 point for oTher causes). The likelihood that this patient has HIT is approximately 14%. Further heparin exposure should be avoided in order to avoid the potential for thrombosis. HIT antibody assay should be sent to confirm the diagnosis. Anticoagulation should be continued with a nonheparin anticoagulant such as argatroban or bivalirudin. Vitamin K antagonists should be avoided in patients with HIT until platelet count recovers because they cause depletion of protein C, which may lead to venous limb gangrene. If a patient is taking a vitamin K antagonist at the time of HIT diagnosis, it should be discontinued immediately and reversed with vitamin K.

Keywords: Diagnosis; Platelet abnormalities; Thrombocytopenia; HIT

REFERENCES

Cuker A, Gimotty PA, Crowther MA, Warkentin TE. Predictive value of the 4Ts scoring system for heparin-induced thrombocytopenia: a systematic review and meta-analysis. *Blood* 2012;120(20):4160–4167.

Srinivasan AF, Rice L, Bartholomew JR et al. Warfarin-induced skin necrosis and venous limb gangrene in the setting of heparin-induced thrombocytopenia. *Arch Intern Med* 2004;164(1):66.

Warkentin TE, Greinacher A, Koster A, Lincoff AM. Treatment and prevention of heparin-induced thrombocytopenia: American College of Chest Physicians evidence-based clinical practice guidelines. *Chest* 2008;133(6):340S–380S.

15. ANSWER: C

With no other obvious cause, this patient's thrombocytopenia is likely drug induced, with vancomycin and famotidine as possible causes.

Thrombocytopenia has a reported prevalence of 8 to 67% and an incidence of 12 to 44% in critically ill patients. The cause of thrombocytopenia is often multifactorial. It may be from increased platelet consumption, seen in tissue trauma, bleeding, or DIC; or from increased platelet destruction due to extracorporeal circulation or immune mechanisms. Hemodilution may also play a role.

Thrombocytopenia has been associated with major bleeding and has been found to be an independent risk factor for mortality. With this in mind, it is important to find and correct reversible causes of thrombocytopenia among the critically ill.

Drug-induced immune thrombocytopenia (DIT), including immune thrombocytopenia and TTP, has been reported to account for up to 25% of all drug-related blood dyscrasias. Some studies estimate the incidence is 10 cases per million per year, but this value may be underestimated because DIT is a diagnosis of exclusion and often goes unrecognized. DIT is a prevalent, reversible cause of thrombocytopenia in the critically ill.

This patient has no other obvious cause of platelet consumption or destruction, so DIT must be considered. Sepsis may cause thrombocytopenia, but this patient does not have systemic inflammatory response or hemodynamic instability characteristic of sepsis. Disseminated intravascular coagulopathy is ruled out by normal fibrinogen level. While bone marrow suppression can be a cause of thrombocytopenia, normal WBC count and hemoglobin level make this diagnosis less likely.

More than 30 drugs have been associated with thrombocytopenia through either published case reports or based on drug-dependent, platelet-reactive antibodies identified by flow cytometry. The most notable of these are linezolid, vancomycin, trimethoprim-sulfamethoxazole, carbamazepine, and many of the penicillins. Famotidine and pantoprazole have also been implicated.

Keywords: Diagnosis; Platelet abnormalities; Other; Drug-induced thrombocytopenia

REFERENCES

Andersohn F, Bronder E, Klimpel A, Garbe E. Proportion of drug-related serious rare blood dyscrasias: estimates from the Berlin Case-Control Surveillance Study. *Am J Hematol* 2004;77(3):316–318.

Hui P, Cook DJ, Lim W et al. The frequency and clinical significance of thrombocytopenia complicating critical illness: a systematic review. *Chest* 2011;139:271–278.

Williamson DR, Lesur O, Tetrault JP et al. Thrombocytopenia in the critically ill: prevalence, incidence, risk factors, and clinical outcomes. *Can J Anesth* 2013;60(7):641–651.

16. ANSWER: A

This patient most likely has PCV, as determined by the high hemoglobin and hematocrit levels, but normal EPO level.

In PCV, there is hyperplasia of all hematologic cell lines, but the hallmark of the disease is red cell hyperplasia. These cells grow in vitro in the absence of EPO. The diagnosis of PCV is made clinically. Bone marrow abnormalities, such as an increase in megakaryocytes and cellular hyperplasia with a loss of the fat spaces, while characteristic, can never alone be diagnostic for PCV.

EPO levels can help distinguish PCV from secondary erythrocytosis, with the latter associated with high levels of EPO. It is important to be able to differentiate between primary and secondary erythrocytosis. In secondary erythrocytosis, it is important to reverse any modifiable risk factors like smoking.

There are no other signs or symptoms of malignancy in this question stem, making that answer choice unlikely.

While it is important to test for pregnancy in this patient of childbearing age, pregnancy typically leads to a physiologic anemia rather than the polycythemia seen in the question stem.

Keywords: Diagnosis; Hemoglobin abnormalities; Polycythemia

REFERENCE

Spivak JL. Polycythemia vera: myths, mechanisms, and management. *Blood* 2002;100(13):4272–4290.

17. Answer: D

Idarucizumab is a direct reversal agent for dabigatran and should be administered to this bleeding, unstable patient.

Oral thrombin inhibitors are non–vitamin K oral anticoagulants. They are associated with less serious bleeding than warfarin and require no laboratory monitoring or dose adjustment. The safety profile and ease of administration have led to oral thrombin inhibitors becoming increasingly popular for outpatient anticoagulant for atrial fibrillation as well as venous thromboembolism.

The Randomized Evaluation of Long-Term Anticoagulation Therapy (RE-LY) Trial was a randomized, double-blind, open-label, noninferiority trial that compared blinded fixed doses of dabigatran, 100 and 150 mg twice daily, with open-label use of warfarin with a target INR of 2 to 3. Patients who received the higher dose of dabigatran had the lowest incidence of stroke or systemic embolization at 2-year follow-up. Major bleeding occurred more often in the warfarin group (3.36% vs. 2.71% in the 100-mg dabigatran group and 3.11% in the 150-mg dabigatran group), but GI bleeding was significantly higher in the 150-mg dabigatran group (1.51% per year) than the warfarin group (1.02% per year).

The results of the RE-LY study favor the use of dabigatran for prevention of stroke or systemic embolization. Even though bleeding is reduced, major bleeding events still occur, specifically GI bleeding. In addition, patients taking direct thrombin inhibitors may require emergency surgery and reversal of anticoagulation, so reversal of these agents is imperative.

Until recently, there was no effective reversal agent for oral thrombin inhibitors, posing increased risk to bleeding patients taking these novel agents. Idarucizumab is a monoclonal antibody fragment and binds dabigatran at much higher affinity than thrombin, thus allowing for removal of the dabigatran molecule from circulation. In the RE-VERSE AD study, patients taking dabigatran who had serious bleeding or required urgent procedures were given idarucizumab in an attempt to reverse the anticoagulant action of dabigatran. In this trial, idarucizumab completely reversed the anticoagulant effect of dabigatran within minutes, as determined by normalization of dilute thrombin time. Intraoperative hemostasis was reported in 33 out of 36 patients who were taking dabigatran and received idarucizumab before emergency surgery. As a result of this trial, idarucizumab is a widely available and important reversal agent for patients needing immediate reversal of dabigatran.

Before the availability of idarucizumab, patients taking dabigatran requiring immediate reversal of anticoagulation were given FFP and possibly concentrated clotting factors such as protein complex concentrates. This imprecise therapy relies on competitive reversal, rather than targeted therapy, for reversal of anticoagulation. This is a less favorable option than the precise reversal that idarucizumab offers.

Dabigatran has a large volume of distribution and thus may not be effectively removed by dialysis. Some case reports show decreasing levels with dialysis administration, so it is not the most reliable option.

Keywords: Management strategies, anticoagulants, thrombin inhibitors

REFERENCES

Chang DN, Dager WE, Chin AI. Removal of dabigatran by hemodialysis. *Am J Kidney Dis* 2013;61(3):487–489.

Connolly SJ, Ezekowitz MD, Yusuf S et al. Dabigatran versus warfarin in patients with atrial fibrillation. *N Engl J Med* 2009;361(12):1139–1151.

Ezekowitz MD, Connolly SJ, Parekh A et al. Rationale and design of RE-LY: randomized evaluation of long-term anticoagulant therapy, warfarin, compared with dabigatran. *Am Heart J* 2009;157:805–810.

Pollack Jr CV, Reilly PA, Eikelboom J et al. Idarucizumab for dabigatran reversal. *N Engl J Med* 2015;373(6):511–520.

18. ANSWER: B

This patient was given enoxaparin dose based on total body weight, which is a significant overdose for a patient.

Enoxaparin has been used safely and effectively for many conditions, including venous thromboembolism (VTE), atrial fibrillation, valvulopathy, and acute coronary syndrome. It is also used in lower doses for prophylaxis against VTE. Enoxaparin 1 mg/kg subcutaneously twice daily and enoxaparin 1.5 mg/kg subcutaneously once daily are both US Food and Drug Administration (FDA)-approved regimens for the treatment of DVT with or without pulmonary embolism. Using enoxaparin may confer benefit, specifically for patients who suffer VTE in the setting of cancer, where recurrence is particularly high.

The volume of distribution of enoxaparin is roughly equivalent to plasma—the drug does not distribute into adipose tissue. This pharmacokinetic characteristic may increase the antithrombotic activity of enoxaparin in extremely obese patients compared with nonobese patients with the risk for elevated antifactor Xa levels, which are associated with increased bleeding events. This patient was given a dose of enoxaparin that was likely too high, given that it was dosed at his full body weight.

The incidence of obesity has grown to more than 33% in the United States, and hospital admissions of obese patients have proportionally increased. The American Association of Colleges of Pharmacy and American College of Physicians recommend monitoring the antithrombotic effect of low-molecular-weight heparins in special populations, including patients with obesity, using anti–factor Xa assay with a target peak therapeutic range of 0.6 to 1 IU/mL for twice-daily enoxaparin treatment dosing. Lower doses are often prescribed in obese patients. Despite this trend toward underdosing obese patients, factor Xa levels may be elevated in up to half of morbidly obese patients, although these increased levels were not associated with a significant difference in bleeding. This increase in Xa levels may still be significant because they are associated with higher levels of bleeding.

Malignancy may cause ischemic stroke by increasing risk for VTE or, in some cases, may cause hemorrhagic stroke as a result of severe thrombocytopenia. There is no evidence in this question stem that malignancy played a role in this patient's bleed. There is also no evidence that the patient is hypertensive or that he is suffering from acute liver failure.

Keywords: Management strategies, anticoagulants, heparin, low-molecular-weight heparin

REFERENCES

Petersen JL, Mahaffey KW, Hasselblad V et al. Efficacy and bleeding complications among patients randomized to enoxaparin or unfractionated heparin for antithrombin therapy in non–ST-segment elevation acute coronary syndromes: a systematic overview. *JAMA* 2004;292(1):89–96.

Wang TF, Milligan PE, Wong CA et al. Efficacy and safety of high-dose thromboprophylaxis in morbidly obese inpatients. *Thromb Haemost* 2014;111(1):88.

19. ANSWER: D

A TEG can be a very useful tool when standard lab work is unrevealing for the cause of acute coagulopathy. A small amount of clotted blood from the patient is spun in a small cup. Changes in the clot strength are recorded in graphs like the one in this question stem. Important variables are summarized in Table 3.3 and in the following image.

The patient's TEG reveals a low K value and low maximal amplitude (MA)—this is the classic finding of a patient with platelet dysfunction. Low MA and inadequate alpha-angle can also be the result of DIC, but DIC is unlikely given the normal fibrinogen level and normal INR.

Table 3.3 IMPORTANT VARIABLES FROM A THROMBOELASTOGRAM

VALUE	WHAT IT REPRESENTS	VARIABLES THAT AFFECT THE VALUE
R time	Time of latency from initial clot formation	Factor VIIIa and tissue factor
K value	Amplification of clot or clot strength	Thrombin and platelet activation
Alpha angle	Propagation of clot formation	Fibrin and fibrinogen
MA	Maximum amplitude	Platelet bonding and fibrinogen
LY 30	Clot stability	Fibrinolysis

In addition, there is no obvious inciting event that may have initiated the dysregulated coagulopathy seen in DIC. The most likely scenario for this patient is that he suffered a hemorrhagic stroke as a result of platelet dysfunction. With very little information about the patient in the question stem, it is unclear whether this patient was taking antiplatelet agents, but the TEG reveals the likely etiology of the hemorrhage. One clue is the presence of a sternotomy scar, which identifies this patient as someone who has CAD, so it is possible that he takes antiplatelet agents for stents or simply to reduce cardiac risk. It is also likely that he suffers from peripheral artery disease and may take antiplatelet agents for this.

Aspirin irreversibly binds to cyclo-oxygenase-1 enzyme and subsequently inhibits production of thromboxane A2, a potent eicosanoid involved in platelet aggregation. Clopidogrel and ticlopidine both selectively and irreversibly inhibit the P2Y12 adenosine diphosphate receptor. These agents have been used effectively to treat a wide range of cardiovascular and cerebrovascular diseases, such as for prophylaxis after coronary or intracranial stent placement. Because of an active metabolite, clopidogrel in particular persists after cessation of the medication. Some studies have demonstrated a higher incidence of postoperative bleeding

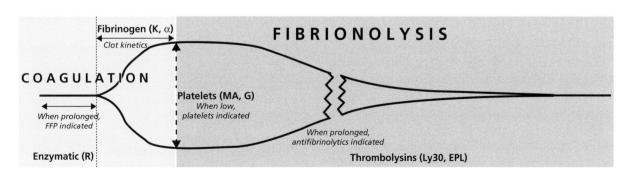

Figure A19.1

with clopidogrel compared with aspirin. Some experts recommend aggressive antiplatelet reversal for up to 4 days after the last known dose.

Prophylactic treatment with anticoagulants and antiplatelet agents has clear benefits in select patients with cardiac and vascular diseases. Over the previous decade, there has been a significant increase in the use of these agents, so the intensivist must be aware of their use and adverse effects. Patients experiencing ICH while taking antiplatelet agents have been reported to present with larger hematomas and suffer a worse prognosis compared with control groups. Many institutions have established protocols and guidelines to "reverse" the impairment of platelet aggregation.

It is unclear whether "reversal" of antiplatelet agents is beneficial for patients with ICH. Although there is no specific antidote, the aspirin effect is believed to be reversed by one platelet transfusion. Desmopressin seems capable of correcting aspirin-induced platelet dysfunction. Because of the active metabolite of clopidogrel that persists after cessation of the medication, some experts recommend continued platelet transfusion for 4 to 5 days after the last dose of the medication. Desmopressin may also be useful for the reversal of clopidogrel.

This patient likely would receive platelet transfusion and desmopressin to help reverse the bleeding effects of possible antiplatelet therapy. Repeat TEG shortly after administration of platelets and desmopressin would likely show normalization of MA and alpha-angle.

Keywords: Management strategies, anticoagulants, antiplatelet agents

REFERENCES

Hunt H, Stanworth S, Curry N et al. Thromboelastography (TEG) and rotational thromboelastometry (ROTEM) for trauma-induced coagulopathy in adult trauma patients with bleeding. *Cochrane Database Syst Rev* 2015;(2):CD004896.
Ivascu FA, Howells GA, Junn FS et al. Predictors of mortality in trauma patients with intracranial hemorrhage on preinjury aspirin or clopidogrel. *J Trauma Acute Care Surg* 2008;65(4):785–788.
Yende S, Wunderink RG. Effect of clopidogrel on bleeding after coronary artery bypass surgery. *Crit Care Med* 2001;29(12):2271–2275.

20. Answer: A

IVC filters are implantable devices designed to intercept thrombus that has broken free from the lower extremities or pelvis and prevent its migration to the lungs. There are two types of IVC filters: permanent and retrievable. There are also temporary IVC filters that show promise for very short-term prevention of pulmonary embolism and may be beneficial for patients with short-term pulmonary embolism prevention needs, such as trauma patents.

IVC filters are not benign, and caval thrombus can occur as a result of the filter trapping a large thrombus. In addition, recurrent thrombus formation inside the filter and propagating can lead to caval stenosis or occlusion. There is some evidence that caval thrombus after IVC filter placement occurs at a rate of 2.8%. There is currently no consensus on the recommendation for anticoagulation following IVC filter placement, but there is some evidence to suggest that patients with an IVC filter who remain on anticoagulation have lower rates of recurrent VTE and are less likely to form thrombus within the filter.

In 2010 and again in 2014, the FDA issued a safety communication urging all physicians who place IVC filters to take an active role in ensuring proper follow-up for patients who have received an IVC filter. The goal is to ensure that patients who no longer have an indication for IVC filtration have their filters evaluated for removal in a timely manner. Many IVC filter practices have now adopted dedicated IVC filter clinics to follow these patients.

For this patient, the benefit of anticoagulation must be weighed against the risk for bleeding. Her laboratory values show significant coagulopathy (INR 2.2) and moderate thrombocytopenia (platelet count 32), making anticoagulation with unfractionated heparin or low-molecular-weight heparin risky. In patients with VTE and contraindication to anticoagulation, an IVC filter may be considered. While placement of IVC filters is a widely accepted therapy, it is unclear whether IVC filters portend benefit to the patient. Several controlled trials, including the PREPIC II trial and the RIETE trial, found that IVC filter placement reduces the risk for pulmonary embolism but increases the risk for DVT and has no effect on mortality.

Keywords: Management strategies, IVC filters, other mechanical devices

REFERENCES

Angel LF, Tapson V, Galgon RE et al. Systematic review of the use of retrievable inferior vena cava filters. *J Vasc Intervent Radiol* 2011;22(11):1522–1530.
Kearon C, Akl EA, Ornelas J et al. Antithrombotic therapy for VTE disease: CHEST guideline and expert panel report. *Chest* 2016;149:315–352.
Muriel A, Jiménez D, Aujesky D et al. Survival effects of inferior vena cava filter in patients with acute symptomatic venous thromboembolism and a significant bleeding risk. *J Am Coll Cardiol* 2014;63(16):1675–1683.
Ray CE, Mitchell E, Zipser S et al. Outcomes with retrievable inferior vena cava filters: a multicenter study. *J Vasc Intervent Radiol* 2006;17(10):1595–1604.
PREPIC Study Group. Eight-year follow-up of patients with permanent vena cava filters in the prevention of pulmonary embolism: the PREPIC (Prévention du Risque d'Embolie Pulmonaire par Interruption Cave) randomized study. *Circulation* 2005;112:416–422.

4.

GASTROENTEROLOGY

Naveen Kukreja

QUESTIONS

1. A 73-year-old female presents to the intensive care unit (ICU) with a diagnosis of acute ischemic colitis and no other past medical history. Upon arrival, her blood pressure (BP) is 71/32 mm Hg, heart rate (HR) 122 bpm, respiratory rate (RR) 32 breaths/minute, and O_2 saturation 91% on a 100% non-rebreather mask. She is intubated for respiratory distress, resuscitated, and taken to the operating room, where she has a subtotal colectomy with end-colostomy creation. She remains intubated postoperatively and arrives to the ICU on 6 µg/minute of norepinephrine with a BP of 109/44 mm Hg, HR 92 bpm, RR 22 breaths/minute, and O_2 saturation 95% on volume control ventilation There are no obvious signs of bleeding. Laboratory values are as follows:

White blood cell (WBC) count: 13.3 K/µL
Platelets: 130 K/µL
International normalized ratio (INR): 2.7
Aspartate aminotransferase (AST): 1007 U/L
Alanine aminotransferase (ALT): 1597 U/L
Alkaline phosphatase: 84 U/L
Total bilirubin: 2 mg/dL
Direct bilirubin: 1.4 mg/dL
Indirect bilirubin: 0.5 mg/dL
Sodium: 139 mEq/L
CO_2: 19 mEq/L
Blood urea nitrogen (BUN): 31 mg/dL
Creatinine: 2.1 mg/dL

What is the MOST likely etiology of her coagulopathy?

A. Sepsis
B. Hypoxic hepatitis
C. Preexisting cirrhosis of the liver
D. Vitamin K deficiency

2. What is the MOST appropriate treatment for the coagulopathy in the patient in question 1?

A. Vitamin K
B. Cryoprecipitate
C. Supportive care and time
D. *N*-acetylcysteine

3. A 33-year-old male arrived to the hospital by ambulance with a gunshot wound to the abdomen. He is brought to the operating room, where he undergoes a damage-control laparotomy with small bowel resection. Intraoperatively, he receives 4 units of type-specific packed red blood cells and 2 units of fresh frozen plasma. His abdomen is closed, and he is brought to the ICU intubated. The next day, he is noted to be jaundiced. His labs are as follows:

Total bilirubin: 6.2 mg/dL
Direct bilirubin: 1 mg/dL
Indirect bilirubin: 5.2 mg/dL
Alkaline phosphatase: 109 U/L
AST: 104 U/L
ALT: 97 U/L
INR: 1.3
Albumin: 3.3 g/dL
Lactate dehydrogenase (LDH): 2000 U/L
Haptoglobin: 10 mg/dL

What is the MOST likely reason for this patient's hyperbilirubinemia?

A. Acute-on-chronic hepatic dysfunction
B. Choledocholithiasis
C. Hemolytic transfusion reaction
D. Cholestasis

4. A 54-year-old male with a history of alcoholic cirrhosis presents with profuse hematemesis and confusion. He is intubated a short time after his arrival to the emergency department (ED). He receives 3 units of packed red blood cells, 3 units of fresh frozen plasma, and 1 unit of platelets in the ED. He arrives to the ICU hemodynamically stable after having multiple esophageal varices banded endoscopically by the gastroenterology team in the ED while intubated. His ventilatory requirements are minimal. Which antibiotic is MOST appropriate for the prevention of spontaneous bacterial peritonitis?

A. Ceftriaxone
B. Vancomycin
C. Fluconazole
D. No antibiotic is indicated

5. A 24-year-old female ingested a toxic amount of Tylenol and is subsequently brought to the ED after being found by her family. Upon arrival to the ICU, she is difficult to arouse. Her BP is 82/42 mm Hg, HR 101 bpm, RR 25 breaths/minute, and O_2 saturation 98% on 6 L/minute via nasal cannula. Her INR is 4.1, and her pH is 7.21. What is the MOST common cause of death in this scenario?

A. Infection
B. Bleeding
C. Thromboembolism
D. Cerebral edema

6. A 43-year-old female presents with increasing abdominal girth. She has unintentionally lost 15 pounds over the last year and denies smoking, alcohol, and drug use. The patient has no significant travel history or sick contacts. On physical exam, her abdomen is uniformly protuberant, nontender, and tympanic on percussion. She has no jaundice or caput medusa and no palpable masses appreciated. Abdominal ultrasound demonstrates significant ascites with normal blood flow in the hepatic and portal venous systems. Her INR is 1.3, and her serum albumin is 3. She is uncomfortable with the distention, so she is sent for diagnostic and therapeutic paracentesis while waiting for the appropriate workup to ensue. What is the MOST likely finding on analysis of the ascitic fluid?

A. Serum ascites-albumin gradient (SAAG) >1.1 with polymorphonuclear neutrophils (PMNs) >250 with no malignant cell lines appreciated
B. SAAG <1.1 with PMNs <250 with no malignant cell lines appreciated
C. SAAG >1.1 with cytology revealing malignant cell lines
D. SAAG <1.1 with cytology revealing malignant cell lines

7. A 49-year-old male presents to the ED by ambulance. The patient was found on lying unconscious on the sidewalk in a pool of blood. There was copious bloody vomitus soaking his shirt. He smells of alcohol. He has a protuberant abdomen with visible distended veins around his umbilicus. When palpating his abdomen, he moans. His BP is 84/33 mm Hg, HR 98 bpm, RR 21 breaths/minute, O_2 saturation 93% on a non-rebreather mask, and axillary temperature 38.5° C. He is intubated for airway protection, two large bore intravenous (IV) lines are started, a type and screen are sent to the laboratory, and a request to crossmatch 2 units of blood is sent to the blood bank. His blood pressure corrects with the fluid challenge. He is given a dose of ceftriaxone. What is the MOST important medication to give this patient to minimize his chance of bleeding while waiting for the gastroenterology team?

A. Vitamin K
B. Pantoprazole
C. Octreotide
D. Desmopressin (DDAVP)

8. A 67-year-old male with hepatitis C virus (HCV) cirrhosis of the liver presents to the ICU with refractory hypoxemia. He originally presented to the hospital with spontaneous bacterial peritonitis 2 days prior. He has been being treated with broad-spectrum antibiotics while ascitic fluid cultures are pending. At home, he receives 4 L/minute of oxygen by nasal cannula. He is now on 60% venti-mask with an O_2 saturation of 90%. His O_2 saturation reproducibly improves when he lay supine in bed. Blood gas analysis demonstrates a PaO_2 of 50 mm Hg. Subsequent right heart catheterization demonstrates a mean pulmonary artery pressure of 20 mm Hg with a pulmonary capillary wedge pressure of 12 mm Hg. Contrasted echocardiography demonstrates a positive right-to-left shunt in five cardiac cycles. What therapy is MOST likely to reverse this patient's hypoxemia long term?

A. No available treatment
B. Liver transplantation
C. Tadalafil
D. Transjugular intrahepatic portosystemic shunt (TIPS)

9. Which of the following contributes the MOST to a patient's Model for End-Stage Liver Disease (MELD) score?

A. Bilirubin
B. Sodium
C. INR
D. Creatinine

10. A 47-year-old male with a history of alcohol abuse presents to the ED with delirium tremens. He is complaining of abdominal pain and nausea. He is confused and combative. He has the following laboratory values:

Prothrombin time: 22.3 seconds
INR: 1.9
Direct bilirubin: >10 mg/dL
Total bilirubin: 42.3 mg/dL
Platelets: 150 K/μL

Assuming a control prothrombin time of 12 seconds, which of the following BEST represents this patient's Maddrey Discrimination Score and indicated therapy?

A. 88 with glucocorticoids indicated
B. 111 with liver transplantation indicated
C. 30 with hemodialysis indicated
D. 31 with octreotide infusion indicated

11. A 52-year-old male with a past medical history of cirrhosis of the liver presents to ED with active hematemesis. He is intubated for airway protection. He is given fresh frozen plasma, platelets, and cryoprecipitate to correct his medical coagulopathy and given ceftriaxone for spontaneous bacterial peritonitis prophylaxis. He is started on octreotide and pantoprazole infusions. His hepatologist performs an esophagogastroduodenoscopy at bedside and attempts banding of two varices at the gastroesophageal junction, but immediately the varices begin to bleed again. This is the second time this year he has presented for a variceal bleed. Previously, the varices were banded with successful control of the bleeding. A Sengstaken-Blakemore tube is inserted. The gastric balloon is inflated and put on tension with successful control of the active bleeding. At this point, what is the next BEST management to prevent further rebleeding of the varices?

A. TIPS
B. Liver transplantation
C. Supportive care and time
D. Emergent esophagectomy

12. A 42-year-old female with a history of alcohol-induced cirrhosis of the liver, portal hypertension with refractory ascites, and hepatic hydrothorax presents to the ICU for postprocedural hemodynamic monitoring after TIPS. A preoperative echocardiogram demonstrated a mean pulmonary artery pressure of 47 and an ejection fraction of 35%. Her pre-TIPS MELD score was 14. Her pre-TIPS portosystemic gradient (PSG) was 15 mm Hg, and her post-TIPS PSG was 3 mm Hg. Which of the following is this patient LEAST at risk for after the procedure?

A. Portosystemic encephalopathy
B. Cor pulmonale
C. Hepatic ischemia
D. Hepatorenal syndrome

13. A 30-year-old female with no prior medical history presents to the hospital with a 2-week history of worsening abdominal pain, distention, weakness, right upper quadrant pain, and jaundice. She denies recent travel history or sick contacts. Her only home medication is an oral contraceptive. She is afebrile with a normal BP and HR. On physical exam, she has marked ascites without any signs of peritonitis and has palpable hepatosplenomegaly. She does not have jugular venous distention. She receives a paracentesis with improvement but not complete resolution of her abdominal pain. Her laboratory work shows:

WBC: 13,000 L/μL	Hepatitis A virus (HAV)
Hemoglobin: 12.2 mg/dL	anti–immunoglobulin M
Hematocrit: 34%	(IgM) negative
Platelet count: 1001 K/μL	HAV anti-IgG negative
Alkaline phosphatase:	Hepatitis B surface antigen
302 U/L	(HBsAg) negative
AST: 700 U/L	HBV IgM anti–hepatitis B
ALT: 692 U/L	core antigen (HBcAg)
LDH: 210 U/L	negative
Total bilirubin: 3.9 mg/dL	HBV IgG anti-HBcAg
Direct bilirubin: 3.1 mg/dL	negative
INR: 2.7	HBV hepatitis B early
Serum albumin: 2.9 g/dL	antigen (HBeAg)
Ascitic albumin: 0.9 g/dL	negative
Ascitic WBC count:	HCV polymerase
120/mm³	chain reaction (PCR)
Ascitic LDH: 91 U/L	negative

Which is the MOST appropriate test to establish the underlying diagnosis?

A. Liver biopsy
B. Ultrasound Doppler study of the liver and its vasculature
C. CA-19-9 level
D. Transthoracic echocardiogram

14. A 44-year-old female presents with a 3-day history of fever, abdominal pain, anorexia, malaise, and vomiting. She was recently diagnosed with cholangiocarcinoma. She underwent an endoscopic retrograde cholangiopancreatography (ERCP) with

common bile duct (CBD) stent placement 3 days prior for biliary obstruction. She is febrile to 38.9° C, HR 110 bpm, RR 31 breaths/minute, and BP 99/47 mm Hg. On exam, she has right upper quadrant tenderness and is confused and emaciated. A right upper quadrant ultrasound is performed of the abdomen and is notable for absence of biliary dilation and a 3 × 3 cm cystic lesion of the right lobe of the liver. Contrast computed tomography (CT) scan of the abdomen demonstrated a cystic hypodense lesion with peripheral enhancement and an air-fluid level inside the lesion. Her laboratory values are as follows:

WBC: 18.9 K/μL
Platelets: 127 K/μL
AST: 210 U/L
ALT: 189 U/L
Alkaline phosphatase: 301 U/L
Total bilirubin: 4.7 mg/dL
Direct bilirubin: 3.1 mg/dL

What is the next BEST step in the management?

A. Repeat ERCP with repeat CBD stent placement
B. Magnetic resonance cholangiopancreatography (MRCP)
C. Aspiration of lesion, culture of the aspirate, and 14 days of ampicillin
D. Aspiration of lesion, culture of the aspirate, and 8 weeks of piperacillin/tazobactam

15. Which of the following is NOT a variable in the Child-Turcotte-Pugh scoring system?

A. Bilirubin
B. Albumin
C. INR
D. Platelet count

16. A 48-year-old female with a history of alcoholic cirrhosis of the liver presents to the ED with profuse hematemesis. She is immediately intubated, and massive blood product resuscitation is administered. Infusions of pantoprazole and octreotide are initiated, and the patient is given a dose of ceftriaxone for spontaneous bacterial peritonitis prophylaxis. The gastroenterologist performs an esophagogastroduodenoscopy and is unsuccessful at banding an actively bleeding varix at the gastroesophageal junction. What is the next BEST step?

A. Place Minnesota tube
B. Emergent TIPS
C. Transfer to ICU for ongoing resuscitation
D. Vasopressin

17. A 69-year-old male with a history of hypertension, hyperlipidemia, atrial fibrillation, and obstructive sleep apnea presents to the ICU with acute-onset abdominal pain. He has no prior surgical history. He was initially admitted to the hospital for an influenza infection, which began 3 days prior and has been being treated with oseltamivir. The pain began suddenly. It is dull, diffuse, worsening, and nonradiating. On physical exam, his abdomen is nondistended and soft without rebound tenderness or guarding. There are no masses appreciated. His HR is 131 bpm, narrow complex, and irregular without discernable P waves on the telemetry strip. BP is 99/41 mm Hg, RR is 28 breaths/minute, temperature is 38.2° C. His WBC count is 17,000/μL. Lactic acid is 7.7 mmol/L. A free-air series of plain films performed at the bedside is negative for free air. What is the MOST likely diagnosis?

A. Bowel obstruction
B. Bowel perforation
C. Mesenteric ischemia
D. *Clostridium difficile* colitis

18. A 73-year-old male with a history of alcoholic cirrhosis of the liver and metastatic hepatocellular carcinoma is found lying on the ground unconscious in his home by his daughter. It is unknown how long he had being lying there. He is brought to the ED and found to have aspiration pneumonia for which he is started on meropenem. On physical exam, he demonstrates bitemporal muscle wasting and protuberant nontender abdomen. A nasoenteric feeding tube is inserted. Before the institution of enteric nutrition, which management strategies should be LEAST appropriate?

A. Monitor electrolytes
B. Supplement thiamine
C. Slow incremental increase in tube feedings
D. Parenteral nutrition

19. A 48-year-old female with a history of colon cancer undergoes a left hemicolectomy with primary anastomosis. She begins taking enteric nutrition on postoperative day 2. She is discharged the next day. Three days later, she develops abdominal pain and fever, and vomits with food intake. She reports normal bowel movements. She is admitted to the ICU with a temperature of 39° C, HR 125 bp, RR 31 breaths/minute, and BP 85/31 mm Hg. On physical exam, her abdomen is nondistended and grossly tender to palpation with rebound tenderness. There are no palpable masses. Her incision looks

to be healing appropriately without erythema, edema, or drainage. Her labs are as follows:

WBC: 17 K/μL
Hematocrit: 30%
Platelets: 171,000/μL
Sodium: 141 mEq/L
Chloride: 98 mEq/L
CO_2: 21 mEq/L
BUN: 28 mg/dL
Creatinine: 1.5 mg/dL
Lactic acid: 6 mmol/L

What is the MOST likely diagnosis?

    A. Anastomotic leak
    B. Incarcerated hernia
    C. Bowel ischemia
    D. *Clostridium difficile* infection

20. A 69-year-old male with a history of type 2 diabetes, hypertension, and obstructive sleep apnea is admitted with diverticulitis. He is treated with ertapenem, hydration, and IV pain medicine. Three days later, he is much improved. He is tolerating a diet, and his pain is controlled. His discharge is being planned when you are called by his nurse to his bedside. His temperature is 39.1°C, RR 26 breaths/minute, and HR 122 bpm, and he is encephalopathic. His WBC count is 20 K/μL. His abdominal exam is benign. He is able to tell you that his back hurts. When he is not stimulated, he lays supine, favoring flexing his left hip, bending his left knee, and externally rotating his left thigh. He has point tenderness of his left lumbar paraspinal area. What is the MOST appropriate treatment for this patient's problem?

    A. Antibiotics and drainage
    B. Antibiotics and emergent exploratory laparotomy
    C. Nasogastric tube decompression
    D. Antibiotics, narcotic pain medications, and acetaminophen

21. A 55-year-old male with a history of alcohol abuse and type 2 diabetes presents with acute alcoholic pancreatitis. He is admitted and treated with pain medicine, nasoenteric feedings, and bowel rest. A contrast enhanced CT scan demonstrates areas of necrosis. Six weeks go by, at which point imaging is repeated and demonstrates organized fluid collections suggestive of pseudocyst formation. Two days later, he develops a fever and abdominal pain. He has a WBC count of 18 K/μL. He is tachycardic, tachypneic, and hypotensive. He is intubated and resuscitated, and further workup reveals that the most likely source for his sepsis is an infected pseudocyst. Which antibiotic regimen is the BEST empiric therapy to administer until the fluid collection can be aspirated and cultured?

    A. Cefazolin
    B. Fluconazole
    C. Vancomycin
    D. Imipenem and cilastin

22. A 78-year-old male with a history of atrial fibrillation and hypertension is emergently taken to the operating room for acute mesenteric ischemia. Revascularization is successful, and mesenteric perfusion is restored. He is kept intubated overnight because he was given significant resuscitation before and during the operation. Overnight, his becomes anuric, and his peak airway pressures climb. On exam, his abdomen is tense and distended. He is not dyssynchronous with the ventilator. What is the next BEST step in evaluation of this patient?

    A. Measure bladder pressure
    B. Return to operating room emergently
    C. Immediate CT of the abdomen with IV contrast
    D. Trial of neuromuscular blockade

23. A 43-year-old female with a past medical history of morbid obesity and type 2 diabetes presents to the ICU after being admitted for severe pancreatitis and cholangitis. She is intubated for encephalopathy with inability to protect her airway as well as refractory hypoxemia. Her current ventilator settings on assist control are tidal volume 6 mL/kg ideal body weight, RR 16 breaths/minute, positive end-expiratory pressure 12 cm H_2O, and forced inspiratory oxygen (FiO_2) 60%. Her PaO_2 is 65 mm Hg with an SaO_2 of 94%. She is given intravenous fluids for resuscitation. She is requiring 10 μg/minute of norepinephrine to maintain her mean arterial pressure (MAP) higher than 65 mm Hg. Right upper quadrant ultrasound demonstrates a dilated CBD approximately 8 mm in diameter with visible stones with intrahepatic biliary ductal dilation. Blood work reveals:

WBC: 21 K/μL
Glucose: 212 mg/dL
AST: 301 U/L
ALT: 320 U/L
Alkaline phosphatase: 1058 U/L
Lipase: 765 U/L
Amylase: 599 U/L
Lactic acid: 5.1 mmol/L
Total bilirubin: 4.9 mg/dL
INR: 2.1
Platelets: 41 K/μL

What is the next BEST step in management?

  A. Continue resuscitation for 2 days, then laparoscopic cholecystectomy

  B. ERCP and placement of nasobiliary catheter

  C. Broad-spectrum antibiotics and fluid resuscitation

  D. Percutaneous biliary drainage

24. Which of the following statements is LEAST correct with regard to acute pancreatitis?

  A. Early ERCP (within 24–48 hours) is only indicated if there is concomitant cholangitis

  B. Gallstones are the most common cause

  C. Prophylactic antibiotics are not recommended

  D. Requires parenteral nutrition

25. An 83-year-old female presents to the ICU after a car accident. She was a restrained passenger and suffered blunt force trauma to the chest resulting in multiple ribs fracture and a right-sided pneumothorax, a left femoral fracture, and fracture of the right hand. She had been kept intubated because she needed two consecutive orthopedic operations. During this time, she was sedated with dexmedetomidine and fentanyl infusions. She is extubated on hospital day 4 and was having considerable pain for which she was being given scheduled acetaminophen, celecoxib, and hydromorphone. On hospital day 6, she complains of severe abdominal pain. She had been receiving continuous tube feeds as well a supplemental regular diet for comfort during this time period. CT of the abdomen and pelvis with oral and IV contrast demonstrates a colonic diameter of 13 cm with air going all the way down to the rectum on the scout film. There are no indications of bowel obstruction on the CT scan. What is the next BEST step?

  A. Administer neostigmine with continuous cardiac monitoring

  B. Administer senna and docusate

  C. Nasogastric tube feeding and nothing by mouth (NPO)

  D. Administer metoclopramide

ANSWERS

1. ANSWER: B

This patient has likely hypoperfused her liver before resuscitation. Her AST and ALT are elevated to more than 20 times the upper limit of normal in the context of hemodynamic instability. The patient exhibits physiology similar to sepsis and has systemic inflammatory response syndrome, but the underlying etiology is likely not infectious in etiology. Cirrhosis and vitamin K deficiency, while they may be contributing factors, are both unlikely to be the main underlying etiology given what appears to be an acute rise in AST and ALT suggesting recent hepatocyte insult.

Hemodynamic instability is usually present before evidence of liver injury is apparent. In most cases, the ischemic injury is detected after an episode of hypotension or other circulatory disturbances like systemic inflammatory responses. The usual pattern is elevation of liver aminotransferase associated with marked rise in LDH levels. AST and ALT levels can rise 25 to 150 times the normal values, within 1 to 3 days after liver injury. Serum bilirubin is often elevated but starts after the AST and ALT levels have started to normalize. If the hemodynamic instability is corrected, the levels will normalize within 7 to 10 days. Hepatopulmonary syndrome occurs in many patients but is found to be reversible after the hepatic function improves. The pathophysiology is postulated to be related to intrapulmonary vasodilation and shunting.

Ischemic hepatitis is almost always self-limited but is associated with a mortality rate of up to 25%. The extent of liver injury correlates with the nature and duration of hemodynamic instability and jaundice. Prognosis is poor in patients with need for vasopressor therapy, presence of septic shock, hepatorenal syndrome, and coagulopathy.

Keywords: Hepatic dysfunction/failure (acute and chronic)

REFERENCES

Lightsey JM, Rockey DC. Current concepts in ischemic hepatitis. *Curr Opin Gastroenterol* 2017;33(3):158.
Waseem N, Chen P. Hypoxic hepatitis: a review and clinical update. *J Clin Transl Hepatol* 2016;4(3): 263–268.

2. ANSWER: D

The treatment for hypoxic hepatitis is correction of the underlying reason of inadequate oxygen delivery to the liver and time. In this case, the patient needed to be resuscitated and have the underlying reason for illness—her ischemic colon—resolved. Following correction of the underlying cause, correction of the coagulopathy can take up to 1 week in patients with hypoxic hepatitis. The goal for the management of ischemic hepatitis is always to improve cardiac output and hence prevent end-organ hypoperfusion. In the absence of specific therapy, maintenance of hemodynamic stability and other supportive measure to correct the underlying etiology have been found to be more useful in improvement of liver function. Vitamin K is used to correct vitamin K deficiency leading to coagulopathy or to reverse the effects of warfarin anticoagulation in nonemergent situations. Oral vitamin K is generally preferred when possible in the critical care setting because IV vitamin K has the potential to cause an anaphylactic response; this is now seen less frequently than the previously reported incidence of 1 in 5000 owing to a change in the preservative used in IV vitamin K.

Cryoprecipitate is administered when there are concerns of hypofibrinogenemia, which can be seen in consumptive coagulopathies, dilutional coagulopathies, and hepatic coagulopathies. *N*-acetylcysteine is used intravenously to treat hepatic injury related to acetaminophen overdose and in nebulized form to loosen mucous plugs in patients with cystic fibrosis or chronic obstructive pulmonary disease. Acetylcysteine has hepatoprotective effects by restoring glutathione and helping with nontoxic conjugation of acetaminophen. It also has mucolytic effects through its sulfhydryl group, which lowers the mucus viscosity. It has also been used to treat a variety of other medical problems; however, the data for these other uses are inconclusive.

Keywords: Hepatic dysfunction/failure (acute and chronic)

REFERENCES

Tapper EB, Sengupta N, Bonder A. The incidence and outcomes of ischemic hepatitis: a systematic review with meta-analysis. *Am J Med* 2015;128(12):1314.
Waseem N, Chen P. Hypoxic hepatitis: a review and clinical update. *J Clin Transl Hepatol* 2016;4(3): 263–268.

3. ANSWER: C

Hemolytic transfusion reaction should be suspected in the context of the patient receiving significant amounts of blood products followed by acute onset of indirect hyperbilirubinemia, elevated LDH, and decreased haptoglobin. Acute-on-chronic hepatic dysfunction is not supported by the normal INR and serum albumin, which imply normal hepatic synthetic function. Sepsis can lead to hypoxic hepatitis, which would be characterized by hemodynamic instability, heart failure, or respiratory insufficiency followed by increases in the AST and ALT to greater than 20 times the upper limit of normal and worsened hepatic synthetic function. This patient received type-specific blood (as implied in the stem), which had not been cross-matched (excluded from the stem). The incidence of transfusion reaction is 1 in 1000 with type-specific blood transfusions. It is characterized by indirect (unconjugated) acute hyperbilirubinemia, increase in LDH, decreased haptoglobin, and increased reticulocyte count. Cholestasis is unlikely in a previously healthy male with no history of hepatobiliary trauma or manipulation. It would be characterized by direct hyperbilirubinemia and increased alkaline phosphatase out of proportion to serum transaminases, with or without impaired hepatic synthetic function. Choledocholithiasis would have a similar pattern on liver function tests because it is a reason for cholestasis. It would be considered by findings on right upper quadrant ultrasound or MRCP suggestive of gallstones in the CBD. Cholestasis, acute-on-chronic liver failure, and choledocholithiasis all would present with direct hyperbilirubinemia.

Keywords: Laboratory studies, coagulation parameters; Laboratory studies, additional relevant studies (e.g., amylase, lipase)

REFERENCES

Carson JL, Guyatt G, Heddle NM et al. Clinical practice guidelines from AABB: red blood cell transfusion thresholds and storage. *JAMA* 2016;316(19):2025.

Davenport RD. Pathophysiology of hemolytic transfusion reactions. *Semin Hematol* 2005;42(3):16.

Dhaliwal G, Cornett P, Tierney L. Hemolytic anemia. *Am Fam Physician* 2004;69(11):2599–2607.

4. ANSWER: A

Bacterial infections are a frequent complication in patients with cirrhosis and upper gastrointestinal bleeding. Antibiotic prophylaxis has been found to decrease the incidence of bacterial infections and mortality. The risk factors associated with high risk for spontaneous bacterial peritonitis include ascitic fluid protein concentration <1 g/dL, variceal hemorrhage, or prior episode of spontaneous bacterial peritonitis. Also, antibiotic prophylaxis has been noted to increase blood pressure and systemic vascular resistance, and by doing so may delay the onset of hepatorenal syndrome. Antibiotics active against enteric bacteria have been commonly used as antibiotic prophylaxis in patients with cirrhosis and upper gastrointestinal bleeding. The American Association for the Study of Liver Disease and the Baveno V consensus recommended antibiotic prophylaxis for cirrhotic patients with upper gastrointestinal bleeding. Oral norfloxacin (400 mg twice daily),

intravenous ciprofloxacin, and intravenous ceftriaxone (1 g/day) are preferred. Recently, quinolone-resistant gram-negative organisms have become more prevalent, and thus, ceftriaxone is considered to be one of the drugs of choice for prevention of spontaneous bacterial peritonitis after a variceal bleed. Because the organisms of concern are gram negative, vancomycin would be inappropriate. Because fungal infections are not nearly as common infectious causes postvariceal bleed, fluconazole would be inappropriate.

Keywords: Pharmacologic management, antimicrobials; Pharmacologic management, antimicrobials

REFERENCES

Fernández J, Navasa M, Planas R et al. Primary prophylaxis of spontaneous bacterial peritonitis delays hepatorenal syndrome and improves survival in cirrhosis. *Gastroenterology* 2007;133(3):818.

Fernández J, Ruiz del Arbol L, Gomez C et al. Norfloxacin vs ceftriaxone in the prophylaxis of infection in patients with advanced cirrhosis and hemorrhage. *Gastroenterology* 2006;131(4):1049–1056.

Garcia-Tsao G, Sanyal AJ, Grace ND, Carey W. Prevention and management of gastroesophageal varices and variceal hemorrhage in cirrhosis. *Hepatology* 2007;46: 922–938.

Saab S, Hernandez JC, Chi AC, Tong MJ. Oral antibiotic prophylaxis reduces spontaneous bacterial peritonitis occurrence and improves short-term survival in cirrhosis: a meta-analysis. *Am J Gastroenterol* 2009;104(4):993.

5. ANSWER: D

This patient has acute liver failure (ALF). ALF is defined as the onset of hepatic encephalopathy and coagulopathy within 26 weeks of jaundice in a patient without preexisting liver disease. The most common cause of death in ALF is cerebral edema with resultant brainstem herniation. The typical signs of cerebral edema include systemic hypertension and bradycardia. Neurological exam may reveal hyperreflexia and altered pupillary reactiveness. Cerebral edema should be treated with typical strategies for malignant intracranial hypertension with the addition of lactulose (aggressive bowel cleansing) and rifaximin for ammonia clearance. IV indomethacin and total hepatectomy have been used in refractory situations in which the patient has been allocated a liver graft. Infection, while common in ALF, is not the most common cause of death. It is recommended that patients be treated with antibiotics prophylactically while in ALF because infections are common, frequently patients will not have all of the signs of an infection when they are infected, and infection can preclude transplantation if one becomes necessary. Bleeding is common in ALF as a result of impaired clotting factor production in the context of decreased hepatic synthetic capability and ongoing inflammation from hepatic insult. This derangement also increases the risk for thromboembolism; however, neither bleeding nor thromboembolism is the leading cause of death in ALF.

Keywords: Hepatic dysfunction/failure (acute and chronic)

REFERENCES

Bernal W, Wendon J. Acute liver failure: a review. *N Engl J Med* 2013;369:2525–2534.

Stravitz RT. Critical management decisions in patients with acute liver failure. *Chest* 2008;134(5):1092.

6. ANSWER: D

This patient has history and findings concerning for peritoneal carcinomatosis. Ascitic fluid, when obtained in the context of having an unclear etiology, should have the SAAG calculated. SAAG = (albumin concentration of serum) − (albumin concentration of ascitic fluid). SAAG is used to diagnose portal hypertension and is more useful than protein ratios used in the exudate/transudate concept. Transudates have SAAG greater than 1.1, which suggests portal hypertension as the etiology for the ascites. Exudates have SAAG less than 1.1, which suggests etiologies other than those associated with portal hypertension. Transudates can be found in diagnoses such a cirrhosis, Budd-Chiari syndrome, congestive heart failure, or constrictive pericarditis. SAAG less than 1.1 (exudative fluid) is found in peritoneal carcinomatosis (so long as there is not concomitant portal hypertension) with malignant ascites, pancreatitis, nephrotic syndrome, and tuberculosis spontaneous bacterial peritonitis. Having PMNs of more than 250/μL suggests spontaneous bacterial peritonitis, and antibiotic treatment should be considered. While the nature of this question is challenging, the elements of the SAAG score are useful to know.

Keywords: Laboratory diagnosis, hepatic dysfunction; Laboratory studies, nutritional assessment (albumin, prealbumin); Diagnostic modalities, paracentesis, diagnostic

REFERENCES

Ginès P, Cárdenas A, Arroyo V, Rodés J. Management of cirrhosis and ascites. *N Engl J Med* 2004;350:1646–1654.

Runyon BA, Montano AA, Akriviadis EA et al. The serum-ascites albumin gradient is superior to the exudate-transudate concept in the differential diagnosis of ascites. *Ann Intern Med* 1992;117(3):215.

7. ANSWER: C

This patient has findings consistent with portal hypertension (ascites and caput medusae). The scent of alcohol provides a reason to think that the patient has cirrhosis of the liver, which could account for the portal hypertension. The blood-soaked shirt and hemodynamic instability that responded to a volume challenge are consistent with an upper gastrointestinal bleed. In the context of portal hypertension, this must be presumed a variceal bleed until proved otherwise. An octreotide infusion would decrease the risk for a variceal bleed most in this patient. Pantoprazole, a proton pump inhibitor, impairs acid secretion in the stomach, which would decrease the risk of ulcer bleeding over the course of the day. While proton pump inhibitors are commonly coadministered in this scenario, the most important medication to administer is octreotide because the patient is at greater risk for a variceal bleed than a peptic ulcer bleed. DDAVP is commonly given to bleeding patients with uremia-induced platelet dysfunction to improve hemostasis. Vitamin K is given to patients who have coagulopathy secondary to vitamin K deficiency, such as those with severe malnourishment, with impaired gastrointestinal absorption, or on warfarin therapy. While this patient may be coagulopathic and giving him vitamin K may slightly decrease this coagulopathy, vitamin K is thought to take 8 hours to work when given orally and 6 hours when given parenterally. Vitamin K may be given in this context but would take at least 6 hours to improve vitamin K–clotting factor production if it were to improve at all. It is not the next most important medication for the patient to receive to minimize his chances of rebleeding for the time it takes for the gastroenterology team to arrive to perform an endoscopic evaluation and potential treatment.

The initials step in the management of an acute variceal bleed include hemodynamic stability, protecting the patient's airway, and correcting any coagulopathies. The first management modality is initiating an octreotide bolus followed by a infusion. It should be started in all patients suspected of having a variceal bleed while awaiting endoscopic confirmation and subsequent sclerotherapy and ligation.

Keywords: Stomach—GI hemorrhage, lower; Stomach—GI hemorrhage, upper

REFERENCES

Garcia-Tsao G, Sanyal AJ, Grace ND, Carey W. Prevention and management of gastroesophageal varices and variceal hemorrhage in cirrhosis. *Hepatology* 2007;46:922–938.

Ludwig D, Schädel S, Brüning A et al. 48-hour hemodynamic effects of octreotide on postprandial splanchnic hyperemia in patients with liver cirrhosis and portal hypertension: double-blind, placebo-controlled study. *Dig Dis Sci* 2000;45(5):1019.

McCormick PA, Biagini MR, Dick R et al. Octreotide inhibits the meal-induced increases in the portal venous pressure of cirrhotic patients with portal hypertension: a double-blind, placebo-controlled study. *Hepatology* 1992;16(5):1180.

Wells M, Chande N, Adams P et al. Meta-analysis: vasoactive medications for the management of acute variceal bleeds. *Aliment Pharmacol Ther* 2012;35(11):1267–1278.

8. ANSWER: B

This patient has hepatopulmonary syndrome. Hepatopulmonary syndrome has a poorly understood pathogenesis but is thought to be secondary to inappropriate precapillary and capillary dilations of pulmonary vasculature secondary to inappropriately elevated increased levels of nitric oxide leading to increase ventilation-perfusion mismatch, modest intrapulmonary shunting, and decreased DL_{CO}. Of note, there is an increased incidence of hepatopulmonary syndrome in patients with cutaneous spider nevi, which are typically found on the face, neck, upper trunk, and arms. Portopulmonary syndrome, commonly confused with hepatopulmonary syndrome, also has a poorly understood pathogenesis and is thought to result from imbalances of vasodilatory and vasoconstricting mediators, similar in concept to hepatopulmonary syndrome; however, the exact mediator cascade differs. Portopulmonary syndrome requires that the patient have portal hypertension. Typically, the development of portopulmonary syndrome is years after the diagnosis of portal hypertension. On right heart catheterization, the mean pulmonary artery pressure is higher than 25 mm Hg, with a pulmonary capillary wedge pressure less than 15 mm Hg in the absence of other causes of pulmonary hypertension. This patient demonstrates orthodeoxia (improvement of oxygenation when supine). He has a right-to-left shunt on contrasted echocardiography that takes more than two cardiac cycles, suggestive of an intrapulmonary shunt. He has a relatively normal mean pulmonary artery pressure, differentiating it from portopulmonary syndrome, which is not amenable to liver transplantation. It is of note that liver transplantation may still be considered in these patients if mean pulmonary artery pressure is less than 35 mm Hg. Patients with hepatopulmonary syndrome tolerate mild hypoxemia remarkably well. Oxygenation in patients with hepatopulmonary syndrome improves after liver transplantation. It normally takes months for the oxygenation to normalize, which allows for more permissive oxygenation requirements after transplantation when determining whether or not to extubate a patient with hepatopulmonary syndrome. Other treatments for hepatopulmonary syndrome are supplemental oxygenation and rarely coiling of intrapulmonary vascular dilations. Treatment options for portopulmonary syndrome include inhaled epoprostenol, bosentan, calcium channel blockers, nitric oxide, and anticoagulation.

Keywords: Hepatic dysfunction/failure (acute and chronic); Liver transplantation, rejection, complications

REFERENCES

Rodriguez-Roisin R, Roca J, Agusti AG et al. Gas exchange and pulmonary vascular reactivity in patients with liver cirrhosis. *Am Rev Respir Dis* 1987;135(5):1085.

Younis I, Sarwar S, Butt Z et al. Clinical characteristics, predictors, and survival among patients with hepatopulmonary syndrome. *Ann Hepatol* 2015;14(3):354–360.

9. ANSWER: C

The equation for the calculation of a patient's MELD is MELD = $3.78 \times \ln[$serum bilirubin (mg/dL)$] + 11.2 \times \ln[$INR$] + 9.57 \times \ln[$serum creatinine (mg/dL)$] + 6.43$. The multiplier of natural log of the INR is 11.2, which is higher than that of the other two determinants. Sodium level is only considered in the MELD-Na. The MELD-Na predicts waiting list mortality better than MELD alone. The equation for the MELD-Na is MELD-Na = MELD – Na (mEq/L) – [$0.025 \times$ MELD $\times$ (140 – Na mEq/L)] + 140. Serum albumin is not considered in either of the two calculations.

Keywords: Laboratory studies; Coagulation parameters; Hepatorenal syndrome; Liver transplantation, rejection, complications

REFERENCES

Leise MD, Kim WR, Kremers WK et al. A revised model for end-stage liver disease optimizes prediction of mortality among patients awaiting liver transplantation. *Gastroenterology* 2011;140(7):1952.

Luca A, Angermayr B, Bertolini G et al. An integrated MELD model including serum sodium and age improves the prediction of early mortality in patients with cirrhosis. *Liver Transpl* 2007;13(8):1174.

Ruf AE, Kremers WK, Chavez LL et al. Addition of serum sodium into the MELD score predicts waiting list mortality better than MELD alone. *Liver Transpl* 2005;11:336.

10. ANSWER: A

Severity and mortality risk in patients with hepatitis secondary to alcohol may be estimated using the Maddrey discriminant function. Patients with scores greater than 32 have higher short-term mortality and may benefit from treatment with glucocorticoids. Patients with scores lower than 32 have lower short-term mortality and do not benefit from steroids. Other potential scoring systems for the degree of alcohol hepatitis include the MELD score (see question 9), Glasgow Alcoholic Hepatitis (GAH) score (based on age, WBC count, urea, INR, and bilirubin), and the Hepatic Histology Score (requires biopsy). Patients with a GAH score greater than 9 gain a survival benefit from glucocorticoids.

Keywords: Hepatic; Hepatitis

REFERENCE

Lucey M, Mathurin P, Morgan T. Alcoholic hepatitis. *N Engl J Med* 2009;360:2758–2769.

11. ANSWER: A

Two of the few recognized, widely accepted indications for TIPS are recurrent variceal hemorrhage despite adequate endoscopic therapy and active hemorrhage despite emergent endoscopic treatment. This patient fits both of these indications. Other relative indications for TIPS are refractory ascites, bleeding varices at the gastric fundus, Budd-Chiari syndrome, hepatorenal syndrome, hepatic hydrothorax, and protein-losing enteropathy due to portal hypertension. Liver transplantation would require workup and listing, which may take time that the patient does not have. This patient may qualify for a liver transplantation, which may ultimately fix this problem, but this is not the immediate next step to stop this patient from bleeding again. Supportive care and time are going to be part of this patient's ultimate care plan; however, it is likely that without a TIPS this patient will rebleed, especially because this had been trialed for him in the past. Emergent esophagectomies have been performed in the past for esophageal perforations but not for bleeding varices at the gastroesophageal junction.

Keywords: Stomach, GI hemorrhage, lower; Stomach, GI hemorrhage, upper; Liver transplantation, rejection, complications; Hepatic dysfunction/failure (acute and chronic)

REFERENCES

Boyer TD, Haskal ZJ, American Association for the Study of Liver Diseases. The role of transjugular intrahepatic portosystemic shunt (TIPS) in the management of portal hypertension: update 2009. *Hepatology* 2010;51(1):306.

Garcia-Pagán JC, Di Pascoli M, Caca K et al. Use of early-TIPS for high-risk variceal bleeding: results of a post-RCT surveillance study. *J Hepatol* 2013;58(1):45.

Garcia-Tsao G, Sanyal AJ, Grace ND, Carey W. Prevention and management of gastroesophageal varices and variceal hemorrhage in cirrhosis. *Hepatology* 2007;46:922–938.

12. ANSWER: D

TIPS procedures have been associated with a variety of potential postprocedure complications. Risk for these complications is reduced with careful patient selection. Absolute contraindications for TIPS include heart failure, severe tricuspid regurgitation, pulmonary hypertension with a mean pulmonary artery pressure greater than 45 mm Hg, multiple hepatic cysts, uncontrolled systemic infection, and unrelieved biliary obstruction. Given this patient's mean pulmonary artery pressure, she is at risk for developing right heart failure after the shunting of the portal circulations into the systemic circulation with relatively sudden increase in venous return. This increase in systemic blood volume can also exacerbate left ventricular dysfunction with resultant pulmonary edema and potential cardiogenic shock. In normal patients, the main oxygen supply to the liver is through the portal vein. A TIPS shunts part of this blood past the liver, decreasing its blood supply and placing the patient at risk for hepatic ischemia. Patients are thought to be at risk when the postprocedure PSG is less than 5 mm Hg. Post-TIPS hepatic encephalopathy is a risk for any patient undergoing TIPS. The incidence of new-onset or worsened hepatic encephalopathy is approximately 20 to 31% of all patients undergoing TIPS. Risk factors for post-TIPS hepatic encephalopathy are age, prior hepatic encephalopathy, Child-Pugh class, and large decrease in PSG. While hepatorenal syndrome may be seen in patients with TIPS, renal function has been demonstrated to improve after the TIPS procedure as opposed to worsening.

Keywords: Hepatorenal syndrome; Endoscopy, upper, lower with therapeutic intervention

REFERENCES

Chung HH, Razavi MK, Sze DY et al. Portosystemic pressure gradient during transjugular intrahepatic portosystemic shunt with Viatorr stent graft: what is the critical low threshold to avoid medically uncontrolled low pressure gradient related complications? *J Gastroenterol Hepatol* 2008;23:95–101.

Gaba RC, Khiatani VL, Knuttinen MG et al. Comprehensive review of TIPS technical complications and how to avoid them. *Am J Roentgenol* 2011;196(3):675–685.

13. ANSWER: B

This patient has a history of present illness and clinical features suggestive of Budd-Chiari syndrome. Budd-Chiari syndrome is venous outflow obstruction of the hepatic venous outflow tracts. The obstruction can be anywhere from the venules themselves all the way up to the right atrium. Budd-Chiari syndrome frequently presents in females around the age of 30 years who have an undiagnosed history of myeloproliferative disorders. In this case, the patient has a thrombocytosis, the etiology of which needs to be ascertained, that places her at increased thrombotic risk. She is also taking oral contraceptives, a risk factor known to predispose patients to thrombosis as well. The relatively short onset and worsening symptoms are consistent with hepatic venous obstruction, the diagnosis of which can be confirmed with ultrasound Doppler imaging demonstrating the paucity or absence of blood flow in the hepatic vein as well a congested enlarged liver. At this time, the portal and splenic veins should be assess for concomitant portal or splenic vein thrombosis. While liver biopsy may show findings consistent with obstructive venopathy, it is invasive and poses a bleeding risk to a coagulopathic patient who has a process that may require further anticoagulation. The findings may be patchy locality throughout the liver, thus making them unreliable. This test poses a high risk with minimal diagnostic benefit to the patient. CA 19-9 levels may be elevated in the pancreatic and ovarian malignancies. Patients with Budd-Chiari syndrome may have an underlying malignancy; however, the assessment of this would take place during the search for a cause by means of a hypercoagulation workup after the primary reason for her symptoms had been ascertained. With the absence of jugular venous distention, right and left heart failure and outflow obstruction would be unlikely; thus, cardiac anatomic assessment is not likely to be of value at this time.

Keywords: Diagnostic modalities; Imaging (ultrasound)

REFERENCES

DeLeve LD, Valla DC, Garcia-Tsao G; American Association for the Study Liver Diseases. Vascular disorders of the liver. *Hepatology* 2009;49(5):1729.

Menon KV, Shah V, Kamath PS. The Budd-Chiari syndrome. *N Engl J Med* 2004;350:578.

Plessier A, Valla DC. Budd-Chiari syndrome. *Semin Liver Dis* 2008;28(3):259–269.

14. ANSWER: D

This patient has a history and clinical findings suggestive of a pyogenic liver abscess. Pyogenic liver abscesses can be the result of various abdominal infections with involvement of the portal circulation (e.g., appendicitis, diverticulitis, ulcerative colitis). Another predisposing factor to development of pyogenic liver abscess is the history of biliary obstruction, which this patient was recently treated for. The presence of an air-fluid level inside a peripherally enhancing cystic lesion on CT is suggestive of gas-producing infection. The treatment of these abscesses consists of drainage and culture of the drainable contents followed by antibiotic therapy for at least 8 weeks. Antibiotics are generally started with broad-spectrum therapy covering gram-negative and anaerobic organisms. Frequently, the contents of these cystic lesions are viscous, so leaving a percutaneous drain for continued drainage is not frequently done. Two thirds of these lesions are culture-positive for *Escherichia coli*. *Streptococcus faecalis*, *Klebsiella* species, and *Proteus vulgaris* are also common.

Keywords: Management strategies; Infectious pyogenic liver abscess

REFERENCES

Branum GD, Tyson GS, Branum MA, Meyers WC. Hepatic abscess: changes in etiology, diagnosis, and management. *Ann Surg* 1990;212(6):655–662.

Seeto RK, Rockey DC. Pyogenic liver abscess: changes in etiology, management, and outcome. *Medicine (Balt)* 1996;75(2):99–113.

Stain SC, Yellin AE, Donovan AJ et al. Pyogenic liver abscess. modern treatment. *Arch Surg* 1991;126(8):991–996.

15. ANSWER: D

The Child-Turcotte-Pugh scoring system was originally developed to evaluate the risk of the portocaval shunt procedure secondary to portal hypertension but is currently being used to describe perioperative risk and overall severity of liver disease. Overall perioperative mortality rates have been described as 10% for class A, 30% for class B, and 75 to 80% for class C. The score is calculated on a 15-point scale. The variables considered are bilirubin level (1 point for <2 mg/dL, 2 points for 2–3 mg/dL, and 3 points for >3 mg/dL), albumin level (1 point for >3.5 g/dL, 2 points for 2.8–3.5 g/dL, and 3 points for <2.8 g/dL), INR (1 point for <1.7, 2 points for 1.7–2.2, and 3 points for >2.2), encephalopathy (1 point for none, 2 points for controlled, and 3 points for uncontrolled), and ascites (1 point for none, 2 points for controlled, and 3 points for uncontrolled). Class A is 5 to 6 points, class B is 7 to 9 points, and class C is 10 to 15 points.

Keywords: Diagnostic criteria; Portal hypertension; Laboratory studies

REFERENCES

Child CG, Turcotte JG. Surgery and portal hypertension. In: Child CG, ed. *The liver and portal hypertension*. Philadelphia: Saunders; 1964, pp. 50–64.

Mansour A, Watson W, Shayani V, Pickleman J. Abdominal operations in patients with cirrhosis: still a major surgical challenge. *Surgery* 1997;122(4):730.

Telem DA, Schiano T, Goldstone R et al. Factors that predict outcome of abdominal operations in patients with advanced cirrhosis. *Clin Gastroenterol Hepatol* 2010;8(5):451.

16. ANSWER: A

Patients who have an acute variceal bleed should receive medical therapy aimed at reducing splanchnic pressure. This can be achieved by the administration of octreotide, vasopressin, or terlipressin. Endoscopy is the next step in attempting to control bleeding with attempts at either band ligation or sclerotherapy. If endoscopic control of bleeding is attempted and fails, placement of a balloon tamponade device is indicated for bleeding control, and then emergent TIPS should be considered. Vasopressin can be used to decrease splanchnic pressure if octreotide and terlipressin are not feasible. Frequently, the dose of vasopressin required is higher than what is used for other indications. This infusion rate (0.4-unit bolus followed by 0.4–1 units/minute) can precipitate bowel, cerebral, and myocardial ischemia and is frequently administered with a concomitant infusion of nitroglycerine to offset this. This patient should be transferred to the ICU for ongoing blood product resuscitation if emergent TIPS after balloon tamponade placement is not feasible. Administering factor VII is considered when all other measure to correct medical coagulopathy have been exhausted, given its highly prothrombotic properties. It should not be used before optimization of invasive strategies, and thus it would not be appropriate at this stage. Of note, endoscopic therapy fails in 20% of patients and will require procedural intervention; TIPS results in 90 to 100% resolution of bleeding when applied.

Keywords: Gastrointestinal hemorrhage; Management strategies

REFERENCES

Balachandran V, Eachempati S. Liver failure, gastrointestinal bleeding, and acute pancreatitis. *Comprehens Crit Care Adult* 2012:511–523.
Chojkier M, Conn: esophageal tamponade in the treatment of bleeding varices. A decade progress report. *HO Dig Dis Sci* 1980;25(4):267.
Fort E, Sautereau D, Silvain C et al. A randomized trial of terlipressin plus nitroglycerin vs. balloon tamponade in the control of acute variceal hemorrhage. *Hepatology* 1990;11(4):678.
Hunt PS, Korman MG, Hansky J, Parkin WG. An 8-year prospective experience with balloon tamponade in emergency control of bleeding esophageal varices. *Dig Dis Sci* 1982;27(5):413.

17. ANSWER: C

This patient is presenting with sudden-onset abdominal pain in the presence of rapid atrial fibrillation. He has pain out of proportion to exam, describing visceral pain (dull and diffuse) without findings suggestive of peritonitis (rigidity, guarding, rebound tenderness). He has an elevated lactic acid level, which suggests some sort of malperfusion. Bowel obstruction, while it certainly could present in such a fashion, is less likely without a history of prior operations or nausea and vomiting. Bowel perforation would be unlikely given the lack of exam findings consistent with peritoneal irritation. If mesenteric ischemia persists, bowel perforation or infarction may ensue. *C. difficile* colitis is unlikely given the lack of history of diarrhea and the sudden onset of this patient's symptoms. Intra-abdominal abscess findings can be subtle with a great variety of presentations. This patient's sudden onset of extreme abdominal pain without peritoneal irritation should raise suspicion for mesenteric ischemia long before raising suspicion for intra-abdominal abscess, given the lack of risk factors for an abscess (i.e., diabetes, recent surgery, recent trauma, inflammatory bowel disease, history of diverticular disease).

Keywords: Infectious; Perforations; Volvulus; Vascular diseases

REFERENCES

Clair D, Beach J. Mesenteric ischemia. *N Engl J Med* 2016;374:959–968.
Cudnik MT, Darbha S, Jones J et al. The diagnosis of acute mesenteric ischemia: a systematic review and meta-analysis. *Acad Emerg Med* 2013;20(11):1087.

18. ANSWER: D

This patient has multiple characteristics that should alert the provider to the risk for refeeding syndrome. He is elderly with a history of alcoholism and cancer. He demonstrates physical exam findings consistent with malnutrition (i.e., bitemporal muscle wasting). Other patient characteristics that are associated with refeeding syndrome are anorexia nervosa, poorly controlled diabetes, chronic malabsorption disease states (Crohn disease, cystic fibrosis, short bowel syndrome), long-term diuretic use (electrolyte depletion), and long-term antacid users (phosphate binders). Objective risk factors include body mass index less than 18.5 kg/m², unintentional weight loss of more than 10% in the previous 3 to 6 months, and little or no nutritional intake for more than 5 days. Patients perceived to be at risk for refeeding syndrome should have their nutrition begun slowly at 10 kcal/kg per day and slowly increased to goal over 4 to 7 days. They should be carefully rehydrated and should receive 2 to 4 mmol/kg per day of potassium supplementation, 0.3 to 0.6 mmol/kg per day of phosphorus supplementation, and 0.3 mmol/kg per day of IV magnesium supplementation. This should be adjusted for disease processes and preexisting electrolyte imbalances. They should have their potassium, phosphorus, calcium, and magnesium levels followed closely because they frequently need aggressive replacement. Close coordination with a dietitian or experienced provider is recommended. Thiamine deficiency is sometimes seen in this population; therefore, supplementation would be reasonable, although not universally given. While parenteral nutrition would theoretically be well tolerated, its cost and the risk for complications make it the least likely to be helpful in this case, particularly taking into consideration that simply reducing intake to 500 kcal/day makes feeding safe in this population.

Keywords: Refeeding syndrome; Nutrition; Malabsorption

REFERENCES

National Institute for Clinical Excellence. Nutrition support for adults: clinical guidelines. CG32. 2006;1–176.

Walmsley R. Refeeding syndrome: screening, incidence, and treatment during parenteral nutrition. J Gastroenterol Hepatol 2013;28(Suppl 4):113–117.

19. ANSWER: A

This patient is presenting with an acute abdomen on postoperative day 6 after colorectal surgery with a primary anastomosis. This presentation is suggestive of an anastomotic leak. Anastomotic leaks are dreaded complications of colorectal surgery. The average time to manifestation of leaks is generally thought of as being 5 to 7 days after surgery but in some studies has peaked to as long as 13 days. The risk factors for anastomotic leaks are depend on the site of anastomosis (extraperitoneal vs. intraperitoneal).

The major risk factors for extraperitoneal leaks include distance from anal verge, anastomotic ischemia, male gender, and obesity. The major risk factors for intraperitoneal leaks include American Society of Anesthesiologists score of III to V, emergent surgery, prolonged operative time, and hand-sewn ileocolic anastomosis. Neither male gender nor obesity have been found to be risk factors for intraperitoneal leaks. Anastomotic leaks generally presents with fever and abdominal pain. This patient is unlikely to have an incarcerated hernia without palpable masses as long as the mesenteric fat defect was closed intraoperatively (risk for internal hernia). While this patient certainly could present with bowel ischemia, peritoneal signs tend to be absent in bowel ischemia until late in the course of the ischemia. This patient is at risk for *C. difficile* infection given that she had been hospitalized recently; however, a lack of history of diarrhea makes this diagnosis unlikely. Volvulus is traditionally thought of as being associated with chronic constipation and is unlikely in someone who is reporting no change in bowel movements.

Keywords: Infectious complications; Bowel disorders; Volvulus

REFERENCES

Hyman N, Manchester TL, Osler T, Cataldo PA. Anastomotic leaks after intestinal anastomosis: it's later than you think. *Ann Surg* 2007;245(2):254.

Kingham TP, Pachter HL. Colonic anastomotic leak: risk factors, diagnosis, and treatment. *J Am Coll Surg* 2009;208(2):269.

Platell C, Barwood N, Dorfmann G, Makin G. The incidence of anastomotic leaks in patients undergoing colorectal surgery. *Colorectal Dis* 2007;9(1):71.

20. ANSWER: A

This patient has a history and physical exam findings suggestive of a psoas abscess. Psoas abscesses historically were most commonly secondary to mycobacterial infections. With tuberculosis infections relatively uncommon these days, abscess formation is secondary to gastrointestinal and pelvic infections by spreading along the fascial sheath around the psoas muscle. Psoas abscess has been found to occur in patients with Crohn disease, ulcerative colitis, appendicitis, colorectal surgery, and other abdominal surgeries. Hip pain after these surgeries should raise the suspicion for psoas abscess. Findings tend to include fever, back pain, and patient preference of flexing and externally rotating the ipsilateral hip while flexing the knee. Diagnosis can be made with ultrasound, contrast-enhanced CT scan, or magnetic resonance imaging. Treatment is with drainage of the abscess and antibiotics based on the culture results of the abscess drainage. *Staphylococcus* species are the most common causative organisms, but in this case, when the primary infection was the diverticular infection, enteric organisms (both aerobic and anaerobic) and gram-negative organisms should be covered as well because these are also frequently polymicrobial.

Keywords: Infectious complications; Psoas abscess; Management strategies

REFERENCES

Hsieh MS, Huang SC, Loh el-W et al. Features and treatment modality of iliopsoas abscess and its outcome: a 6-year hospital-based study. *BMC Infect Dis* 2013;13:578.

Mallick IH, Thoufeeq MH, Rajendran TP. Iliopsoas abscesses. *Postgrad Med J* 2004;80(946):459.

Shields D, Robinson P, Crowley TP. Iliopsoas abscess: a review and update on the literature. *Int J Surg* 2012;10(9):466–469.

Yacoub WN, Sohn HJ, Chan S et al. Psoas abscess rarely requires surgical intervention. *Am J Surg* 2008;196(2):223.

21. ANSWER: D

Antibiotic therapy for infected pseudocysts should be geared toward coverage of gram-negative and anaerobic enteric bacteria. If the infected collection has had surgical manipulation, fungal infections can be considered as well. The ideal antibiotic in the context of a septic patient would be a bactericidal broad-spectrum antibiotic that covers many enteric gram-negative bacteria. Imipenem and cilastin cover many gram-negative bacteria, including *Pseudomonas* species. They also cover anaerobes, have adequate pancreatic penetration, and are bactericidal. Many studies have been done regarding the use of prophylactic antibiotics and necrotizing pancreatitis. Results have discouraged the use of prophylactic antibiotics, however, in this case, the patient is no longer in the initial inflammatory phase of acute pancreatitis but rather is in the second stage of pancreatitis with pseudocyst formation. He was previously not demonstrating signs of systemic inflammation but now is, and thus infection of the pancreatic fluid collection must be considered. Cefazolin covers primarily gram-positive infections and thus would not be appropriate. This is the case for vancomycin as well. Fluconazole is an antifungal drug that could be considered if the necrotizing collection were manipulated surgically but should be used in conjunction with antibacterial antibiotics until cultures suggest that it would be adequate to use as monotherapy because of culture data. Clindamycin has good gram-positive and anaerobic bacterial coverage but does not have adequate gram-negative coverage and thus should not be used as monotherapy in the treatment of infected pancreatic fluid collections. Other drugs that could be considered for use would be fluoroquinolones with metronidazole and fourth-generation cephalosporins.

Keywords: Pharmacologic management; Antimicrobials

REFERENCES

De Vries A, Besselink MG, Buskens E et al. Randomized controlled trials of antibiotic prophylaxis in severe acute pancreatitis: relationship between methodologic quality and outcome. *Pancreatology* 2007;7:531–538.

Jafri NS, Mahid SS, Idstein SR et al. Antibiotic prophylaxis is not protective in severe acute pancreatitis: a systemic review and meta-analysis. *Am J Surg* 2009;197:806–813.

Pederzoli P, Bassi C, Vesontini S et al. A randomized multicenter clinical trial of antibiotic prophylaxis of septic complications in acute necrotizing pancreatitis with imipenem. *Surg Gynecol Obstet* 1993;176:480–483.

Tenner S, Bailie J, Dewitt J, Vege S. American College of Gastroenterology guideline: management of acute pancreatitis. *Am J Gastroenterol* 2013;108(9):1400–1415.

Villatoro E, Bassi C, Larvin M. Antibiotic therapy for prophylaxis against infection of pancreatic necrosis in acute pancreatitis. *Cochrane Database Syst Rev* 2006;(4):CD002941.

22. ANSWER: A

This patient has a clinical scenario and exam findings that are concerning for abdominal compartment syndrome. Abdominal perfusion pressure = mean arterial pressure – intra-abdominal pressure. It is usually heralded by multiple organ failure with bladder pressures (intra-abdominal pressure) above 25 mm Hg. Abdominal hypertension is defined as an intra-abdominal pressure above 12 mm Hg. Upward displacement of the diaphragm results in decrease in pulmonary compliance, which leads to increased peak airway pressures and ventilation-perfusion mismatch. Compression of the inferior vena cava causes decreased cardiac venous return, decreased cardiac output, and increased peripheral vascular resistance. Direct compression of the kidneys causes an obstruction of venous outflow and decreases glomerular filtration rate and urine output. Compression of the mesenteric vasculature leads to decreases in splanchnic perfusion, mesenteric venous hypertension, intestinal edema, and visceral edema. Risk factors are massive resuscitation, intra-abdominal hemorrhage, bowel distention, ascites, abdominal masses, pregnancy, and abdominal closure under tension. Previous pregnancy, cirrhosis, and morbid obesity can chronically increase abdominal wall compliance and may be protective. Bladder pressure is an estimate of intra-abdominal pressure, which should be measured after a large resuscitation in a patient who has stopped making urine and is having pulmonary compliance issues to assess for intra-abdominal hypertension. Returning to the operating room emergently for decompressive laparotomy may preclude being needed later in the patient's hospital course, but it is not the first thing to do to evaluate what is wrong with this patient. At least an attempt should be made at evaluating and confirming the underlying problem so as to not expose the patient to more invasive procedures unnecessarily. An immediate CT scan could be considered if one were concerned about perforation with signs of free air under the diaphragm or re-establishment of mesenteric ischemia. It requires the patient to travel, and the patient is having ventilatory problems, which should be evaluated and addressed beforehand. Trial of neuromuscular blockade may in fact help this patient's condition, but neuromuscular blockade should be given with a diagnosis in hand if time permits. Measuring a bladder pressure is done at the bedside and is noninvasive, which would confirm the diagnosis of this patient's underlying problem. Mesenteric Doppler can be considered in patients in whom mesenteric ischemia is a consideration (as in this patient). It can be technically challenging in some patients who are significantly edematous and is operator dependent. Its use should be reserved for patients who cannot receive IV contrast or those who are too unstable to undergo CT scanning. This patient has other stigmata of another problem that should not be overlooked and that should be identified and treated quickly, and thus CT is not the next best step.

Keywords: Diagnostic modalities; Abdominal pressure measurement (bladder pressure, other); Abdominal compartment syndrome

REFERENCES

Malbrain ML, Cheatham ML, Kirkpatrick A et al. Results from the International Conference of Experts on Intra-abdominal Hypertension and Abdominal Compartment Syndrome. I. Definitions. *Intensive Care Med* 2006;32(11):1722.

Sheri S, Bittner E, Kasotakis G. Gastrointestinal: abdominal compartment syndrome. *MGH Rev Crit Care Med* 2014:85–86.

Van Mook WN, Huslewe-Evers RP, Ramsay G. Abdominal compartment syndrome. *Lancet* 2002;360(9344):1502.

Vidal MG, Ruiz Weisser J, Gonzalez F et al. Incidence and clinical effects of intra-abdominal hypertension in critically ill patients. *Crit Care Med* 2008;36(6):1823.

23. ANSWER: B

This patient is presenting with gallstone pancreatitis and cholangitis and should undergo ERCP in the first 24 hours of admission. The patient should likely have her gallbladder removed in the future after she is no longer critically ill to prevent recurrence. This patient would benefit from CBD decompression. This patient is coagulopathic and thus would not be a candidate for sphincterotomy. She is also too unstable to leave the ICU to receive fluoroscopic guidance for instrumentation. She could receive percutaneous CBD drainage transhepatically but would need her coagulopathy corrected. Percutaneous drainage is associated with longer hospital stays and is more uncomfortable for the patient. ERCP is the first-line preferred method of drainage when feasible. ERCP with nasobiliary tube placement would allow for CBD irrigation and decompression, can be performed at the bedside, and, while frequently performed with fluoroscopy, can be performed in critically ill patients without fluoroscopy. Broad-spectrum antibiotics and fluids are already being given to the patient, and owing to the signs of cholangitis and severe acute pancreatitis secondary to CBD obstruction, relieving the obstruction is indicated. Continuing without ERCP would be inappropriate. If this patient had only biliary pancreatitis without signs of cholangitis, the role of ERCP would be controversial and at the discretion of the consulting gastroenterologist.

Keywords: Gallbladder disease (stones, cholecystitis); Management strategies; Endoscopy—upper, lower; ERCP

REFERENCES

Mosler P. Management of acute cholangitis. *Gastroenterol Hepatol (NY)* 2011;7(2):121–123.

Tenner S, Bailie J, Dewitt J, Vege S. American College of Gastroenterology guideline: management of acute pancreatitis. *Am J Gastroenterol* 2013;108(9):1400–1415.

Wang HP, Huang SP, Sun MS et al. Urgent endoscopic nasobiliary drainage without fluoroscopic guidance: a useful treatment for critically ill patients with biliary obstruction. *Gastrointest Endosc* 2000;52(6):741–744.

24. ANSWER: D

Enteral nutritional support is the preferred method of nutrition in patients with acute pancreatitis. Patients who received enteric feeds demonstrated a significant reduction in overall mortality and the rate of multiple organ failure. Prophylactic antibiotics are not recommended irrespective of the type or severity of pancreatitis. In patients with suspected infected necrotizing pancreatitis, carbapenems alone or a quinolone combined with metronidazole is recommended because these are known to have good pancreatic penetration. Most infections are derived from the gut (like *E. coli* and *Pseudomonas, Klebsiella,* and *Enterococcus* species). Gallstones are the most common culprit in causing pancreatitis, and if they are found to be associated with cholangitis, early ERCP within 24 hours of admission is recommended.

Keywords: Pancreatitis; Nutrition; Antimicrobials

REFERENCES

Berg S, Bittner E. Gastrointestinal: acute pancreatitis. *MGH Rev Crit Care Med* 2014:86–89.

McClave SA, Chang W K, Dhaliwal R, Heyland DK. Nutrition support in acute pancreatitis: a systematic review of the literature. *JPEN J Parenter Enteral Nutr* 2006;30(2):143.

Petrov MS, Pylypchuk RD, Emelyanov NV. Systematic review: nutritional support in acute pancreatitis. *Aliment Pharmacol Ther* 2008;28(6):704.

Yao H, He C, Deng L, Liao G. Enteral versus parenteral nutrition in critically ill patients with severe pancreatitis: a meta-analysis. *Eur J Clin Nutr* 2018;72(1):66–68.

25. ANSWER: A

This patient has Ogilvie syndrome (colonic pseudo-obstruction). Ogilvie syndrome is defined as colonic dilation to greater than 9 cm in the absence of obstruction. Acute colonic pseudo-obstruction usually occurs in association with chronic illnesses, after surgery, in association with metabolic disturbances. Elderly, inactive patients who are taking narcotics are at risk. As per data from a national database, the incidence of acute colonic pseudo-obstruction is approximately 100 per 100,00 inpatient admissions per year. These patients are at risk for colonic perforation and ischemia and the associated high mortality. Colonic decompression is a priority, and the mode to achieve that can be with a single dose of neostigmine or endoscopic decompression. This patient should be monitored with serial abdominal exams and serial plain abdominal radiographs every 12 to 24 hours. Conservative management works in nearly 50% of these patients without significant abdominal pain. Single-dose neostigmine leads to resolution in 80 to 90% of patients with cecal diameter greater than 12 cm, significant abdominal pain, or other signs of peritonitis. This patient should receive neostigmine because it is the first-line treatment for Ogilvie syndrome.

Senna, docusate, and metoclopramide would be ineffective in this scenario. They could be trialed if the diameter were less than the 12-cm threshold, but at this point, the patient should receive neostigmine. The patient should be made NPO, but nasogastric decompression only helps if the patient is complaining of nausea. This patient is not complaining of nausea. Continued observation may be considered in more mild cases, but this patient is has severe dilation of the colon (>12 cm) and thus should be treated more acutely.

Keywords: Toxic mega colon; Surgical intervention (timing, therapeutic options); Pharmacologic management

REFERENCES

Ponec R, Saunders M, Kimmey M. Neostigmine for the treatment of colonic pseudo-obstruction. *N Engl J Med* 1999;341:137–141.

Ross SW, Oommen B, Wormer BA et al. Acute colonic pseudo-obstruction: defining the epidemiology, treatment, and adverse outcomes of Ogilvie's syndrome. *Am Surg* 2016;82(2):102.

Saunders MD. Acute colonic pseudo-obstruction. *Best Pract Res Clin Gastroenterol* 2007;21(4):671.

Valle RG, Godoy FL. Neostigmine for acute colonic pseudo-obstruction: a meta-analysis. *Ann Med Surg (Lond)* 2014;3(3):60.

5.

TRAUMA AND DISASTER MANAGEMENT

Joshua Person and Lillian S. Kao

QUESTIONS

1. Your hospital facility is notified that multiple bus passengers are suspected to have been exposed to a terrorist chemical attack involving a nerve agent (sarin). In addition to activating a disaster response, your hospital is preparing the medical decontamination area and is transferring non–critically ill patients out of intensive care in anticipation of receiving multiple patients. In addition to atropine, which of the following first-line antidotes should be on hand to treat exposure to the nerve agent?

A. Pralidoxime
B. Phentolamine
C. Diazepam
D. Magnesium

2. A 10-year-old male is swimming at the beach in rough waters when he suffers a drowning event. Bystanders bring him ashore within 10 minutes, and he is found to be apneic and without a pulse. What is the best first step in resuscitation?

A. Perform a Heimlich maneuver
B. Start chest compressions immediately
C. Place him in a prone position
D. Deliver two rescue breaths

3. A 21-year-old male is admitted to the intensive care unit (ICU) after a near-drowning event in a freshwater lake. He is neurologically intact and hemodynamically stable. He is intubated in the emergency department (ED) secondary to hypoxia and hypercapnia. His chest radiograph is shown here. Current ventilator settings are as follows: tidal volume 800 mL (12 mL/kg), respiratory rate (RR) 16 breaths/minute, positive end-expiratory pressure (PEEP) 8, and forced inspiratory

oxygen (FiO_2) 0.9. Arterial blood gas (ABG) analysis shows pH of 7.32, $PaCO_2$ of 52, and O_2 of 92.

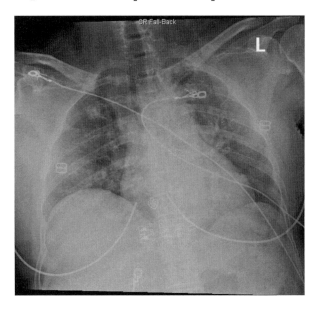

Which of the following is the best next step in management?

A. Exogenous surfactant administration
B. Lung protective ventilation
C. Renal replacement therapy
D. Extracorporeal membrane oxygenation (ECMO)

4. A 25-year-old female presents to the ED after she was found with altered mental status by her roommate. She has a history of depression and previous suicide attempts. She was last seen normal 6 hours prior. Vitals include blood pressure (BP) 87/54 mm Hg, heart rate (HR) 128 bpm, RR 20 breaths/minute and shallow, O_2 saturation 99%, and temperature 39° C. On exam, she is minimally responsive to painful stimulus, pupils are 8 mm and slowly reactive, mucous membranes are dry, and bowel sounds are absent. Glucose level is normal. She is intubated for airway protection. An electrocardiogram (ECG) shows a monomorphic wide-complex tachycardia with a prolonged QRS interval of 110 milliseconds. Administration of which of the following is the next best step in her management?

A. Sodium bicarbonate
B. Acetylcysteine
C. Naloxone
D. Calcium

5. A 25-year-old man is stabbed in the left flank. On arrival to the ED, his Glasgow Coma Scale (GCS) score is 14. His vital signs are as follows: HR 120 bpm, BP 85/43 mm Hg, RR 28 breaths/minute, and O_2 saturation 98%. He receives 1 L of crystalloid to which he has a transient response. His chest radiograph shows no pneumothorax or hemothorax. Focused assessment with sonography for trauma (FAST) exam is positive in the left upper quadrant. He is planned for emergent laparotomy. Which of the following is the most appropriate next step in resuscitating this patient in the interim?

A. Another 1-L bolus of crystalloid
B. Transfuse 1 unit each of red cells, plasma, and platelets
C. Norepinephrine infusion
D. No fluid therapy at this time

6. A 52-year-old man sustains a gunshot wound to the right upper quadrant and is intubated in the field. His vital signs on presentation are: GCS 3T, BP 65/palpable mm Hg, HR 145 bpm, and RR 14 breaths/minute (mechanically ventilated). He is taken emergently to the operating room, and massive transfusion protocol is initiated. He is transfused 2 units of packed red blood cells and 2 units of fresh frozen plasma. A retrohepatic caval injury is identified, and significant bleeding is ongoing. Which of the following should be employed in the initial decision to transfuse platelets?

A. Platelet count less than 100,000/μL
B. Activated clotting time of thromboelastography ≥140 seconds
C. Abnormal bleeding time >15 minutes
D. Empiric transfusion to maintain a balanced ratio

7. A 42-year-old male presents after a high-speed motor vehicle collision. FAST exam is negative, and cross-sectional imaging demonstrates multiple bilateral rib fractures and a nondisplaced sternal fracture. Vital signs include BP 128/86 mm Hg, HR 114 bpm, RR 14 breaths/minute, and O_2 saturation 97% on 2-L nasal

cannula. He has no other injuries. Which of the following rules out the diagnosis of cardiac contusion?

A. Normal echocardiogram
B. Absence of cardiac murmur on physical exam
C. Normal ECG and troponin I level
D. Absence of hemopericardium on FAST exam

8. A 40-year-old man is brought to the ED intubated after an explosive device is detonated in an underground passageway at a major commuter hub. Chest radiograph reveals bilateral perihilar infiltrates. No pneumothorax or hemothorax is seen. Over the next several days, he requires increased positive pressure ventilation and PEEP. On postinjury day 4, he develops an arrhythmia and hypotension leading to cardiopulmonary arrest. Which of the following is the most likely cause of the arrest?

A. Mitral valve rupture
B. Chemical pneumonitis
C. Pulmonary hemorrhage
D. Air embolism

9. A 32-year-old male is admitted to the ICU after a fall from 20 feet. He underwent a complete trauma evaluation and was found to have multiple bilateral rib fractures and pulmonary contusions, which were apparent on chest radiograph and confirmed on computed tomography (CT). He is hemodynamically stable but appears to be in moderate respiratory distress. RR is 20 breaths/minute, and O_2 saturation is 96% on 8 L via nasal cannula. ABG analysis shows pH 7.32, $PaCO_2$ 51, and PaO_2 114. Which of the following interventions is most likely to avoid mechanical ventilation?

A. Corticosteroid administration
B. Epidural placement for analgesia
C. Empiric treatment with antibiotics
D. Aggressive fluid resuscitation

10. A 24-year-old male presents to the ED after being stabbed. Vitals signs are as follows: BP 85/50 mm Hg, HR 138 bpm, RR 24 breaths/minute, and SpO_2 100% on 2-L nasal cannula. Physical exam is significant for a single 2-cm stab wound to the right flank without active bleeding. He is intoxicated but arouses to voice and follows simple commands in all extremities. Two large-bore intravenous (IV) lines are established, and resuscitation with balanced blood products is started. Chest radiograph is unremarkable, and FAST exam is negative in all views. Gross hematuria is noted after placement of a Foley catheter. Despite ongoing transfusions, he remains hypotensive. Which of the following is the MOST appropriate next step in management?

A. CT scan of the abdomen
B. Repeat FAST exam
C. Renal angiogram and embolization
D. Emergent laparotomy

11. A 58-year-old male presents after an all-terrain vehicle (ATV) accident. He is hemodynamically stable, and CT demonstrates right sacroiliac joint widening and comminuted fractures of bilateral inferior and superior pubic rami. He complains of inability to void when asked to provide a urine sample. What is the best next step in management?

A. Place a transurethral catheter
B. Place a suprapubic catheter
C. Perform a CT cystogram
D. Obtain a retrograde urethrogram (RUG)

12. A 46-year-old female was the restrained driver in a high-speed motor vehicle collision. She was intubated for airway protection. Vital signs on arrival are as follows: BP 95/60 mm Hg, HR 128 bpm, SpO$_2$ 100% on, FiO$_2$ 1, and GCS 5T (E1 V1T M3). FAST exam is positive in the right upper quadrant and pelvis. Initial labs include hemoglobin 12.9, platelets 248, international normalized ratio (INR) 1.2, base excess –7, and lactate 5.8. BP improves with initial resuscitation, and CT demonstrates multiple cerebral contusions, bilateral rib fractures, and a grade IV liver laceration with active arterial extravasation and hemoperitoneum. She is admitted to the ICU, and an intracranial pressure (ICP) monitoring device is placed. Four hours after admission, her neurological exam is unchanged, and repeat labs show hemoglobin 8.1, base excess –6, lactate 4.6, and INR 1.5. Her mean arterial pressure (MAP) is 63 mm Hg, HR 119 bpm, and ICP 16 mm Hg. What is the MOST appropriate plan of care?

A. Hepatic angioembolization
B. Emergent laparotomy
C. Norepinephrine infusion
D. No intervention

13. A middle-aged male is transported to the ER following a gunshot wound. BP is 80/40 mm Hg, HR is 138 bpm, and SpO$_2$ is 100% on a non-rebreather mask. He is lethargic with minimal response to commands but is protecting his airway. There are decreased breath sounds on the left and a single left thoracoabdominal ballistic injury in the mid-axillary line at the level of the sixth intercostal space. Chest radiograph shows a moderate left pleural effusion, and the projectile is visualized overlying T12. FAST exam is negative. Left tube thoracostomy is performed with immediate

return of 500 mL of blood. What is the best next step in management?

A. Endotracheal intubation
B. Pericardial window
C. Exploratory laparotomy
D. Left thoracotomy

14. An 18-year-old male is a restrained back-seat passenger in a high-speed motor vehicle collision. On exam, he is intubated and unresponsive. HR is 90 bpm, systolic BP is 110 mm Hg, and GCS is 3T. He has an abdominal wall contusion (or a "seat belt" sign). On CT imaging, he has a subarachnoid hemorrhage, multiple rib fractures, pulmonary contusions, a small amount of free fluid in the pelvis, and a mesenteric contusion with associated bowel wall thickening. His white blood cell count is 16,000/mm³. Which of the following would be the most appropriate next step?

A. Serial abdominal exams
B. FAST exam
C. Diagnostic peritoneal lavage (DPL)
D. Exploratory laparotomy

15. A 38-year-old woman is admitted to the ICU after a high-speed motor vehicle collision. She was intubated, and a right-sided chest tube was placed for a tension pneumothorax. Additional injuries include subarachnoid hemorrhage, bilateral rib fractures, sternal fracture, pneumomediastinum, and pulmonary contusions. The chest tube is on suction, and there is a continuous air leak. She is on assist control ventilation with a rate of 15, delivered tidal volume 500 mL (8 mL/kg), exhaled tidal volume 350 mL, PEEP 8 cm H$_2$O, and FiO$_2$ 60%. An ABG is obtained: pH 7.29, pCO$_2$ 56, pO$_2$ 85. Repeat chest radiograph demonstrates extensive subcutaneous emphysema and a moderate-sized pneumothorax despite an appropriately positioned chest tube. What is the best next step?

A. Flexible bronchoscopy
B. Selective ventilation of the left lung with a double-lumen tube
C. Right anterolateral thoracotomy
D. ECMO

16. A 56-year-old female was involved in an ATV accident in which she suffered a complex (Schatzker V) tibial plateau fracture. On initial presentation, she has a normal neurovascular exam. Four hours after admission, she complains of severe leg pain despite multiple doses of pain medications. On exam, she has intact dorsalis pedis and posterior tibial pulses, firm swelling of her calf, severe pain to palpation of her lower leg, and

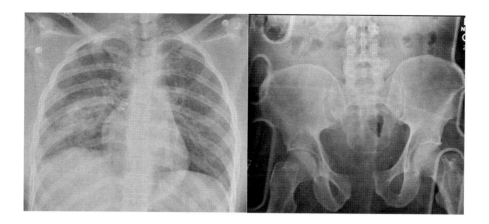

Figure Q17.1

severe pain with passive dorsiflexion of her foot. She has a normal motor exam but has an ill-defined paresthesia on the dorsal aspect of her foot. What is the MOST appropriate next step in management?

A. Measure compartment pressures
B. Magnetic resonance imaging (MRI) of the left lower extremity
C. Angiography of the left lower extremity
D. Emergent four-compartment fasciotomy

17. A 27-year-old male presents to the ED after a high-speed motorcycle collision. He veered into an embankment while traveling at approximately 65 mph and was thrown from the vehicle. He was wearing a helmet and did not lose consciousness. Arrival vital signs are as follow: BP 95/60 mm Hg, HR 129 bpm, RR 20 breaths/minute, and SpO₂ 94% on 4-L nasal cannula. He has adequate IV access, and FAST exam is negative. Chest radiograph and pelvic radiograph are shown here. What is the BEST next immediate step in management?

A. 2 L of crystalloid
B. Pelvic binder
C. Pelvic angiography
D. Emergent laparotomy

18. A 29-year-old male is involved in a high-speed motorcycle collision resulting in multiple rib fractures, pelvic fractures, and a right femur fracture. After several days, he is noted to have an area of ecchymosis and soft tissue swelling that develops along his right thigh and gluteus. He is afebrile and hemodynamically normal. He has no tenderness to palpation. His white blood cell count is 9000/mm³. Which of the following is the best next step for definitive diagnosis?

A. Ultrasonography
B. CT scan

C. MRI
D. Angiography

19. An 18-year-old male presents to the ER after a high-speed MVC. He has an intact airway with bilateral breath sounds, BP 80/30 mm Hg, HR 145 bpm, RR 16 breaths/minute, and SpO₂ 100% on non-rebreather face mask. Chest radiograph shows multiple rib fractures and is otherwise unremarkable. Pelvic radiograph demonstrates widening of the pubic symphysis. FAST exam is positive in bilateral upper quadrants and negative for pericardial fluid. A pelvic binder is placed, and massive transfusion protocol is initiated. After rapid transfusion of 3 units of red blood cells and 3 units of fresh frozen plasma, the BP is 75/40 mm Hg and HR is 138 bpm. You plan to take the patient to the operating room for emergent laparotomy but suspect he will experience cardiovascular collapse owing to massive hemorrhage before your proposed intervention. Which of the following is the best next step in management?

A. Placement of resuscitative endovascular balloon occlusion of the aorta (REBOA) in zone 1
B. Placement of REBOA in zone 2
C. Placement of REBOA in zone 3
D. Resuscitative left thoracotomy

20. An 18-year-old male presents hemodynamically stable to the ED following a stab wound to the medial left upper arm. Physical exam demonstrates a single 2-cm wound just distal to the left axilla without active bleeding or hematoma. He has a palpable left radial pulse and no neurological deficits. Chest radiograph is normal. Which of the following is the most appropriate screening test to evaluate for arterial injury?

A. Injured extremity index (IEI)
B. Conventional angiography
C. CT angiography
D. Operative exploration

ANSWERS

1. Answer: A

Nerve agents, such as sarin, are organophosphate compounds. They are generally odorless and colorless; they are liquids at room temperature, but they can be aerosolized, vaporized, or dispersed by evaporation. For example, in a 1996 attack on a Tokyo subway, plastic bags containing liquid sarin were punctured, and the nerve agent was allowed to evaporate. Nerve agents can be absorbed either through the skin and mucous membranes or by ingestion or inhalation.

The mechanism of action of nerve agents is irreversible inhibition of acetylcholinesterase at nicotinic and muscarinic receptors, both centrally and peripherally. Nerve agents can affect multiple systems (Table 5.1). Symptoms of nerve agent poisoning can be easily remembered by the mnemonic DUMBBELS, which stands for: Diarrhea, Urination, Miosis, Bronchorrhea/Bronchospasm, Emesis, Lacrimation, and Salivation. The toxicity of nerve agents depends on the dosing and the exposure.

The treatment of nerve agent poisoning begins with decontamination; in particular, any contaminated clothing must be removed and stored in a plastic bag. The skin should be decontaminated with soap and water; dilute hypochlorite solution may inactive the agents as well. Personal protective gear should be worn by healthcare personnel until decontamination has been completed, at which time exposure risk becomes minimal. Patients should be supported from a cardiorespiratory standpoint until the antidote can be administered. The antidote consists of atropine and pralidoxime chloride (2-PAM), which is an oxime. Atropine is a competitive antagonist of acetylcholine, while 2-PAM works by breaking the bond between the nerve agent and the anticholinesterase enzyme. Atropine should be administered in 2-mg doses and can be repeated until life-threatening symptoms are controlled. Pralidoxime is administered intravenously at a dose of 15 to 25 mg/kg.

Adjunctive treatments may include a benzodiazepine such as diazepam for fasciculations or seizures, phentolamine for pralidoxime-induced hypertension, or treatment for arrhythmias such as torsades de pointes.

Keywords: Specialized areas; Disaster management; Biologic, chemical, and nuclear exposures

Table 5.1 SYMPTOMS OF NERVE AGENT POISONING BY SYSTEM

SYSTEM	SYMPTOMS
Central nervous system	Headache Confusion Seizures Irritability Lethargy Ataxia Coma Permanent brain damage
Cardiovascular system	Variable heart rate disturbances (initial tachycardia followed by bradycardia) Blood pressure changes (initial hypertension followed by hypotension) Heart block Prolonged QT interval Arrhythmias
Respiratory system	Bronchospasm Pulmonary edema Bronchorrhea
Gastrointestinal system	Nausea/vomiting Abdominal cramping Diarrhea
Genitourinary system	Urinary incontinence
Musculoskeletal system	Fasciculations Muscle weakness Flaccid paralysis
Ocular	Reduced vision Miosis
Other systems	Salivation Lacrimation Perspiration Rhinorrhea

REFERENCES

American College of Surgeons. *Disaster management and emergency preparedness course*, 2nd edition. Chicago: American College of Surgeons; 2018.

Candiotti K. A primer on nerve agents: what the emergency responder, anesthesiologist, and intensivist needs to know. *Can J Anaesth* 2017;64(10):1059–1070.

2. ANSWER: D

Drowning is the third most common cause of accidental death in the United States, accounting for approximately 4000 fatalities annually. Most drowning events are preventable and can be avoided by simple means such as adequate supervision of swimming children, fencing around pools, swimming with a partner, use of flotation devices, and avoidance of alcohol or drug use while swimming. Although there is variation in the literature regarding the definition of drowning, it is the process resulting in primary respiratory impairment from submersion or immersion in a liquid medium. Aspiration of a significant volume can lead to washout of surfactant, hypoxemia, noncardiogenic pulmonary edema, and acute respiratory distress syndrome (ARDS).

Initial management in the prehospital setting is one of the most important factors affecting patient outcome. Poor neurological outcomes are associated with submersion for longer than 5 minutes (most important determinant), time to initiation of basic life support more than 10 minutes, age more than 14 years, GCS less than 5, apnea or ongoing cardiopulmonary resuscitation (CPR) at ED presentation, and arterial pH less than 7.1. Rapid rescue and initiation of resuscitation by bystanders is crucial. Ventilation is most important (vs. a nondrowning cardiac arrest), and initial treatment with rescue breathing should be started as soon as the patient is moved to shallow water or a stable surface. The need for CPR is determined, and if there is no response to two adequate rescue breaths, chest compressions should be initiated. CPR and application of an external defibrillator should be done according to standard guidelines. Hypothermic patients should be actively rewarmed and prolonged resuscitation efforts continued until euthermia is achieved. If the drowning event was preceded by a dive into shallow water, a spinal cord injury should be considered and spinal precautions maintained. Heimlich maneuver and postural drainage techniques are of no benefit and should be avoided.

Keywords: Specialized areas; Drowning, fatal, near-drowning; Salt water

REFERENCES

Lavonas EJ, Drennan IR, Gabrielli A et al. Part 10. Special circumstances of resuscitation: 2015 American Heart Association Guidelines for cardiopulmonary resuscitation and emergency cardiovascular care. *Circulation*. 2015;132(18 Suppl 2):S501–S518.

Quan L, Bierens JJ, Lis R et al. Predicting outcome of drowning at the scene: a systematic review and meta-analyses. *Resuscitation* 2016;104:63–75.

Orlowski JP, Szpilman D. Drowning: rescue, resuscitation, and reanimation. *Pediatr Clin North Am* 2001;48(3):627.

Salomez F, Vincent JL. Drowning: a review of epidemiology, pathophysiology, treatment and prevention. *Resuscitation* 2004;63(3):261.

Venema AM, Groothoff JW, Bierens JJ. The role of bystanders during rescue and resuscitation of drowning victims. *Resuscitation* 2010;81(4):434.

3: ANSWER: B

Patients who suffer a drowning event or significant aspiration should be evaluated in a hospital setting. Presentations can vary widely, from patients with no symptoms to those with severe hypoxia and cardiovascular collapse. Most symptoms will develop within 7 hours of the incident, and symptomless patients should be observed in a monitored setting during this period. Basic workup should include a chest radiograph, ECG, electrolytes, complete blood count, and coagulation parameters. If the event was preceded by a dive into shallow water, a trauma evaluation is performed. The degree of hypoxemia should be assessed and supplemental oxygen administered. Bronchospasm is relatively common and should be treated with a beta-agonist. The need for intubation and mechanical ventilation should follow standard indications, and a lung-protective ventilation strategy should be employed. There is no quality evidence for exogenous surfactant administration, and if refractory hypoxia develops, ECMO can be considered. There is also no evidence for the use of glucocorticoids or prophylactic antibiotics unless the water is grossly contaminated. If clinical infection develops, then water-borne pathogens such *as Aeromonas, Proteus,* and *Pseudomonas* species should be considered.

In the past, an emphasis was placed on the physiologic differences between freshwater and salt-water drowning. The hypertonicity of salt water was thought to create an osmotic gradient, drawing plasma into the pulmonary interstitium and alveoli and causing massive pulmonary edema and serum hypertonicity. Aspiration of freshwater was thought to have the opposite effect, resulting in fluid shifts into the intravascular compartment, causing massive fluid overload. Further investigation revealed that drowning survivors do not aspirate large enough volumes to cause these changes; therefore, the distinction between salt water and freshwater is no longer considered clinically relevant.

Keywords: Specialized areas; Drowning, fatal, near-drowning, freshwater

REFERENCES

Lavonas EJ, Drennan IR, Gabrielli A et al. Part 10. Special circumstances of resuscitation: 2015 American Heart Association Guidelines for cardiopulmonary resuscitation and emergency cardiovascular care. *Circulation*. 2015;132(18 Suppl 2):S501–S518.

Orlowski JP, Szpilman D. Drowning: rescue, resuscitation, and reanimation. *Pediatr Clin North Am* 2001;48(3):627.

Quan L, Bierens JJ, Lis R et al. Predicting outcome of drowning at the scene: A systematic review and meta-analyses. *Resuscitation* 2016;104:63–75.

Salomez F, Vincent JL. Drowning: a review of epidemiology, pathophysiology, treatment and prevention. *Resuscitation* 2004;63(3):261.

Venema AM, Groothoff JW, Bierens JJ et al. The role of bystanders during rescue and resuscitation of drowning victims. *Resuscitation* 2010;81(4):434.

4. ANSWER: A

This patient presents with signs and symptoms of tricyclic antidepressant (TCA) overdose. An ECG should be obtained, and the finding of a prolonged QRS longer than 100 milliseconds prompts treatment with IV sodium bicarbonate.

Overdose has become the leading cause of injury-related death in the United States. This brief review will focus on the initial evaluation and management of the critically ill patient with an unknown overdose. Frequently, the critically ill overdose patient presents without the ability or willingness to provide a reliable history, and the offending agent is unknown to the medical team. For this reason, an organized and targeted approach is required for optimal care. Advanced cardiac life support (ACLS) protocols intended for cardiac patients may be suboptimal or even harmful, leading to missed opportunities for specific life-saving interventions.

Readily available information from first responders, family, and medical records should be sought to help determine the offending agent. A rapid "toxidrome-oriented" physical exam should be performed, focusing on characteristic findings associated with specific substances. This includes vital signs, mental status, pupillary status, mucous membranes, temperature, bowel sounds, and motor tone. Basic laboratory testing should include blood glucose, complete blood count, renal panel, lactate, ABG analysis including carboxyhemoglobin and methemoglobin levels, serum acetaminophen and salicylate levels, ECG, and urine drug screen.

As with all critically ill patients, initial management focuses on airway, breathing, and circulation. Many toxins interfere with oxygenation and ventilation, and high-flow oxygen should be administered to all critically ill overdose patients. Patients who cannot protect their airway should be intubated. If the clinical presentation is suggestive of an opioid overdose, reversal with the administration of naloxone can be attempted before intubation. Administration of flumazenil should be avoided in all cases because of fear of withdrawal seizures. Poisoning with aspirin leads to initial tachypnea owing to direct effects on the respiratory center of the brain. Intubation should be avoided if possible because hyperventilation is beneficial and high minute ventilation may be difficult to maintain with mechanical ventilation and sedation. Toxin-mediated development of profound metabolic acidosis will lead to a compensatory respiratory alkalosis with very high minute ventilation. Despite a $PaCO_2$ near 10 mm Hg, these patients can remain significantly acidotic. If minute ventilation slows because of sedation, seizures, or fatigue, arterial pH will fall abruptly, leading to rapid decompensation. IV sodium bicarbonate should be administered immediately before intubation, and strategies to maximize minute ventilation should be used. If a dialyzable toxin is suspected (e.g., aspirin, methanol, ethylene glycol), hemodialysis should be initiated as soon as possible. Hypotension should initially be treated with rapid infusion of 2 L of crystalloid. Persistent hypotension is treated with a vasopressor infusion such as norepinephrine or phenylephrine. Selected antidotes can be administered empirically to hypotensive patients if a specific etiology is suspected. Asystole and ventricular fibrillation is managed according to ACLS protocols. Hypotension with bradycardia suggests overdose with digoxin, calcium channel blocker, or beta-blocker, and specific therapy for each agent is available. Monomorphic wide-complex tachycardia is associated with TCAs, antihistamines, cocaine, and type IA antiarrhythmics. Treatment with sodium bicarbonate boluses should be administered until the QRS is less than 100 milliseconds or arterial pH reaches 7.55. Polymorphic ventricular tachycardia (torsades de pointes) is treated with magnesium sulfate.

After the ABCs have been assessed and treated accordingly, the patient should be fully exposed and examined. Any external contaminants, including transdermal medication patches, should be removed, and alterations in temperature should be aggressively treated. Strategies aimed at elimination of poisons such as gastric lavage, activated charcoal, bowel irrigation, and hemodialysis may be helpful in select patients. Consultation with poison control centers or a toxicologist may be helpful if the clinical picture is unclear.

Keywords: Specialized areas; Poisonings; Toxic ingestion; Overdoses

REFERENCES

Albertson TE, Dawson A, de Latorre F et al. TOX-ACLS: toxicological-oriented advanced cardiac life support. *Ann Emerg Med* 2001;37(Suppl 4):S78.

Erickson TB, Thompson TM, Lu JJ. The approach to the patient with an unknown overdose. *Emerg Med Clin North Am* 2007;25(2):249–281.

5: ANSWER: D

This patient has class III or IV hemorrhagic shock as evidenced by increased HR, decreased BP, increased RR, and decreased GCS. Based on his transient response to a 1-L crystalloid infusion before arrival, he has moderate and ongoing blood loss (15–40%). Although he has a moderate to high risk for requiring blood transfusion, aggressive fluid resuscitation before hemorrhage source control may exacerbate additional bleeding. Furthermore, crystalloid infusions and even balanced blood product transfusions can cause dilutional coagulopathy.

The strategy of limiting fluid and blood product resuscitation, resulting in a lower than normal BP, until hemorrhage control can be achieved in a traumatically injured patient is known by several names, including hypotensive resuscitation, permissive resuscitation, permissive hypotension, and controlled resuscitation. There have been several randomized trials comparing restricted to aggressive fluid administration in traumatically injured patients. There was significant heterogeneity between trials in terms of patient populations, fluid resuscitation protocols, setting (i.e., prehospital or hospital), and outcomes measured. Therefore, definitive conclusions regarding a mortality benefit of permissive hypotension cannot be made. Nonetheless, advanced trauma life support (ATLS), 10th edition, no longer recommends a second liter of crystalloid, and ATLS acknowledges that delaying aggressive fluid resuscitation until definitive hemorrhage control in penetrating trauma may prevent additional bleeding. The European guideline on management of major bleeding and coagulopathy following trauma recommends a target systolic BP of 80 to 90 mm Hg until definitive hemorrhage control in patients without a traumatic brain injury (TBI).

The combination of permissive hypotension, hemostatic resuscitation (or early empiric use of blood and clotting products), and damage-control surgery is known as damage-control resuscitation. Balanced or hemostatic resuscitation refers to the transfusion of blood components in a balanced ratio so as to minimize coagulopathy. Damage control surgery refers to limiting of operative procedures to life-saving interventions and source control—both hemorrhage control to stop bleeding (i.e., packing of solid organ injuries, ligation of vessels) and temporary control of hollow viscus injuries to minimize contamination (i.e., resection of perforated small bowel without anastomosis). Temporary abdominal closure is performed, and the patient is taken to the ICU for correction of the lethal triad of hypothermia, coagulopathy, and metabolic acidosis.

Although the European guidelines recommend vasopressors to support a target BP in hemorrhagic shock, there are insufficient data to recommend the use of vasopressors in early trauma resuscitation. Furthermore, in this clinical scenario, the patient is maintaining an adequate, although lower than normal, BP and is en route to receiving definitive hemorrhage control.

Keywords: Specialized areas; Life support and resuscitation, ATLS

6. ANSWER: D

Massive transfusion is defined by ATLS as greater than 10 units of packed red blood cells within the first 24 hours or more than 4 units within an hour after injury. Hemostatic resuscitation or early empiric use of blood and clotting products is one component of damage-control resuscitation of traumatically injured patients requiring massive transfusion. Balanced or hemostatic resuscitation refers to the transfusion of blood components in a balanced ratio so as to minimize coagulopathy. The Pragmatic Randomized Optimal Platelet and Plasma Ratios (PROPPR) trial compared two different ratios (1:1:1 vs. 1:1:2) for transfusion of plasma, platelets, and red blood cells in traumatically injured patients who were predicted to require massive transfusion. The results of the trial demonstrated no difference in mortality; however, patients receiving blood products in a 1:1:1 ratio were more likely to achieve hemostasis and less likely to die from exsanguination within 24 hours. Thus, this patient who is receiving massive transfusion should undergo 1:1:1 transfusion of blood components without consideration initially for coagulation studies.

In patients who are not receiving massive transfusion or after this patient is no longer requiring massive transfusion, use of platelets should be guided by coagulation studies. A Cochrane Review comparing conventional coagulation studies (i.e., prothrombin time, partial thromboplastin time, and platelet count) to thromboelastography (TEG) or rotational thromboelastometry (ROTEM) did not make any recommendations based on a small number of studies and concerns about risk for bias. However, a single-center randomized trial of conventional coagulation studies versus TEG in traumatically injured patients found that TEG-based resuscitation resulted in improved survival and fewer platelet and plasma transfusions. The triggers for transfusion were platelets less than $100,000/\mu L$ in the conventional group and activated clotting time 140 seconds or longer in the TEG group. Bleeding time is not routinely used in resuscitation of traumatically injured patients with hemorrhagic shock.

Keywords: Specialized areas; Life support and resuscitation; Other (trauma-induced coagulopathy)

REFERENCES

American College of Surgeons. *Advanced trauma life support: student course manual*, 10th edition. Chicago: American College of Surgeons; 2018.

Carrick MM, Leonard J, Slone DS et al. Hypotensive resuscitation among trauma patients. *Biomed Res Int* 2016;2016:8901938 [Epub 2016 Aug 9].

Harris T, Davenport R, Mak M, Brohi K. The evolving science of trauma resuscitation. *Emerg Med Clin North Am* 2018;36(1);85–106.

Rossaint R, Bouillon B, Cerny V et al. The European guideline on management of major bleeding and coagulopathy following trauma: fourth edition. *Crit Care* 2016;20:100.

REFERENCES

American College of Surgeons. *Advanced trauma life support: student course manual*, 10th edition. Chicago: American College of Surgeons; 2018.

Gonzalez E, Moore EE, Moore HB et al. Goal-directed hemostatic resuscitation of trauma-induced coagulopathy: a pragmatic randomized clinical trial comparing a viscoelastic assay to conventional coagulation assays. *Ann Surg* 2016;263(6):1051–1059.

Harris T, Davenport R, Mak M, Brohi K. The evolving science of trauma resuscitation. *Emerg Med Clin North Am* 2018;36(1);85–106.

Holcomb JB, Tilley BC, Baraniuk S et al. Transfusion of plasma, platelets, and red blood cells in a 1:1:1 vs a 1:1:2 ratio and mortality in patients with severe trauma: the PROPPR randomized clinical trial. *JAMA* 2015;313(5):471–482.

Hunt H, Stanworth S, Curry N et al. Thromboelastography (TEG) and rotational thromboelastometry (ROTEM) for trauma induced coagulopathy in adult trauma patients with bleeding. *Cochrane Database Syst Rev* 2015;(2):CD010438.

Ismailov RM, Ness RB, Redmond CK et al. Trauma associated with cardiac dysrhythmias: results from a large matched case-control study. *J Trauma* 2007;62(5):1186.

Nagy KK, Krosner SM, Roberts RR et al. Determining which patients require evaluation for blunt cardiac injury following blunt chest trauma. *World J Surg* 2001;25(1):108.

Velmahos GC, Karaiskakis M, Salim A et al. Normal electrocardiography and serum troponin I levels preclude the presence of clinically significant blunt cardiac injury. *J Trauma* 2003;54(1):45.

7. ANSWER: C

Blunt cardiac injury (BCI) is the term used to describe a wide variety of traumatic myocardial abnormalities ranging from asymptomatic self-limited arrhythmias to rapidly fatal cardiac wall rupture. The most common form of BCI is known as "cardiac contusion" and represents a nonspecific myocardial injury. Diagnosis is difficult because of the lack of a clear definition of the condition or a gold standard diagnostic modality. Complications related to BCI include arrhythmia, cardiac wall motion abnormality, decreased contractility with potential progression to cardiogenic shock, and valvular, septal, or atrioventricular wall rupture. Although no specific injury patterns, such as sternal fracture, have been reliably associated with diagnosis of BCI, it is recommended that patients with significant blunt trauma to the anterior chest be screened for the condition. This is especially important in patients who present without other indications for continuous cardiac monitoring before admission to a nonmonitored unit or discharge home. An admission ECG and troponin I should be obtained in patients in whom BCI is suspected. If the ECG and troponin I level are normal, then BCI is ruled out. If the initial ECG reveals a new abnormality (e.g., arrhythmia, ST changes, ischemia, heart block), the patient should be admitted for continuous cardiac monitoring. If the initial troponin I level is elevated, admission to a monitored unit with serial troponin levels is indicated. Patients with hemodynamic instability (after other traumatic causes of hypotension have been ruled out) or persistent new arrhythmia should have an echocardiogram performed. Clinical or echocardiographic evidence of severe cardiac injury (tamponade; ruptured valve, septum, or ventricular wall) require emergent surgical consultation and intervention. Acute coronary syndrome is rare in this setting, and cardiology and cardiovascular surgery consultation should be obtained. Systemic thrombolysis is generally avoided because of bleeding risk. Cardiac arrhythmias are generally treated according to standard ACLS guidelines.

Keywords: Basic pathophysiology; Cardiovascular; Trauma; Other (e.g., cardiac contusion)

REFERENCES

Clancy K, Velopulos C, Bilaniuk JW et al. Screening for blunt cardiac injury: an Eastern Association for the Surgery of Trauma practice management guideline. *J Trauma Acute Care Surg* 2012;73(5 Suppl 4):S301–S306.

8. ANSWER: D

The patient has primary-blast lung injury from a high-order explosive; these contain the fuel and oxidizer within the same chemical compound. When these high-order explosives detonate, they generate a high-pressure blast wave. There are four mechanisms of blast injury: primary, secondary, tertiary, and quaternary (Table 5.2). Gas-filled structures such as the lungs are particularly susceptible to primary-blast injury, which results from the shock front of the blast wave.

Symptoms from primary-blast lung injury usually occur within 90 minutes and can include dyspnea, cough, chest pain, hemoptysis, and hypoxia. Imaging usually reveals a classic "butterfly" or "bat-wing" pattern of perihilar infiltrates. Additional injuries from secondary and tertiary blast injury may also be present, such as pulmonary contusions. Chest tubes are indicated in the presence of pneumothoraces or hemothoraces and can be considered prophylactically before transport. Judicious fluid administration and respiratory support are the mainstays of therapy. In patients who require mechanical ventilation,

Table 5.2 **CATEGORIES OF BLAST INJURY**

CATEGORY	BODY PARTS AFFECTED	CHARACTERISTIC TYPE OF INJURY
Primary	Gas-filled structures such as lungs, gastrointestinal tract, and middle ear	Results from exposure to an explosive shock wave
Secondary	Any body part	Results from injury from flying debris and bomb fragments
Tertiary	Any body part	Results from being displaced bodily by the blast wind
Quaternary	Any body part	All other explosion-related sequelae not related to the other mechanisms (i.e., burn injury and inhalation of toxic substances); includes exacerbation of existing conditions

a lung-protective ventilation strategy should be used. High PEEP should be used cautiously because there is a risk for air embolism; patients may have alveolar-arterial fistulas as a result of the blast injury. Air embolism may manifest as sudden death, as in this scenario. Adjunctive treatments such as alternative forms of ventilation, inhaled nitric oxide, and ECMO have been reported, but data are limited.

Other pulmonary complications can occur after primary-blast lung injury, including tension pneumothorax, pulmonary contusions, ARDS, and pulmonary hemorrhage. Quaternary blast injury can result in exacerbation of underlying pulmonary disorders such as asthma and chronic obstructive pulmonary disease.

Keywords: Basic pathophysiology; Pulmonary; Blast injury

REFERENCES

American College of Surgeons. Disaster management and emergency preparedness course, 2nd edition. Chicago: American College of Surgeons; 2018.

Scott TE, Kirkman E, Haque M et al. Primary blast lung injury—a review. *Br J Anaesth* 2017;118(3):311–316.

Yeh DD, Schecter WP. Primary blast injuries—an updated concise review. *World J Surg* 2012;36(5):966–972.

9. ANSWER: B

This patient presents with a significant chest wall injury and associated pulmonary contusions. Pain associated with thoracic wall injury contributes significantly to hypoventilation and should be treated aggressively. Of the available options, adequate analgesia represents the best option to optimize ventilation and avoid intubation.

Significant blunt injury to the chest frequently results in bony thoracic injury and pulmonary contusion. Respiratory compromise due to alveolar hemorrhage and pulmonary parenchymal disruption usually presents within hours of the initial injury. Symptoms secondary to hypoxemia and hypercarbia peak around 72 hours after injury and usually resolve within 7 days. The diagnosis should be considered in patients following rapid deceleration injuries, such as those associated with high-level falls and vehicular collisions. It can also occur following blast injuries due to the shock wave produced by explosions.

There are three basic mechanisms that account for these injuries. The spalling effect involves the shearing force that occurs at the interface between a gas and a liquid. When air-containing organs such as the lungs are exposed to this force, there is disruption of the alveolus at the point of initial contact with the shock wave. The inertial effect occurs when the low-density alveolar tissue is stripped from

heavier hilar and bronchial tissues owing to different rates of acceleration in response to the insult. The implosion effect results from rebound or overexpansion of gas bubbles as pressure waves pass. In addition to these mechanisms, pulmonary parenchymal trauma may result from direct injury from deformity of the adjacent chest wall.

The diagnosis of parenchymal lung injury is usually confirmed with a CT scan of the chest. Frequently, contusions identified on CT will not be apparent on initial chest radiograph. CT is both highly sensitive for diagnosis and highly predictive of the need for subsequent mechanical ventilation. Clinically relevant pulmonary contusions are associated with increased mucus production, decreased mucus clearance from the airways, decreased surfactant production, ventilation-perfusion mismatch, increased intrapulmonary shunt, and loss of lung compliance. These patients are at increased risk for complications such as pneumonia, ARDS, and long-term pulmonary disability. Management is primarily supportive and should focus on judicious fluid administration, pain control of associated bony thoracic injuries to optimize pulmonary toilet, and close monitoring for respiratory decline. Intubation is indicated for respiratory failure, and select patients may benefit from noninvasive positive pressure ventilation. Patients with significantly displaced rib fractures or flail chest may benefit from early surgical fracture stabilization to restore chest wall mechanics. Although these patients are at increased risk for the development of pneumonia, the use of empiric antibiotics or glucocorticoids have shown no benefit. Severe hypoxia and ARDS should be treated according to standard guidelines utilizing a lung-protective ventilation strategy, alveolar recruitment, permissive hypercapnia, and prone positioning. If refractory hypoxemia persists, consideration can be made for ECMO.

Keywords: Basic pathophysiology; Pulmonary; Chest trauma (e.g., pulmonary contusion, flail chest)

REFERENCES

Battle CE, Evans PA. Predictors of mortality in patient with flail chest: a systematic review. *Emerg Med J* 2015;32:961–965.

Bulger EM, Edwards T, Klotz P, Jurkovich GJ. Epidural analgesia improves outcome after multiple rib fractures. *Surgery* 2004;136:426–430.

Cohn SM, Dubose, JJ. Pulmonary contusion: an update on recent advances in clinical management. *World J Surg* 2010;34:1959–1970.

Deunk J, Poels T, Brink M et al. The clinical outcome of occult pulmonary contusion on multidetector-row computed tomography in blunt trauma patients. *J Trauma* 2010;68:387–394.

Ganie FA, Lone H, Lone GN et al. Lung contusion: a clinic-pathological entity with unpredictable clinical course. *Bull Emerg Trauma* 2013;1(1):7–16.

Voggenreiter G, Neudeck F, Aufmkolk M et al. Operative chest wall stabilization in flail chest—outcomes of patient with or without pulmonary contusion. *J Am Coll Surg* 1998;187:130–138.

10. ANSWER: D

The patient presents with hemorrhagic shock in the setting of penetrating trauma. Initial resuscitation with blood products in a balanced ratio by a massive transfusion protocol is ideal. This patient is a nonresponder to initial resuscitation indicating ongoing bleeding and should be taken immediately to the operating room for definitive hemorrhage control by laparotomy.

A CT scan in penetrating trauma can be considered for stable patients or those with a favorable response to initial resuscitation. CT scans should include IV contrast administration and delayed-phase imaging to evaluate for arterial contrast extravasation and genitourinary collecting system injuries. Nonoperative management of penetrating renal trauma is an accepted treatment modality in stable patients without other indications for surgical exploration. Angiography and embolization by interventional radiology is an option for stable patients with arterial contrast extravasation on CT or ongoing transfusion requirements.

In this question stem, gross hematuria after placing a urinary catheter indicates the source of bleeding may include the genitourinary tract. The abdominal portion of the FAST exam is used to identify intraperitoneal free fluid. In an unstable trauma patient, free peritoneal fluid is assumed to represent blood and an abdominal source of bleeding. Patients with isolated injury to retroperitoneal structures (e.g., the kidneys, inferior vena cava, aorta, pancreas) will usually have a negative FAST exam because bleeding is confined to the retroperitoneum. Further transfusion and repeating the FAST exam represent a delay to definitive hemorrhage control, which is associated with increased mortality.

Keywords: Critical illness diagnosis and management; Renal; Diagnoses; Renal trauma

REFERENCES

Barbosa RR, Rowell SE, Fox EE et al. Increasing time to operation is associated with decreased survival in patients with a positive FAST exam requiring emergent laparotomy. *J Trauma Acute Care Surg* 2013;75(101):S48–S52.

Demetriades D, Hadjuzacharia P, Constantinou C et al. Selective nonoperative management of penetrating abdominal solid organ injuries. *Ann Surg* 2006;244(4):620–628.

Holevar M, Ebert J et al. Practice management guidelines for the management of genitourinary trauma. 2004.

11. ANSWER: D

This patient presents with multiple pelvic fractures and inability to void. RUG should be performed to evaluate for urethral injury before urinary catheter placement.

Blunt traumatic urethral injuries are more common in males and most associated with pelvic fractures, especially displaced anterior arch fractures. Clinical signs of urethral injury include blood at the urethral meatus, gross hematuria, urinary retention, inability to pass a urinary catheter, perineal hematoma, and displacement of the prostate on rectal exam. Successful passage of a urinary catheter does not exclude urethral injury, and attempts at blind placement should be avoided because this may worsen the injury. Because clinical findings are not reliably present, a high index of suspicion is required to make the diagnosis, and a urethral injury should be suspected when a pubic arch fracture exists.

RUG is the gold standard for diagnosis of urethral injuries and characterizes the injury location (anterior or posterior) and extent of the injury (partial or complete). If an injury is confirmed on RUG, a cystogram should then be performed because 10 to 20% of posterior urethral injuries will have a concomitant bladder injury. Urologic consultation should be obtained, with the primary objective being establishment of prompt and reliable bladder drainage to prevent complications associated with urinary extravasation and facilitate stabilization of associated injuries.

Keywords: Critical illness diagnosis and management; Renal; Diagnoses; Urethral injury

REFERENCES

Figler B, Hoffler CE, Reisman W et al. Multi-disciplinary update on pelvic fracture associated bladder and urethral injuries. *Injury* 2012;43:1242–1249.

Holevar M, DiGiacomo JC et al. Practice management guidelines for the evaluation of genitourinary trauma: Eastern Association for the Surgery of Trauma. 2003.

Holevar M, Ebert J et al. Practice management guidelines for the management of genitourinary trauma: Eastern Association for the Surgery of Trauma. 2004.

12. ANSWER: A

This patient presents in hemorrhagic shock after blunt trauma with severe TBI and a high-grade liver laceration with active bleeding. She had an adequate response to initial resuscitation and remains hemodynamically stable but has findings consistent with ongoing bleeding (decreasing hemoglobin and mild hypotension). Hemorrhage control is essential in the injured patient with severe TBI to prevent ongoing hypotension and maintain adequate cerebral perfusion. Resuscitation with blood products should continue, and hemorrhage control by angioembolization should be attempted. Hemodynamic instability or failure of embolization would require laparotomy.

The initial management of blunt hepatic injuries is guided by the hemodynamic status of the patient. Hemodynamically unstable patients with evidence of intraperitoneal bleeding (positive FAST exam or DPL) or peritonitis on clinical exam should undergo immediate laparotomy and definitive hemorrhage control without delay. Initial nonoperative management of hemodynamically stable patients is standard of care at most US trauma centers, regardless of injury grade. Nonoperative management has a reported success rate of 82 to 100% and consists of close observation in an ICU setting, serial abdominal exams, serial hemoglobin and hematocrit measurements, and a period of limited activity. Most failures of nonoperative management (75%) are due to hemodynamic instability.

Angioembolization is an important adjunct in the treatment of blunt hepatic injuries with reported efficacy as high as 83%. CT findings that can help identify which patients may benefit from angioembolization include injury grade (American Association for the Surgery of Trauma grade III or higher), evidence of arterial injury (contrast extravasation), and evidence of hepatic venous injury. Hemodynamically stable patients with free intraperitoneal contrast extravasation should be considered for immediate angiography if readily available. Close observation with planned angiographic intervention for ongoing bleeding (e.g., transfusion requirement, drop in hemoglobin or hematocrit) is also acceptable.

The goals of management for TBI involve limiting secondary injury by maintaining adequate oxygenation and perfusion. The Brain Trauma Foundation recommends placement of an ICP monitor in all salvageable patients with a severe TBI (GCS 3–8 after resuscitation) and an abnormal CT scan (hematomas, contusions, swelling, herniation, or compressed basal cisterns). Treatment should be initiated with ICP thresholds greater than 22 mm Hg. Cerebral perfusion pressure (CPP) is defined as the MAP minus the ICP. A CPP of 50 to 70 mm Hg should be targeted. Aggressive attempts to maintain CPP above 70 mm Hg with fluids and vasopressors should be avoided because of an increased risk for ARDS. The patient in the question stem has a CPP of 47 mm Hg and an ICP of 16 mm Hg. The low CPP is due to hypotension secondary to ongoing bleeding and should be treated with prompt hemorrhage control and resuscitation with blood products. The neurological exam is unchanged, and ICP is within an acceptable range. While repeat head CT is likely necessary to monitor her injury, bleeding control is the most critical next step.

Keywords: Critical illness diagnosis and management; Gastrointestinal; Diagnoses; Hepatic trauma

REFERENCES

Bratton SL, Chestnut RM, Ghajar J et al. VI. Indications for intracranial pressure monitoring. *J Neurotrauma* 2007;24(1):S37–S44.

Bratton SL, Chestnut RM, Ghajar J et al. VIII. Intracranial pressure thresholds. *J Neurotrauma* 2007;24(1):S55–S58.

Bratton SL, Chestnut RM, Ghajar J et al. IX. Cerebral perfusion thresholds. *J Neurotrauma* 2007;24(1):S59–S64.

Carney N, Totten AM, O'Reilly C et al. Guidelines for the management of severe traumatic brain injury, 4th edition. *Neurosurgery* 2017;80(1):6–15.

Stassen NA, Bhullar I, Cheng JD et al. Nonoperative management of blunt hepatic injury: an Eastern Association for the Surgery of Trauma practice management guideline. *J Trauma Acute Care Surg* 2012;735(4):S288–S293.

13. ANSWER: B

This patient presents in shock. A diagnostic pericardial window is indicated to evaluate for cardiac injury because pericardial FAST exam is unreliable in the setting of penetrating chest trauma with hemothorax (see later). CT scan is unnecessary and contraindicated because of hemodynamic instability. If possible, intubation should be delayed until the patient is in the operating room because paralytics and sedation will decrease sympathetic tone, causing worsening hypotension and potential cardiovascular collapse. Thoracotomy is not currently indicated owing to the low volume of initial chest tube output and evidence of ongoing intra-abdominal hemorrhage (general indications for immediate thoracotomy include initial chest tube output >1500 mL or >200 mL/hour × 4 hours).

FAST is a key component in the diagnosis and treatment of trauma patients, particularly those who are hemodynamically unstable. It is an accepted standard in the ATLS protocol and a tool that all physicians caring for injured patients should be comfortable rapidly performing and interpreting. The goal of FAST is to identify free fluid (presumed to be blood in the setting of trauma in three distinct body cavities: intraperitoneal, pleural, and pericardial). The exam is performed by obtaining ultrasound images of the pericardium, right upper quadrant, left upper quadrant, and pelvis. A positive result is the appearance of a dark "anechoic" stripe around the heart or in the dependent portions of the peritoneal cavity. In a supine patient, blood will tend to collect in the dependent portions of the abdomen, between the liver and kidney (Morison's pouch), around the spleen, and posterior to the bladder. The extended FAST (eFAST) incorporates views of the anterior chest wall to assess for the presence of pneumothorax (identified by the absence of normal "lung slide"). Although multiple studies have demonstrated FAST to be beneficial in the detection of free fluid in hemodynamically unstable trauma patients, it is important to note that FAST exam has several limitations. The exam is operator dependent and can be difficult in patients who are obese, in those with extensive subcutaneous emphysema, and in the presence of severe pelvic fractures. Bleeding confined to the retroperitoneum, hollow viscous injury, and solid-organ injuries without significant hemoperitoneum are not reliably diagnosed with FAST alone.

Following blunt trauma, a patient with *hemodynamic instability* not responding to initial resuscitation with a positive abdominal FAST has a clear indication for laparotomy, and further workup beyond chest and pelvic radiographs is generally not necessary. Alternatively, an unstable patient with a negative FAST may still have intra-abdominal injury, and further workup or surgical exploration may be indicated. FAST exam in stable patients with abdominal trauma can be used as a screening tool but is not sufficient to exclude injury, and further evaluation with abdominal CT should be obtained if there is clinical suspicion.

In the setting of penetrating trauma with hemodynamic instability, FAST exam has limited utility when the injury is clearly confined to a single body cavity (such as an isolated anterior abdominal stab wound) because operative exploration is nearly always mandatory. However, FAST is a particularly useful triage tool when there is the possibility of bleeding in multiple cavities. Penetrating thoracoabdominal wounds frequently lead to a combination of cardiac, thoracic, and abdominal injuries, and the FAST exam can help the surgeon decide which body cavity to explore first. A positive pericardial FAST after penetrating trauma is a reliable predictor of cardiac injury, and exploration is mandatory. A false-negative pericardial FAST may be encountered when a cardiac injury is accompanied by a defect in the pericardium. Blood will decompress through the pericardial defect into the pleural cavity, causing hemothorax rather than hemopericardium. In this setting, pericardial exploration is indicated despite a negative FAST.

Keywords: Critical illness diagnosis and management; Gastrointestinal; Diagnoses; FAST

REFERENCES

Carter JW, Falco MH, Chopko MS et al. Do we really rely on FAST for decision-making in the management of blunt abdominal trauma? *Injury* 2015;46:817–821.

Matsushima K, Khor D, Berona K et al. Double jeopardy in penetrating trauma: get FAST, get it right. *World J Surg* 2018;42(1):99–106.

Natarajan B, Gupta PK, Cemaj S et al. FAST scan: is it worth doing in hemodynamically stable blunt trauma patients? *Surgery* 2010;148(4);695–701.

Savatmongkorngul S, Wongwaisayawan S, Kaewlai R. Focused assessment with sonography for trauma: current perspectives. *Open Access Emerg Med* 2017;9:57–62.

14. ANSWER: C

This patient has an abdominal wall contusion or "seat belt sign" after motor vehicle collision. Management of these injuries can be challenging because they are often associated with intra-abdominal injuries such as intestinal perforation, mesenteric tear, and pancreatic injuries. Physical exam can be equivocal because patients have tenderness related to the abdominal wall contusion. Furthermore, this patient has a TBI with a decreased level of consciousness.

There are multiple tools for evaluating patients with blunt abdominal trauma. This patient already received a CT scan, which demonstrated findings that can be associated with an intestinal injury such as free fluid and a mesenteric contusion with associated bowel wall thickening. There are no widely validated scoring systems for determining the probability of an intestinal injury, although the Bowel Injury Prediction Score devised by McNutt et al. utilizes admission CT scan grade of mesenteric injury ≥4 (1 point), white blood cell count ≥17,000/mm^3 (1 point), and abdominal tenderness in the emergency room (1 point) to determine suspicion for a bowel injury (see Table 5.3 for CT scan scoring system). A score of 2 or higher was associated with a bowel injury. This patient would receive 1 point for a grade 4 mesenteric injury and 0 points for his white blood cell count; abdominal tenderness was not able to be elicited. Thus, the score is not as helpful in this instance.

A FAST exam would not be helpful in this patient because one of its disadvantages is that it can miss bowel and pancreatic injuries. Furthermore, it is already known that the patient has free fluid in his abdomen. In this scenario, the patient is hemodynamically stable, so the decision for laparotomy must be made by weighing the risks of an operation in the setting of a TBI and hypoxia and the benefits of diagnosing a possible bowel injury. DPL, although not performed frequently, may provide additional information to guide decision making. It can be performed at the bedside using an open or Seldinger technique. The abdominal

Table 5.3 COMPUTED TOMOGRAPHY GRADING SCALE FOR MESENTERIC INJURY

GRADE	DESCRIPTION
1	Isolated mesenteric contusion without associated bowel wall thickening or adjacent interloop fluid collection
2	Mesenteric hematoma <5 cm without associated bowel wall thickening or adjacent interloop fluid collection
3	Mesenteric hematoma >5 cm without associated bowel wall thickening or adjacent interloop fluid collection
4	Mesenteric contusion or hematoma (any size) with associated bowel wall thickening or adjacent interloop fluid collection
5	Active vascular or oral contrast extravasation, bowel transection, or pneumoperitoneum

Source: McNutt MK, Chinapuvvula NR, Beckmann NM et al. Early surgical intervention for blunt bowel injury: the Bowel Injury Prediction Score (BIPS). *J Trauma Acute Care Surg* 2015;78(1):105–111.

cavity is accessed through an infraumbilical approach, although a supraumbilical approach may be used if there is a pelvic fracture. Aspiration of gastrointestinal contents, vegetable fibers, or bile indicates the need for laparotomy. One liter of saline or lactated Ringer's solution is then infused, and the lavage is analyzed. A positive DPL suggesting bowel injury would include a white blood cell count higher than $500/mm^3$ or a positive Gram stain. A positive DPL for hemorrhage would include aspiration of 10 mL of gross blood on initial aspiration or more than $100,000/mm^3$ red blood cells in the lavage.

Keywords: Critical illness diagnosis and management; Gastrointestinal; Diagnoses; DPL

REFERENCES

American College of Surgeons. *Advanced trauma life support: student course manual*, 10th edition. Chicago: American College of Surgeons; 2018.

McNutt MK, Chinapuvvula NR, Beckmann NM et al. Early surgical intervention for blunt bowel injury: the Bowel Injury Prediction Score (BIPS). *J Trauma Acute Care Surg* 2015;78(1):105–111.

Whitehouse JS, Weigelt JA. Diagnostic peritoneal lavage: a review of indications, technique, and interpretation. *Scand J Trauma Resusc Emerg Med* 2009;17:13.

15. ANSWER: A

This patient presents with evidence of a tracheobronchial injury and should undergo bronchoscopy for definitive diagnosis. When the diagnosis is confirmed, this patient will need early operative intervention given the significant air leakage and inability to effectively ventilate.

Tracheobronchial injury is rare and usually associated with other life-threatening injuries. Although it is becoming more frequently encountered because of advances in prehospital trauma care, it is estimated that 80% of patients with blunt tracheobronchial injury die before hospital arrival. Of those who survive to hospital admission, the reported mortality has improved from 36% before 1950 to 9% since 1970. Prognosis is improved with early intervention; thus, a high index of suspicion and liberal use of diagnostic fiberoptic bronchoscopy are warranted if tracheobronchial injury is suspected.

Initial management is guided by ATLS principles. A rapid history and thorough physical exam should be performed, with interventions focused on immediate life-threatening injuries and hemorrhage control. Clinical and radiographic findings concerning for tracheobronchial injury include air leaking from a penetrating wound to the neck or chest, extensive subcutaneous emphysema, pneumomediastinum, air surrounding the mainstem bronchi, and persistent pneumothorax with air leak despite tube thoracostomy. Flexible fiberoptic bronchoscopy is the diagnostic gold standard and should be performed if an injury is suspected. It is important to note that endotracheal intubation in the presence of a proximal tracheobronchial injury can exacerbate the injury and convert an incomplete disruption into a complete transection with inability to ventilate distal to the injury. If possible, intubation should be performed in a controlled setting under bronchoscopic guidance. Findings during bronchoscopy include direct visualization of the injury, blood in the airways, obstruction of the bronchus, and inability to visualize the distal lobar bronchus. A majority of tracheobronchial injuries (76%) suffered as a result of blunt trauma are located within 2 cm of the carina, with the proximal right main bronchus being the most frequently injured (43%). Diagnosis of an incomplete bronchial disruption can be difficult if intact peribronchial tissue allows for ventilation past the area of injury. If this is the case, symptoms related to massive air leakage may be absent. Late presentations are usually related to complications secondary to bronchial stenosis or obstruction (i.e., recurrent pneumothoraces, postobstructive pneumonia, bronchiectasis) because granulation tissue forms at the site of injury over the course of several weeks.

Selective single-lung ventilation is not necessary for the management of this patient. A double-lumen endotracheal tube should be avoided because it may exacerbate an injury because of its rigidity. However, if a bronchial injury is identified, selective single-lung ventilation with a bronchial blocker or a carefully placed double-lumen tube in the operating room may be reasonable. There is no indication for ECMO in this patient.

Accurate anatomic localization of the injury is essential to surgical planning because the operative approach differs based on injury location. Cervical tracheal injuries are usually approached through a collar incision. Distal trachea, carina, and right main bronchial injuries are best approached through a right posterolateral thoracotomy, while the left main bronchus is exposed through a left posterolateral thoracotomy. Debridement of devitalized tissue and end-to-end anastomosis are the preferred method of repair. Lobectomy or pneumonectomy may be required if the injury is associated with lobar destruction or irreparable damage to the major pulmonary vasculature.

Keywords: Critical illness diagnosis and management; Pulmonary; Diagnoses; Tracheal/bronchial injury

REFERENCES

Cassada DC, Munyikwa MP, Moniz MP et al. Acute injuries of the trachea and major bronchi: importance of early diagnosis. *Ann Thoracic Surg* 2000;69:1563–1567.

Cheaito A, Tillou A, Lewis C, Cryer H. Traumatic bronchial injury. *Int J Surg Case Rep* 2016;27:172–175.

Kiser AC, O'Brien SM, Detterbeck FC. Blunt tracheobronchial injuries: treatment and outcomes. *Ann Thoracic Surg* 2001;71:2059–2065.

Keywords: Critical illness diagnosis and management; Orthopedic; Diagnoses; Orthopedic trauma

16. ANSWER: D

This patient presents with compartment syndrome (CS), which is a surgical emergency; definitive therapy is a four-compartment fasciotomy. While direct measurement of compartment pressures can assist in diagnosis, it should not delay surgical intervention when the clinical suspicion is high.

Muscles and neurovascular structures in the extremities are separated into compartments by fascia, creating defined anatomical spaces with low compliance. Acute extremity CS occurs when elevated compartment pressure causes a decrease in perfusion pressure, leading to tissue hypoxia. CS is frequently associated with trauma and is reported to occur in 1 to 10% of tibial fractures. All patients with limb injuries should be assessed for CS. Patients identified as particularly high risk for development of CS include males younger than 35 years and patients with tibia or radius/ulna fractures, high-energy injuries (open fractures, severe soft tissue injury), crush injuries, prolonged limb compression, and coagulopathy.

Recommendations to prevent development of CS in high-risk patients include removing circumferential bandages and splints, maintaining limb position at heart level, and avoiding systemic hypotension and hypoxia.

Diagnosis in an awake patient is primarily made on clinical grounds and requires a high index of suspicion. Clinical signs include swelling or tenseness of the compartment, pain out of proportion to the injury, pain with passive stretch of muscles within the compartment, paresthesia of skin supplied by a nerve traversing the compartment, paresis of muscles supplied by nerves traversing the compartment, and pallor of skin overlying the compartment. Pulses are preserved until late in CS, and their presence does not exclude the diagnosis.

Diagnosis in an unconscious patient is challenging as clinical signs are difficult to obtain. Direct measurement of compartment pressure is recommended in high-risk patients if they are unconscious or have equivocal clinical signs. An absolute compartmental pressure of greater than 30 mm Hg or a perfusion pressure of less than 30 mm Hg (diastolic BP minus compartment pressure) is generally considered diagnostic for acute extremity CS.

The only treatment for CS is surgical fasciotomy, which should be performed as soon as possible after diagnosis. Delay in diagnosis or intervention can lead to severe morbidity, including rhabdomyolysis, extremity neurological deficit, ischemic contractures, and limb amputation.

REFERENCES

Park SD, Ahn J, Gee AO et al. Compartment syndrome in tibial fractures. *J Orthop Trauma* 2009;23(7):514–518.

von Keudell AG, Weaver MJ, Appleton PT et al. Diagnosis and treatment of acute extremity compartment syndrome. *Lancet* 2015;386:1299–1310.

Wall CJ, Lynch J, Harris IA et al. Clinical practice guidelines for the management of acute limb compartment syndrome following trauma. *Aust N Z J Surg* 2010;80:151–156.

17. ANSWER: B

The most appropriate first step in management of a hemodynamically unstable patient with a pelvic ring injury is application of a noninvasive pelvic circumferential compression device (PCCD), such as a pelvic binder and blood product resuscitation. Patients presenting with pelvic fractures associated with hemodynamic instability have a reported mortality rate of up to 40%, and the majority will have concomitant extrapelvic injuries. Prompt hemorrhage control is paramount and requires a multidisciplinary approach with anesthesiologists, trauma surgeons, orthopedic surgeons, and interventional radiologists in a facility designated to care for trauma patients.

Initial evaluation of the unstable patient with pelvic fractures is performed according to ATLS guidelines. Chest radiograph, FAST exam, and anteroposterior pelvic radiograph are the initial imaging modalities used to screen for nonextremity sources of hemorrhage. When a pelvic ring injury is present, a PCCD should be applied to stabilize the pelvis. Pelvic compression is accomplished by circumferentially wrapping the pelvis at the level of the greater trochanters with a commercially available device or even a simple bedsheet secured with clamps. Fracture stabilization allows clot formation and decreases the pelvic volume in certain fracture patterns (e.g., "open-book fracture") to allow tamponade of venous and bony bleeding. A repeat radiograph should be obtained after PCCD placement to ensure adequate reduction (Figure 5.1). Resuscitation is accomplished with a balanced ratio of blood products while avoiding crystalloid fluids. Lower extremity and femoral IV access should be avoided because of potential for pelvic venous injuries. The most common source of pelvic bleeding is the posterior venous plexus, and a majority of patients will stabilize with compression and resuscitation. The PCCD should be left in place until the patient is hemodynamically stable without ongoing transfusion requirements, usually 24 to 48 hours. Prolonged use has been associated with skin

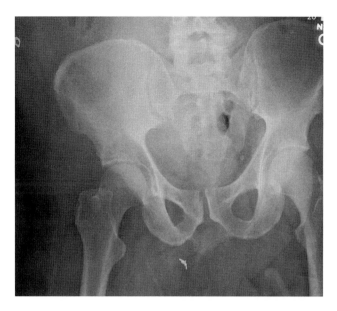

Figure 5.1 Pelvic radiograph demonstrating reduction of pubic symphysis after pelvic circumferential compression device placement.

breakdown over bony prominences, nerve damage, and abdominal or extremity CS.

There are several modalities available for hemorrhage control related to pelvic fractures, and the most appropriate strategy is dictated by the hemodynamic status of the patient, identification of associated injuries, and response to initial resuscitation. Those who respond favorably to initial measures should undergo CT scan with IV contrast for definitive diagnosis. CT evidence of active contrast extravasation related to pelvic fractures should prompt an emergent angiogram and transcatheter arterial embolization regardless of hemodynamic status. Angioembolization is generally performed in a dedicated endovascular suite by an interventional radiologist and has a reported success rate of 85 to 100%. The absence of contrast extravasation on CT does not rule out an arterial source of hemorrhage, and patients with a large associated retroperitoneal hematoma or persistent transfusion requirements after other sources of bleeding have been ruled out should also be considered for angioembolization.

Those who do not respond to initial pelvic compression and resuscitation often have an arterial source of pelvic hemorrhage (most commonly branches of the internal iliac artery) and/or an extrapelvic bleeding source (chest 15%, intra-abdominal 32%, long bones 40%). Chest radiograph and the cardiac portion of the FAST exam are used to screen for intrathoracic hemorrhage. Abdominal FAST exam and/or DPL is used to screen for significant hemoperitoneum. Bleeding related to isolated pelvic fractures is usually confined to the retroperitoneum and will not present with a positive abdominal FAST exam or DPL. Unstable patients with a positive FAST/DPL likely have an associated intra-abdominal injury and should undergo laparotomy for control of intra-abdominal bleeding followed by temporary

pelvic packing. Operative control of bleeding due to severe pelvic fractures is usually accomplished by temporary packing rather than direct repair and ligation of bleeding vessels. Preperitoneal pelvic packing is a procedure in which an incision is made on the lower abdomen from the pubis symphysis directed cranially. Access to the preperitoneal space is obtained by dividing the linea alba while leaving the peritoneum intact. The described procedure includes packing six laparotomy pads into the preperitoneal space (three on each side), followed by temporary closure of the fascia and skin to provide tamponade of bleeding. Postoperative angioembolization can then be performed if indicated for suspected arterial injury or ongoing hemorrhage. Unstable patients with a negative FAST/DPL should undergo emergent angioembolization if resources are immediately available; otherwise, preperitoneal packing can be used as a "bridge" to temporarily stabilize the patient until definitive angioembolization is available. REBOA for temporary hemorrhage control in this scenario is an emerging technique that has been used.

Keywords: Critical illness diagnosis and management; Orthopedic; Management; Pelvic trauma

REFERENCES

Cullinane DC, Schiller HJ, Zielinksi MD et al. Eastern Association for the Surgery of Trauma practice management guidelines for hemorrhage in pelvic fracture—update and systematic review. *J Trauma* 2011;71(6):1850–1868.

Vaidya R, Roth M, Zarling B et al. Application of circumferential compression device (binder) in pelvic injuries: room for improvement. *West J Emerg Med* 2016;17(6):766–774.

White CE, Hsu JR, Holcomb JB. Haemodynamically unstable pelvic fractures. *Injury* 2009;40:1023–1030.

18. ANSWER: C

The differential diagnosis of the ecchymosis and soft tissue swelling includes a Morel-Lavallée lesion, hematoma, seroma, abscess, soft tissue contusion, or neoplasm. Given the acute presentation, neoplasm is less likely. In the setting of trauma, particularly with an associated pelvic fracture, a Morel-Lavallée lesion is high on the differential diagnosis. A Morel-Lavallée lesion is a closed degloving injury whereby the skin and subcutaneous tissue become separated from the underlying fascia. Injury to the capillaries and lymphatics space can cause the resultant space to fill with blood, lymph, and necrotic debris. Over time, a fibrous capsule can develop.

Morel-Lavallée lesions can present as swelling, fluctuance, and pain. The diagnosis can be challenging because the overlying skin may appear normal, although dermal changes such as ecchymosis and necrosis can occur. The diagnosis may be missed on initial presentation, and the lesion may continue to increase slowly in size subsequent to the injury. Multiple imaging modalities may be used to diagnose and characterize a Morel-Lavallée lesion. The imaging modality of choice for definitive diagnosis is MRI. In general, MRI is the diagnostic test of choice for imaging soft tissue tumors as well. Both acute and chronic Morel-Lavallée lesions can be diagnosed. Acute lesions tend to have heterogeneous signal intensity, while chronic lesions appear hypointense on T1-weighted images and hyperintense on T2-weighted images. The latter also have a peripheral hypointense capsule on T1- and T2-weighted images. Ultrasound findings may be nonspecific; acute lesions are often ill-defined with heterogeneous echogenicity. Chronic lesions may show a capsule of varying thickness. Although CT scans are typically performed for trauma patients experiencing significant blunt force trauma, they are not ideal for characterizing soft tissue abnormalities. CT may demonstrate a fluid-fluid level resulting from the mixing of blood and lymph products. Like with ultrasound, acute lesions are often less well defined.

The management of Morel-Lavallée lesions is controversial, and there is no widely accepted algorithm for their management. For small, asymptomatic lesions, observation may be adequate. For symptomatic lesions not associated with a fracture, aspiration with or without percutaneous drainage may be an option. However, aspiration and drainage carry the risk for infecting a sterile fluid collection. Additionally, sclerotherapy has also been suggested to prevent recurrence. Morel-Lavallée lesions that are associated with a fracture may require percutaneous or open drainage; definitive (internal) operative fixation may need to be delayed. Patients with Morel-Lavallée lesions should be observed closely for complications because they can develop significant soft tissue infections, even necrotizing soft tissue infections. Morel-Lavallée lesions associated with infection, necrosis, or an open fracture should undergo surgical intervention.

Keywords: Critical illness diagnosis and management; Musculoskeletal; Diagnoses; Muscular and soft tissue injury (e.g., Morel-Lavallée)

REFERENCES

Diviti S, Gupta N, Hooda K, Sharma K, Lo L. Morel-Lavallee lesions: review of pathophysiology, clinical findings, imaging findings and management. *J Clin Diagn Res* 2017;11(4):TE01–TE04.

Greenhill D, Haydel C, Rehman S. Management of the Morel-Lavallee lesion. *Orthop Clin North Am* 2016;47(1):115–125.

19. ANSWER A

This patient presents in extremis after blunt trauma with intra-abdominal and pelvic sources of hemorrhage. He is a "nonresponder" to initial resuscitation, and you anticipate that cardiovascular collapse will occur before any potential intervention can be performed. Of the provided responses, zone 1 REBOA placement is the best option.

Uncontrolled hemorrhage, if left untreated, will lead to cardiovascular collapse, cerebral and myocardial ischemia, and eventually death. Control of noncompressible hemorrhage (i.e., bleeding within the torso) is challenging because it typically requires an emergent intervention such as angioembolization or surgery to obtain hemostasis.

REBOA for trauma is an emergent procedure used to aid in resuscitation and prevent cardiovascular collapse in the setting of noncompressible hemorrhage originating below the diaphragm. A balloon is advanced into the aorta and inflated, with resultant obstruction of blood flow to the distal circulation. This has the effect of decreasing arterial inflow to the focus of hemorrhage and increasing cardiac afterload and proximal aortic pressure, resulting in an increase in cerebral and myocardial perfusion. The ability to obtain vascular control proximal to the focus of bleeding serves as a bridge for circulatory support until definitive hemorrhage control can be obtained. It is important to note that hemorrhage originating above the diaphragm (i.e., a cardiac, proximal aortic, or great vessel injury) is a contraindication to REBOA because increasing the proximal aortic pressure will lead to increased bleeding. REBOA should be avoided for penetrating chest trauma or if there are signs of thoracic aortic injury (widened mediastinum on chest radiograph).

The technique of placing a REBOA is divided into five steps. Arterial access and sheath insertion (1) are typically obtained in the common femoral artery. Described approaches include percutaneous access, open cutdown, or guidewire exchange over an existing arterial line. To determine the optimal site of balloon position (2), the aorta is divided into three zones. Zone 1 is the descending thoracic aorta from the takeoff of the left subclavian artery to the origin of the celiac artery. Inflation in zone 1 physiologically resembles application of an aortic cross-clamp during a resuscitative left anterolateral thoracotomy and is typically used in the presence of massive intra-abdominal bleeding (i.e., a patient with a positive FAST exam). Zone 2 is the paravisceral aorta from the origin of the celiac artery to the most distal renal artery. Inflation in this zone is not recommended because of the presence of the celiac, mesenteric, and renal arteries. Zone 3 is the infrarenal aorta from the takeoff of the most distal renal artery to the aortic bifurcation. Inflation in this zone is reserved for bleeding associated with severe pelvic fractures or junctional lower extremity hemorrhage not amenable to tourniquet application. Inflation (3) is performed by instilling saline into the balloon after appropriate catheter and balloon location is confirmed, usually by standard radiograph or fluoroscopy. Balloon inflation time should be documented. Balloon deflation (4) is performed after hemorrhage control and volume resuscitation have been achieved. Effective team communication is essential during this step, and significant physiologic derangements should be anticipated. Expected changes include a sudden decrease in circulating volume, increasing acidosis from reperfusion, release of inflammatory mediators, and myocardial rhythm and contractility abnormalities. Deflation is typically performed slowly over the course of several minutes by removing a few milliliters of saline at a time and monitoring for hemodynamic changes. Several cycles of partial deflation and reinflation with continued volume resuscitation may be required before the balloon can be completely removed. Sheath removal (5) is performed as soon as possible after coagulopathy has resolved. The method of removal depends on the size of the sheath; larger sheaths may require cutdown and direct arterial repair, while smaller sheaths can generally be simply removed with application of manual compression. Confirmation of distal arterial perfusion is essential following device removal to prevent complications of lower extremity ischemia and resultant limb loss.

Keywords: Critical illness diagnosis and management; Cardiovascular; Management; REBOA

REFERENCES

Gamberini E, Coccolini F, Tamagnini B et al. Resuscitative endovascular balloon occlusion of the aorta in trauma: a systematic review of the literature. *World J Emerg Surg* 2017;12:42.

Morrison JJ, Galgon RE, Jansen JO et al. A systematic review of the use of resuscitative endovascular balloon occlusion of the aorta in the management of hemorrhagic shock. *J Trauma Acute Care Surg* 2016;80(2):324–334.

Sridhar S, Gumbert SD, Stephens C et al. Resuscitative endovascular balloon occlusion of the aorta: principles, initial clinical experience, and considerations for the anesthesiologist. *Anesth Analg* 2017;125(3):884–890.

20. ANSWER: A

This patient presents with penetrating trauma without signs of vascular injury. An IEI should be performed and, if abnormal, further vascular imaging (usually CT angiogram) obtained. Conventional angiography has largely been replaced by CT angiography for the detection of arterial injury after trauma due to the rapid availability of CT scanners, which provide detailed and accurate identification of vascular injuries. CT angiography can generally be deferred in penetrating trauma without signs of vascular injury and a normal IEI. Immediate operative exploration is reserved for those with hard signs of vascular injury or hemodynamically unstable patients with isolated extremity injury.

Trauma to the extremities, whether by penetrating or blunt mechanism, are commonly encountered in the care of injured patients. Significant extremity hemorrhage should be treated with direct pressure or the liberal use of tourniquets in both the prehospital and ED settings. A brief exam of the extremities should be performed during the primary trauma survey and a more detailed exam obtained after life-threatening injuries have been addressed.

Signs of arterial vascular injury can be split into two groups. "Hard signs" of vascular injury include pulsatile hemorrhage, expanding hematoma, evidence of limb ischemia, presence of a bruit/thrill, and CS. "Soft signs" include a decreased pulse exam compared with the contralateral side, history of substantial hemorrhage at the scene, peripheral nerve deficit, or proximity of injury to a major vessel. Patients with hard signs of vascular injury generally require no further vascular imaging workup and should be taken to the operating room for exploration and repair. The presence of soft signs of vascular injury should prompt further workup, usually a CT angiogram if available. Those patients without signs of vascular injury should have an IEI performed. IEI is a trauma-specific term that is analogous to the ankle-brachial index but can be applied to both the upper and lower extremities. It is the ratio of the highest systolic occlusion pressure in the distal injured extremity (dorsalis pedis/posterior tibial or radial/ulnar) divided by the systolic pressure in a proximal vessel of an uninjured extremity (usually the brachial artery). A normal IEI (>0.9) has a high negative predictive value for arterial injury, allowing the patient to be observed or managed without immediate vascular imaging. An abnormal IEI (<0.9) is predictive of vascular injury that requires further vascular imaging. It is important to note that IEI does not assess for the presence of venous injury, muscle bleeding, non–flow-limiting arterial injury (dissection flap, pseudoaneursym), or injury to a non–end artery (profunda femoris).

Keywords: Critical illness; Cardiovascular; Diagnoses; Subclavian artery injury

REFERENCES

Fox N, Rajani RR, Bokhari F et al. Evaluation and management of penetrating lower extremity arterial trauma: an Eastern Association for the Surgery of Trauma practice management guideline. *J Trauma Acute Care Surg* 2012;73(5):S315–S320.

Gurien LA, Kerwin AJ, Yorkgitis BK et al. Reassessing the utility of CT angiograms in penetrating injuries to the extremities. *Surgery* 2018;163(2):419–422.

Sadjadi J, Cureton EL, Dozier KC et al. Expedited treatment of lower extremity gunshot wounds. 2009;209(6):740–745.

6.

CRITICAL CARE REVIEW
BURNS

James M. Cross, Tonya C. George, and Todd F. Huzar

QUESTIONS

1. A 45-year-old male is admitted to the intensive care unit (ICU) after sustaining 45% second-degree burns in a house fire. The MOST appropriate initial resuscitation for a major burn is which of the following?

A. 2 L of normal saline as a bolus over 1 hour
B. 2 mL/kg body weight/% total body surface area (TBSA) burn of lactated Ringer's solution, with half given over the first 8 hours
C. 2 mL/kg body weight/% TBSA burn of normal saline, with half given over the first 8 hours
D. 125 mL/hour of D_5 ½-normal saline.

2. What complications are LEAST associated with overresuscitation in burn patients?

A. Pulmonary edema
B. Increased interstitial edema
C. Abdominal compartment syndrome
D. Delirium

3. Three days after admission for 40% body surface area burns inflicted in a house fire, a 40-year-old female patient is clinically improving and being weaned from mechanical ventilation. The family suggests that an herbal remedy be applied to the burns on her bilateral lower extremities. Which of the following would be the MOST helpful in improving wound healing in this patient?

A. Polymyxin B
B. Oxandrolone
C. Bacitracin
D. Silver sulfadiazine

4. Which of the following would be the LEAST likely to decrease the hypermetabolic response in patients with large burn injuries?

A. Early excision and grafting of the burn wound
B. Increasing ambient room temperature
C. Use of beta-blockers
D. Intravenous (IV) hydration

5. What is the MOST appropriate prophylaxis against deep vein thrombosis and pulmonary embolism in patients with large burns?

A. Nothing
B. Enoxaparin dosed based on weight and burn size
C. Sequential compression device
D. Enoxaparin 40 mg/day

6. What is the best indicator of adequate resuscitation in patients who sustained large burns?

A. Normal lactate level
B. Normal blood pressure and heart rate
C. Normal hemoglobin level
D. Adequate urine output (0.5 mL/kg per hour)

7. A 22-year-old male presents to your emergency department (ED) with a complaint of pain of the right great toe. He reports being at home with about 20 of his friends watching the Super Bowl when he tripped over a keg of beer, causing a bruise on his toe. The patient noted swelling of his toe close to the end of the game, so he decided to treat the swelling with dry ice that he got from a cooler. He recalled putting the ice into a small plastic bag, placing the bag into his socks, and putting his slippers on for the remainder of the night. He awoke from his couch in the middle of the night with

increased pain in his toe, so he called his girlfriend to bring him to the closest ED. The patient's vital signs are as follows: temperature 97.7° F, heart rate (HR) 102 bpm, blood pressure (BP) 105/67 mm Hg, and respiratory rate (RR) 18. His blood alcohol level is 0.18 g/dL. Upon initial evaluation of the patient, you find him sitting comfortably on a stretcher, fully clothed, with his slippers on and his girlfriend at his bedside. You note areas of subcutaneous tissue death at the distal right foot, including the great toe, and areas of blue-gray discoloration, edema, and small hemorrhagic blistering. What is the most likely cause of this patient's injury?

A. Second-degree contusion
B. Uric acid crystal formation
C. Ice crystal formation
D. Blood clot formation of the great toe

8. The patient discussed in question 7 expresses concern about the viability of the toe and wants to know if anything can be done to save it. What is the most important initial treatment to restore tissue perfusion?

A. Fluid resuscitation
B. Removal of the causative environment
C. Rapid core body temperature warming to 45° C
D. Digital angiography of his great toe

9. A 32-year-old power line worker presents to your ED with a chief complaint of burns to the right hand and forearm after accidentally touching a high-voltage electrical line with a metal pole. At the time of the accident, the patient reports being thrown backward and losing consciousness. Upon awakening, he noticed burns to the right hand and forearm with associated numbness and tingling of his digits. On examination, the patient is noted to have circumferential full-thickness burns of his right forearm with partial-thickness burns of the palmer surface of the right hand. The nurse reports an inability to palpate a radial pulse. You obtain a Doppler ultrasound, but the radial pulse is absent. What is the best next treatment option?

A. Medial and lateral longitudinal incision through the burned skin of the right forearm
B. Medial and lateral longitudinal incision through the burned skin of the right hand
C. Excisional debridement and split-thickness skin grafts of the right forearm burned skin
D. Excisional debridement and split-thickness skin grafts of the right hand burned skin

10. A 32-year-old female with 51% TBSA partial-thickness burns was admitted to your ICU 3 days ago. She was intubated in the field for concerns of inhalation

injury and pain control. Bronchoscopy was performed with no evidence of carbonaceous soot in the airways. Her ventilator settings are as follows: rate 12, tidal volume 450, forced inspiratory oxygen (FiO$_2$) 40%, and PEEP 5. Her dressing care consists of twice-daily application of a topical antimicrobial cream with wet-to-dry gauze bandages. Her arterial blood gas (ABG) analysis shows pH 7.28 PCO$_2$ 33, PO$_2$ 106, HCO$_3$ 17, and O$_2$ saturation 98%. Which of the following topical antimicrobials can be the cause of the patient's metabolic acidosis?

A. Bacitracin/polymyxin B
B. Silver sulfadiazine
C. Mafenide acetate
D. Manuka honey

11. The patient is a 59-year-old woman who was "found down" in a house fire and required extrication from the fire department. The patient was removed from the home and was noted to have 14% TBSA burns on her face, back, chest, and abdomen as well as a significant amount of carbonaceous material in her airway, which prompted intubation on scene. The patient was transported to a level 1 trauma center and evaluated by the trauma service. The patient underwent fiberoptic bronchoscopy and was noted to have a moderate inhalation injury with carbonaceous material throughout her lower airways. Co-oximetry test was done, and she was noted to have a carboxyhemoglobin level of 35%. What is the next MOST appropriate step in managing her carbon monoxide (CO) poisoning?

A. Increase the FiO$_2$ to 100% on the ventilator
B. Wean the ventilator and extubate the patient
C. Start low tidal volume ventilation
D. Consult hyperbaric medicine

12. A 29-year-old man was found trapped in a car that was on fire. The patient was removed from the vehicle and intubated on scene because of respiratory distress. The patient was noted to be hypoxic and hypotensive en route to the hospital, which required the patient being placed on 100% FiO$_2$ and initiation of norepinephrine. On evaluation in the ED, the patient was cyanotic, hypotensive, and significantly hypoxic. ABG analysis showed 6.96/30/60/10/–24/91% on FiO$_2$ of 100% and PEEP of 10. The patient was noted to also have a lactate level of 15. The ED physician is concerned that the patient has acute cyanide toxicity. What is the most appropriate step in management?

A. Send for of a whole blood cyanide level
B. Start fluid resuscitation and give the patient hydroxocobalamin

C. Place femoral cannulas and start venoarterial extracorporeal membrane oxygenation (ECMO)
D. Start the patient on 3% sodium nitrite and 25% sodium thiosulfate infusions

13. A 26-year-old male working at an automobile body shop was using a liquid hydrofluoric acid product to enhance the chrome finish on wheels. After finishing up, the patient noted that he developed a burning sensation in the fingertips of both hands that became more intense over 1 hour, prompting evaluation in your ED. The patient was seen and evaluated, at which time the patient was noted to be complaining of pain in his hands and perioral tingling. An ionized calcium level was sent, which was noted to be 0.95. The patient was started on IV calcium gluconate replacement and admitted to the ICU for observation and monitoring. What is the best course of action?

A. Irrigate his hands with copious amounts of water
B. Start intra-arterial infusion of calcium gluconate
C. Perform emergent excision of the distal fingertips
D. Apply topical 2.5% calcium gluconate to the fingertips as needed until the pain resolves

14. A 47-year-old man was "found down" behind a door in a home that was on fire. The patient's Glasgow Coma Scale (GCS) score on scene was 8, and he was intubated by EMS before being transported to the ED. On presentation, the EMS provider stated that the "patient looked blue" and "his mouth was full of soot" at the time he was intubated. On exam, the patient has scattered second-degree burns on his face and carbonaceous material in his mouth. The patient's chest radiograph was clear, and his ABG was 7.37/50/280/24/0/99% on FiO_2 of 100%. The patient is suspected to have an inhalation injury. What is the best method of diagnosis?

A. Anteroposterior chest radiographs
B. Xenon ventilation-perfusion lung scan
C. Flexible fiberoptic bronchoscopy
D. Computed tomography (CT) scan of the chest with IV contrast

15. A 53-year-old woman was brought by ambulance to the ED after being rescued from a car that was on fire. The patient is seen and examined, at which time she is noted to have some carbonaceous material in her nares and mouth. The patient is also complaining of a severe headache, shortness of breath, blurry vision, and difficulty concentrating. The patient was placed on 100% FiO_2 by a non-rebreather mask, and her pulse oximeter shows a peripheral oxygen saturation (SpO_2) of 92 to 95%. As part of her workup, ABG analysis is performed, and she is noted to have an arterial oxygen saturation (SaO_2) of 79%. What is the most likely explanation of this difference in O_2 saturation?

A. Significantly elevated levels of carboxyhemoglobin
B. Increased ventilation-perfusion mismatching
C. Pulmonary embolism
D. Rapid development of acute respiratory distress syndrome (ARDS)

16. A 65-year-old man is rescued from an apartment fire by firemen about 1 hour ago and brought directly to the ED. On exam, the patient is noted to have about 15% TBSA second-degree burns to the face, torso, and upper extremities. The patient is placed on 100% FiO_2 but becomes tachypneic and short of breath. For this reason, the patient is endotracheally intubated by the ED physicians. The patient is noted to have carbonaceous material in his oropharynx and hypopharynx, which is concerning for inhalation injury. After the patient is transferred to the ICU, the patient undergoes formal bronchoscopy and is noted to have the following findings:

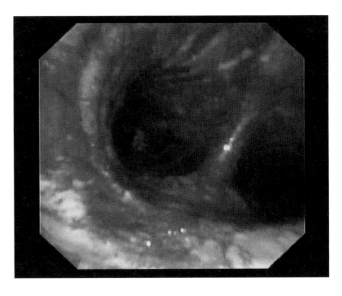

The patient has an obvious severe inhalation injury and is started on a low tidal volume ventilation strategy. Twelve hours later, the patient develops severe hypercapnia and hypoxia. What is the primary cause of the patient's deterioration?

A. Diffuse alveolar damage and lung capillary endothelial injury
B. Occlusion of the distal airways due to cast formation
C. Thromboembolic occlusion of a pulmonary artery
D. Ventilator-associated pneumonia

ANSWERS

1. ANSWER: C

Fluid loss in a major burn (>20% TBSA) is a slow, ongoing process and needs to be corrected in an ongoing fashion. Bolusing with a crystalloid fluid will not improve outcome and will increase the risk for developing pulmonary edema, interstitial edema, and abdominal compartment syndrome. The most effective resuscitation protocols involve replacing the intravascular fluid loss with a balanced electrolyte solution, such as lactated Ringer's, based on the size of the burn and the size of the patient. One of the most widely accepted formulas is the consensus formula, which is 2 mL of lactated Ringer's per kilogram of body weight per % TBSA burn. One half of the fluid is given over the first 8 hours after the burn. The initial resuscitation fluid rate is then altered based on how the patient responds.

Keywords: Burns, management; Fluids and resuscitation

REFERENCES

Demling RH. The burn edema process: current concepts. *J Burn Care Rehabil* 2005;26(5):207–227.

Rae L, Fidler P, Gibran N. The physiologic basis of burn shock and the need for aggressive fluid resuscitation. *Crit Care Clin* 2016;32(4):491–505.

2. ANSWER: D

Overresuscitation has become an increasingly recognized phenomenon in modern burn centers. The reason for overresuscitation is multifactorial and includes overestimation of the burn size, overzealous administration of fluid (including bolusing), and reluctance to titrate fluid based on adequate urine output, among others. This tendency has been termed "fluid creep" and has led to pulmonary edema, increased interstitial edema, and abdominal compartment syndrome. While delirium is not directly associated with overresuscitation, exposure to benzodiazepines during admission has been demonstrated as an independent risk factor for delirium. Furthermore, opiates are associated with improved pain control and reduced delirium.

Keywords: Burns, management; Other therapies (hyperbaric, pharmacologic, surgical)

REFERENCES

Agarwal V, O'Neill PJ, Cotton BA et al. Prevalence and risk factors for development of delirium in burn intensive care unit patients. *J Burn Care Res.* 2010;31(5):706–715.

Chung KK, Wolf SE, Cancio LC et al. Resuscitation of severely burned military casualties: fluid begets more fluid. *J Trauma* 2009;67(2):231–237.

Saffle JL. The phenomenon of "fluid creep" in acute burn resuscitation. *J Burn Care Res* 2007;28(3):382–395.

3. ANSWER: B

Oxandrolone is a testosterone analog with very few virilizing side effects. In a multicenter, randomized, double-blinded, placebo-controlled trial, it was found to improve wound healing in adult burn patients with large (>20% TBSA) burns. Polymyxin B and Bacitracin are topical antimicrobial agents that can be used for application to partial-thickness burns. The advantage with these agents is the ease of application and removal during dressing changes. They are commonly applied to even large and sensitive areas like the face, ears, and perineum. An additional advantage is that they have been found to have minimal systemic absorption and hence a very limited side-effect profile. Silver sulfadiazine cream is the most commonly used agent for burn dressings. Activated silver is notable for having broad-spectrum antimicrobial activity and may also have an anti-inflammatory benefit. It is inexpensive and is the standard of care at many burn centers. Silver sulfadiazine has antimicrobial activity and has been demonstrated to decrease colonization of burn wounds. However, there are no well-designed trials to confirm improved wound healing or a reduced rate of bacterial wound infection.

Keywords: Burns, management; Other therapies (hyperbaric, pharmacologic, surgical)

REFERENCES

Heyneman A, Hoeksema H, Vandekerckhove D et al. The role of silver sulphadiazine in the conservative treatment of partial thickness burn wounds: a systematic review. *Burns* 2016;42(7):1377.

Nadworny PL, Wang J, Tredget EE, Burrell RE. Anti-inflammatory activity of nanocrystalline silver-derived solutions in porcine contact dermatitis. *J Inflamm (Lond)* 2010;7:13.

Norman G, Christie J, Liu Z et al. Antiseptics for burns. *Cochrane Database Syst Rev* 2017;(7):CD011821.

Wolf SE, Edelman LS, Kemalyan N et al. Effects of oxandrolone on outcome measures in the severely burned: a multicenter prospective randomized double-blind trial. *J Burn Care Res* 2006;27(2):131–139.

4. ANSWER: D

The hypermetabolic response after a severe burn injury is greater than with any other condition seen in medicine. It is mediated by large increases in catecholamines, cortisol, and inflammatory cells. This hypermetabolic response, if left unchecked, will lead to muscle wasting, malnutrition, infections, and death. There is evidence that this response may last up to 2 years after injury. There are several interventions, both pharmacologic and nonpharmacologic, that will ameliorate this hypermetabolic response. Keeping the ambient temperature between 28° and 33° C, resting energy expenditure will decrease significantly. Early excision of the burn wound and coverage with either autografts or cadaveric skin have also been shown in many studies to decrease the resting energy expenditure in burn patients. Since catecholamines are known to be one of the major mediators of the postburn hypermetabolic demand, beta-blockers have been used to blunt this response. Multiple clinical trials have shown that propranolol is a safe and effective way to reduce the metabolic response in burn patients. While IV fluid administration may be indicated in thermal injury, it has not been demonstrated to measurably reduced the hypermetabolic state of thermal injury.

Keywords: Burns, management; Fluids and resuscitation

REFERENCES

Porter C, Tompkins RG, Finnerty CC et al. The metabolic stress response to burn injury: current understanding and therapies. *Lancet* 2016;388(10052):1417–1426.

Williams FN, Herndon DN, Jeschke MG. The hypermetabolic response to burn injury and interventions to modify this response. *Clin Plast Surg* 2009;36(4):583–596.

5. ANSWER: B

Patients who suffer from large burns (i.e., >20% TBSA) are at an increased risk for developing deep vein thrombosis and pulmonary embolism. The standard dose of enoxaparin (30 mg twice daily or 40 mg daily), is inadequate in most of these patients, based on measuring anti-Xa levels. Several studies have shown that dosing the enoxaparin based on the size of the burn and the patient's body weight has resulted in appropriate anti-Xa levels and subsequently lower incidence of thromboembolic phenomena. Sequential compression devices may not be effective enough in patients with large burns and may be painful if placed over a burned extremity or donor site.

Keywords: Burns, complications

REFERENCES

Faraklas I, Ghanem M, Brown A, Cochran A. Evaluation of an enoxaparin dosing calculator using burn size and weight. *J Burn Care Res* 2013;34(6):621–627.

Lin H, Faraklas I, Saffle J, Cochran A. Enoxaparin dose adjustment is associated with low incidence of venous thromboembolic events in acute burn patients. *J Trauma* 2011;71(6):1557–1561.

6. ANSWER D

While there is still a search for the perfect end point of resuscitation in burn patients, adequate urine output of 30 to 50 mL/hour (or approximately 0.5 mL/kg per hour) is regarded as the best indicator of resuscitation in most burn patients. Lactate levels tend to resolve more slowly and may be altered by CO and cyanide exposure. HR and BP may be affected by pain and anxiety, and noninvasive BP measurement can be affected by limb edema. Hemoglobin values will be high early on during resuscitation because of intravascular fluid loss and "hemoconcentration" and then be lower than normal as the fluid resuscitation progresses.

Keywords: Burns, management; Fluids and resuscitation

REFERENCE

Caruso DM, Matthews MR. Monitoring end points of burn resuscitation. *Crit Care Clin* 2016;32:525–537.

7. ANSWER: C

Frostbite occurs at the cellular level due to formation of ice crystal, microvascular occlusion, and dehydration within the cells. Frostbite injuries are classified into first-degree, second-degree, third-degree, and fourth-degree injuries. Third-degree frostbite injuries cause subcutaneous and skin necrosis, hemorrhagic blistering, and blue-gray discoloration.

Keywords: Thermoregulation; Hypothermia; Environmental

REFERENCES

Jurkovich GJ. Environmental cold-induced injury. *Surg Clin N Am* 2007;8:247–258.

McIntosh S et al. Wilderness Medical Society practice guidelines for the prevention and treatment of frostbite: 2014 update. *Wilderness Environ Med* 2014;25:S43–S54.

Woo E, Lee JW, Hur G et al. Proposed treatment protocol for frostbite: a retrospective analysis of 17 cases based on a 3-year single-institution experience. Arch Plast Surg 2013;40(5):510–516.

8. ANSWER: B

After the development of a frostbite injury, the initial care and restoration of tissue perfusion start with removing the patient from the offending agent or environment.

Keywords: Thermoregulation; Hypothermia; Environmental

REFERENCES

Ingram B, Raymond T. Recognition and treatment of freezing and nonfreezing cold injuries. *Am Coll Sports Med* 2013;12(2):125–130.

Jurkovich GJ. Environmental cold-induced injury. *Surg Clin N Am* 2007;8:247–258.

9. ANSWER: A

Indications to perform an escharotomy of an extremity include the presence of full-thickness circumferential or near-circumferential burns and the absence of Doppler pulses. Escharotomies are made using medial and lateral longitudinal incisions over the full-thickness burns.

Keywords: Burns, complications

REFERENCES

De Barros M, Coltro PS, Hetem C et al. Revisiting escharotomy in patients with burns in extremities. *J Burn Care Res* 2017;38(4):e691–e698.

Orgill DP, Piccolo N. Escharotomy and decompressive therapies in burns. J Burn Care Res 2009;30(5):759–768.

10. ANSWER: C

Carbonic anhydrase inhibitors such as mafenide acetate inhibit red blood cell carbonic anhydrase and bicarbonate reabsorption within the kidneys. This results in an impairment of carbon dioxide transport within the tissue, subsequent increased tissue PCO_2 levels, a decrease in serum bicarbonate, and subsequent metabolic acidosis.

Keywords: Burns, management; Antimicrobials

REFERENCES

Asch MJ, White MG, Pruitt BA. Acid base changes associated with topical Sulfamylon therapy: retrospective study of 100 burn patients. *Ann Surg* 1970;172(6):946–950.

Black JA, Harris F, Lenton EA et al. Alkalosis in burns in children. *BMJ* 1971;13:387–388.

White G, Asch MJ. Acid-base effects of topical mafenide acetate in the burned patient. N Engl J Med 1971;1284(23):1281–1286

11. ANSWER: A

CO has an approximately 210-times greater affinity than oxygen for hemoglobin. When CO binds to hemoglobin and forms carboxyhemoglobin, it causes the remaining oxygen-binding sites on the hemoglobin molecule to bind the oxygen tighter, thereby decreasing the delivery of oxygen to other tissues. This, in turn, decreases the oxygen-carrying capacity of blood and causes a left shift of the O_2 dissociation curve of the unaffected oxyhemoglobin that decreases the ability to unload O_2 at the tissue level. The management of acute CO poisoning is the administration of humidified, 100% oxygen (O_2) whether by non-rebreather mask (if not intubated) or 100% FiO_2 if the patient is intubated and on mechanical ventilation. The rationale for initiating oxygen therapy is that the O_2 shortens the half-life of carboxyhemoglobin by competing with CO at the hemoglobin-binding sites and subsequently decreasing hypoxia and improving tissue oxygenation. The half-life of CO on room air is approximately 4 to 5 hours, but it can decrease to an hour or less with the addition of 100% normobaric oxygen.

This patient has a moderate inhalation injury and CO poisoning, so weaning the ventilator and extubating the patient would be incorrect (answer B).

There is no evidence at this time to suggest that the patient has developed ARDS; therefore, the initiation of low tidal volume ventilation in not warranted. In addition, there are data in the burn literature to suggest that low tidal volume ventilation is not adequate for ventilation and oxygenation in thermally injured patients (answer C).

Hyperbaric oxygen (HBO) therapy is delivery of 100% oxygen under increased atmospheric pressure, which is recommended to be 2 to 3 atmospheres by the Undersea and Hyperbaric Medicine Society. HBO has been shown to increase the dissolved oxygen content in the blood to a supranormal level and subsequently to decrease the half-life of CO to 20 to 30 minutes. Some clinicians will suggest and advocate the use of HBO in patients with elevated carboxyhemoglobin levels because there are some data to suggest that HBO decreases the incidence of adverse neurological outcomes; however, a Cochrane Review in 2011 demonstrated that the existing randomized control trials do not clearly establish whether HBO therapy in patients with acute CO poisoning reduces the incidence of neurological injury. Furthermore, there is no consensus to date regarding the absolute indications for and the standard duration and intensity of HBO therapy in patients with severe CO poisoning (answer D).

Keywords: Burns, management; Other therapies (hyperbaric, pharmacologic, surgical)

REFERENCES

Buckley NA, Juurlink DN, Isbister G et al. Hyperbaric oxygen for carbon monoxide poisoning. *Cochrane Database Syst Rev* 2011;13(4):CD002041.

Chung KK, Wolf SE, Renz EM et al. High-frequency percussive ventilation and low tidal volume ventilation in burns: a randomized control trial. *Crit Care Med* 2010;38(10): 231–237.

Ernst A, Zibrak JD. Carbon monoxide poisoning. *N Engl J Med* 1998;339(22):1603–1608.

Gorman D, Drewry A, Huang YL, Sames C. The clinical toxicology of carbon monoxide. *Toxicology* 2003;187(1):25–38.

Huzar TF, George T, Cross JM. Carbon monoxide and cyanide toxicity: etiology, pathophysiology, and treatment in inhalation injury. *Expert Rev Respir Med* 2013;7(2):159–170.

Roughton FJW, Darling RC. The effect of carbon monoxide on the oxyhemoglobin dissociation curve. *Am J Physiol* 1944;141:17–31.

12. ANSWER: B

Based on the history, hemodynamic instability, and laboratory findings, the patient likely has acute cyanide poisoning. Since there is no rapid assay to determine whether the patient has cyanide poisoning, the clinician needs to be suspicious of cyanide poisoning in patients with severe lactic acidosis, profound hypoxemia, and hemodynamic instability after prolonged smoke exposure. There are data to suggest that lactate level higher than 10 mmol/L is a sensitive and specific indicator of acute cyanide poisoning. Fluid resuscitation with isotonic IV fluids is appropriate in the setting of shock, followed by the administration of a commercially available antidote, which in this case, would be hydroxocobalamin. This antidote consists of a vitamin B_{12} precursor that has been found not to interfere with tissue oxygenation, unlike some of the other available cyanide antidotes. Cyanide preferentially binds to the cobalt moiety of hydroxocobalamin owing to its higher affinity for cobalt than cytochrome oxidase a₃. After cyanide is bound, it becomes cyanocobalamin, which is no longer toxic, and is removed from the body through the kidneys. The reason hydroxocobalamin has become more frequently used in the management of cyanide poisoning in patients with inhalation injury is that it has minimal adverse reactions and does not affect oxygen utilization and delivery like some of the other commercially available cyanide antidotes (i.e., dicobalt edetate and the combination of amyl nitrite, sodium nitrite, and sodium thiosulfate).

There are no rapid laboratory studies that can determine blood concentrations of cyanide. Also, most currently available whole-blood cyanide tests take hours to complete, and many institutions do not have the equipment to run these tests. In addition, there is some question about the utility of these tests because cyanide rapidly clears from the blood and the specimens are often drawn hours after the exposure. Furthermore, in the time it takes for the results to return, the patient may die as a result of untreated cyanide poisoning (answer A).

The initiation of venoarterial ECMO may help with oxygenation and hemodynamic support, but it will not remove the cyanide that is bound to the cytochromes nor reverse intracellular hypoxia as a result of the mitochondria's inability to utilize oxygen (answer C).

The use of sodium nitrite and sodium thiosulfate in combination with amyl nitrite has been the mainstay of treating cyanide poisoning in the United States for decades. In cases of suspected cyanide poisoning, the patient is given inhaled amyl nitrite followed by administration of IV sodium nitrite. These two medications cause an oxidative reaction with hemoglobin, transforming it to methemoglobin. Cyanide has a high affinity for methemoglobin and will uncouple from cytochrome oxidase a₃, forming cyanomethoglobin. The patient is then given IV sodium thiosulfate, which interacts with cyanomethoglobin and forms thiocyanate, which is excreted from the kidneys. The reason this drug combination is not used in patients with inhalation injury is that the transformation of oxyhemoglobin to methemoglobin may further worsen hypoxemia in patients with lung injury from inhalation injury and CO poisoning. Furthermore, the administration of IV nitrites can worsen hypotension in patients who are already in hypovolemic or distributive shock.

Keywords: Burns, management; Fluids and resuscitation

REFERENCES

Barillo DJ. Diagnosis and treatment of cyanide toxicity. *J Burn Care Res* 2009;30(1):148–152.

Baud FJ. Cyanide: critical issues in diagnosis and treatment. *Hum Exp Toxicol* 2007;26(3):191–201.

Baud FJ, Barriot P, Toffis V et al. Elevated blood cyanide concentrations in victims of smoke inhalation. *N Engl J Med* 1991;325(25):1761–1766.

Baud FJ, Borron SW, Mégarbane B et al. Value of lactic acidosis in the assessment of the severity of acute cyanide poisoning. *Crit Care Med* 2002;30 (9):2044–2050.

Borron SW. Recognition and treatment of acute cyanide poisoning. *J Emerg Nurs* 2006;32(Suppl 4):S12–S18.

Lawson-Smith P, Jansen EC, Hyldegaard O. Cyanide intoxication as part of smoke inhalation—a review on diagnosis and treatment from the emergency perspective. *Scand J Trauma Resusc Emerg Med* 2011;19:14.

Gracia R, Shepherd G. Cyanide poisoning and its treatment. *Pharmacotherapy* 2004;24(10):1358–1365.

Nelson L. Acute cyanide toxicity: mechanisms and manifestations. *J Emerg Nurs* 2006;32(Suppl 4):S8–11.

13. ANSWER: D

Hydrofluoric acid is one of the more common causes of chemical burns that lead to burn center admission. It can be found in many industrial and commercial settings (e.g., cleaning agents). Hydrofluoric acid is a relatively weak acid compared with other acids (e.g., hydrochloric or sulfuric acid), but the morbidity associated with injury is related to the concentration of the hydrofluoric acid and the length of time the patient is exposed to it. Hydrofluoric acid causes morbidity and possibly mortality by two mechanisms: (1) the hydrogen ions can cause a corrosive burn to the skin like other acids, and the fluoride ions cause liquefactive necrosis (cellular death) of deeper tissues, which is the primary cause of the pain associated with hydrofluoric acid burns; and (2) during the process of liquefactive necrosis, the fluoride ions will bind with calcium, which can precipitate life-threatening hypocalcemia. The fluoride ions will remain active until the acid is completely neutralized by a bivalent cation, which is calcium gluconate. Stuke et al, found that the administration of topical 2.5% calcium gluconate neutralized the fluoride ions that are within the wound. The calcium gel is repeatedly applied until the pain is relieved.

Irrigation with copious amounts of water is typically the initial management for chemical burns and exposures; however, in cases of hydrofluoric acid exposure, water will not neutralize the effects of the fluoride ions already within the deeper tissues (answer A).

Intra-arterial infusion of calcium gluconate and surgical excision of burned tissue tend to be the procedures performed in patients who do not respond to topical calcium gluconate therapy. Both procedures carry a higher level of morbidity associated with them (answers B and C).

Keywords: Burns, management, Other therapies (hyperbaric, pharmacologic, surgical)

REFERENCES

Hatzifotis M, Williams A, Muller M, Pegg S. Hydrofluoric acid burns. *Burns* 2004;30:156–159.

Kirkpatrick JJ, Enion DS, Burd DA. Hydrofluoric acid burns: a review. *Burns* 1995;21:483–493.

Stuke LE, Arnoldo BD, Hunt JL, Purdue JF. Hydrofluoric acid burns: a 15 year experience. *J Burn Care Res* 2008;29:893–896.

14. ANSWER: C

The diagnosis of fire-related inhalation injury requires a combination of history-taking and clinical and diagnostic findings. History and physical exam findings can often be nonspecific and misleading; therefore, evaluation of the tracheobronchial tree is essential in establishing the diagnosis of inhalation injury. The use of flexible fiberoptic bronchoscopy allows for evaluation of the lower airways for the presence of carbonaceous material, mucosal edema, erythema, and mucosal sloughing. The advantages of performing fiberoptic bronchoscopy is visualization of the airways and the ability to perform therapeutic maneuvers if needed. The disadvantages include limited evaluation of the tracheobronchial tree, inability to assess the upper airways, difficulty in performing this procedure in nonintubated patients, and risk for lung injury or worsening hypoxia.

Anteroposterior chest radiographs are often normal in patients who present immediately after smoke exposure and associated inhalation injury, except in cases of severe inhalation and early onset of ARDS (answer A).

Xenon-133 ventilation-perfusion scanning was initially studied in the 1970s as a way to diagnosis inhalation injury in the early, acute setting. Schall et al. found that it was "safe, easy, accurate, and sensitive in the early diagnosis of inhalation injury." Other studies have shown similar findings, and xenon scanning has been shown to correlate with other signs of inhalation injury. However, it is not widely used and has fallen out of favor because of logistic difficulty and expense.

A single-center, retrospective study (Oh et al., 2012) evaluated the use of chest CT at admission in patients with suspected inhalation injury and found that it may assist in predicting future lung dysfunction rather than diagnosing inhalation injury (answer D).

Keywords: Burns, inhalation injury

REFERENCES

Agee RN, Long JM 3d, Hunt JL et al. Use of [133]xenon in early diagnosis of inhalation injury. *J Trauma* 1976;16: 218–224.

Cochrane Collaboration. Evidence based surgery-inhalation injury: diagnosis. *J Am Coll Surg* 2003;196:306–312.

Dries DJ, Endorf FW. Inhalation Injury: epidemiology, pathology, treatment strategies. *Scand J Trauma Resusc Emerg Med* 2013;21:31.

Jones SW, Williams FN, Cairns BA, Cartotto R. Inhalation injury: pathophysiology, diagnosis, and treatment. *Clin Plast Surg* 2017;44(3):505–511.

Oh JS, Chung KK, Allen A et al. Admission chest CT complements fiberoptic bronchoscopy in prediction of adverse outcomes in thermally injured patients. *J Burn Care Res* 2012;33(4):532–538.

Schall GL, McDonald HD, Carr LB et al. Xenon ventilation-perfusion scans: the early diagnosis of inhalation injury. *JAMA* 1978;240(22):2441–2445.

Walker PF, Buehner MF, Wood LA et al. Diagnosis and management of inhalation injury: an updated review. *Crit Care* 2015;19:351.

15. ANSWER: A

The patient presents with signs and symptoms of CO poisoning. More important, the patient has a significant difference between her SpO_2 and her SaO_2, which can be attributed to CO poisoning. Carboxyhemoglobin and oxyhemoglobin have similar wavelengths and subsequent extinction coefficients, and most standard pulse oximeters are unable to differentiate between oxyhemoglobin and carboxyhemoglobin, resulting in misleading, falsely high or normal SpO_2 readings in the setting of CO poisoning. Some older studies have shown that pulse oximeters interpret carboxyhemoglobin almost exactly as oxyhemoglobin and that SpO_2, in these cases of CO poisoning, represents the sum of oxyhemoglobin and carboxyhemoglobin. On the other hand, the SaO_2 is decreased owing to the limited amount of oxygen molecules that can bind to an individual hemoglobin molecule (i.e., two binding sites occupied by CO). This will decrease the overall carrying capacity of blood and delivery of oxygen to the tissues. Interestingly enough, the PaO_2 (dissolved oxygen) is not effected by CO poisoning.

In cases of increased ventilation-perfusion mismatching, pulmonary embolism, and ARDS, the clinician would expect both the SpO_2 and the SaO_2 to be decreased as a result of significant hypoxia (answers B, C, and D). In this case, the patient's SpO_2 is decreased, but the SaO_2 is decreased way out of proportion compared with the SpO_2 because of the decreased oxygen-carrying capacity of blood as a result of high carboxyhemoglobin levels.

Keywords: Burns, complications

REFERENCES

Alexander CM, Teller LE, Gross JB. Principles of pulse oximetry: theoretical and practical considerations. *Anesth Analg* 1989;68:368–376.

Barker SJ, Tremper KK. The effect of carbon monoxide inhalation on pulse oximetry and transcutaneous PO_2. *Anesthesiology* 1987;66:677–679.

Buckley RG, Aks SE, Esham JL et al. The pulse oximetry gap in carbon monoxide intoxication. *Ann Emerg Med* 1994;24:252–255.

Gonzalez A, Gomez-Arnau J, Pensado A. Carboxyhemoglobin and pulse oximetry. *Anesthesiology* 1990;73:573.

Hampson NB. Pulse oximetry in severe carbon monoxide poisoning. *Chest* 1998;114:1036–1041.

Vegfors M, Lennmarken C. Carboxyhaemoglobinaemia and pulse oximetry. *Br J Anaesth* 1991;66:625–626.

(nonoccluded) airways due to bronchial obstruction leading to volutrauma and barotrauma of the unaffected lung segments. Furthermore, the release of inflammatory mediators from the direct lung injury causes bronchospasm, and in cases of significant nitric oxide release, there may be loss of hypoxic pulmonary vasoconstriction that increases the shunt fraction and worsens hypoxia.

Diffuse alveolar damage and lung capillary endothelial injury (answer A) is the primary pathophysiology seen in patients who develop ARDS; however, patients with inhalation injury have a similar injury to their lungs like ARDS, but this is not the primary pathophysiology seen after inhalation injury. In addition, inhalation injury can affect the airways from the nasopharynx down to the alveoli, which is something that does not happen in ARDS. Be aware that patients with inhalation injury may progress to ARDS and may present clinically in a similar fashion; however, the timeframe described in the previous scenario would be a little too quick for ARDS to occur. Keeping this in mind, as well as the bronchoscopy finding, ventilator-associated pneumonia is not likely in this case.

There are some similarities in the clinical presentation of pulmonary embolism and progression of inhalation injury, which include increased alveolar dead space and hypoxemia with associated ventilation-perfusion mismatching and intrapulmonary shunts. However, patients with pulmonary embolism are frequently hypocapnic versus patients with inhalation injury typically develop hypercapnia. In addition, the change in the patient's condition regarding developing hypoxia and hypercapnia happened quite quickly after admission and this would be an uncommon event with an incidence of 1.2% in patients admitted to the ICU based upon a study by Pannucci et al. in 2011.

16. ANSWER: B

After inhalation injury, there is a large increase in the amount of blood flow to the lungs. These changes in blood flow are associated with increases in bronchial microvascular permeability, allowing free movement of protein and small molecules. At the same time, the direct injury to the ciliated, bronchial columnar epithelium causes it to slough off and into the airways. The outcome of these two phenomena is the transudation of protein-rich fluid into the airways, which over the ensuing hours combines and hardens, forming casts. These casts typically occur in the distal terminal bronchioles and possibly in some of the smaller but more proximal bronchioles. These casts may completely occlude the airways and subsequently cause atelectasis of alveoli. The final result is development of ventilation-perfusion mismatching causing hypoxia and hypercapnia. In addition, these patients could develop secondary lung injury as a result of developing "preferential"

REFERENCES

Barrow RE, Morris SE, Basadre JO et al. Selective permeability changes in the lungs and airways of sheep after toxic smoke inhalation. *J Appl Physiol* 1990;68:2165–2170.

Cancio LC. Airway management and smoke inhalation injury in the burn patient. *Clin Plast Surg* 2009;36(4):555–567.

Cox RA, Burke AS, Soejima K et al. Airway obstruction in sheep with burn and smoke inhalation injuries. *Am J Respir Cell Mol Biol* 2003;29(3 Pt 1):295–302.

Dries DJ, Endorf FW. Inhalation injury: epidemiology, pathology, treatment strategies. *Scand J Trauma Resusc Emerg Med* 2013;21:31.

Herndon DN, Traber LD, Linares H et al. Etiology of the pulmonary pathophysiology associated with inhalation injury. *Resuscitation* 1986;14:43–59.

Pannucci CJ, Osborne NH, Wahl WL. Venous thromboembolism in thermally injured patients: analysis of the national burn repository. *J Burn Care Res* 2011;32(1):6–12.

Pulmonary embolism. https://emedicine.medscape.com/article/300901-overview#a2. Accessed on April 29, 2018.

Traber DL, Herndon DN, Enkhbaatar P et al. The pathophysiology of inhalation injury. In Herndon DN, ed. *Total burn care,* 4th edition. London: WB Saunders; 2012, pp. 219–228.

7.

SEDATION, PAIN MANAGEMENT, AND PHARMACOLOGY

Sophie Samuel and Jennifer Cortes

QUESTIONS

1. A 59-year-old female with no significant past medical history who presents to the emergency department (ED) with severe shortness of breath, tachypnea, and altered mental status is intubated for hypoxic respiratory failure. Chest radiograph is shown below. Vital signs while on fentanyl 100 mcg/hr, norepinephrine 0.75 mcg/kg per minute, and vasopressin 0.03 units/minute are as follows:

Heart rate (HR): 124 bpm
Blood pressure (BP): 129/84 mm Hg
Respiratory rate (RR): 26 breaths/minute (on
   mechanical ventilation)
Temperature: 102.1° F

The patient is admitted to the intensive care unit (ICU) with metabolic acidosis. During initial assessment of the patient, she is found to have a Behavioral Pain Score (BPS) score of 3 and a Richmond Agitation and Sedation Scale (RASS) score of +2. Which one of the following is the BEST sedative to initiate on admission?

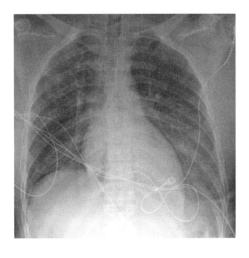

A. Propofol
B. Dexmedetomidine
C. Hydromorphone
D. Midazolam

2. On day 2 of hospitalization, the the same patient as in question 1 remains in septic shock and is now experiencing multiple-organ failure, including acute kidney injury and acute liver failure, and severe acute respiratory distress syndrome (ARDS), with a PaO_2/FiO_2 ratio of 99. The patient is made prone and needs to be paralyzed. What is the MOST appropriate paralytic to initiate?

A. Succinylcholine
B. Rocuronium
C. Vecuronium
D. Cisatracurium

3. On ICU day 13, in the same patient as in questions 1 and 2, the ARDS, septic shock, and multiple-organ failure have resolved. She cannot be extubated due to agitation. During rounds, she has a RASS score of +2 and BPS score of 4, and she nearly self-extubates despite orientation and encouragement from staff and family. The Confusion Assessment Method for the ICU (CAM-ICU) is positive, and she is deemed to have hyperactive delirium. Which of the following is the BEST intervention?

A. Quetiapine
B. Rivastigmine
C. Midazolam
D. Haloperidol

4. A 26-year-old male is transferred to the ICU from an outside hospital after ingestion of 30 sertraline 50-mg tablets approximately 6 hours ago. He is experiencing altered mental status with a Glasgow Coma Scale (GCS)

score of 10, diaphoresis, and muscle rigidity. His vital signs are as follows:

HR: 92 beats/minute
BP: 168/89 mm Hg
RR: 18 breaths/minute
Temperature: 101.4° F

Which of the following are the MOST appropriate intervention?

A. Activated charcoal
B. Ampoule of sodium bicarbonate
C. Cyproheptadine
D. Lorazepam

5. A 19-year-old female is "found down" in her dorm room by her roommate with an empty bottle of amitriptyline next to her. She was transported to the ED by emergency medical services (EMS) and intubated en route. The roommate reports that she last saw the patient normal the previous night and doesn't know how many pills were in the bottle. On physical examination, she has a GSC score of 5 with dry mucous membranes. Her vital signs are as follows:

HR: 114 bpm
BP: 111/68 mm Hg
RR: 16 breaths/minute (on mechanical ventilation)
Temperature: 100.8° F

ECG reveals sinus tachycardia with a QRS of 129 milliseconds. Which of the following is the MOST appropriate initial therapy?

A. 0.9% sodium chloride bolus
B. Sodium bicarbonate
C. Magnesium sulfate
D. Propafenone

6. A patient is transferred to the ICU from the ED with a diagnosis of bipolar disorder. He has been managed by his psychiatrist for 15 years, and his medication reconciliation form demonstrates compliance with his medications up to this point. Which of the following is the MOST likely lab finding?

A. Leukocytopenia
B. Hypernatremia
C. Thrombocytosis
D. Hypokalemia

7. A 44-year-old male with a past medical history of glucose-6-phosphate dehydrogenase (G6PD) deficiency presents to the ED with complaints of shortness of breath, hemoptysis, night sweats, and weight loss. He was released from prison 6 months ago and has a pattern of known drug abuse. On physical examination, he is found to have oral thrush and complains of difficulty swallowing that limits his ability to eat.

Which of the following is the MOST appropriate therapy for the treatment his dysphagia?

A. Nystatin
B. Micafungin
C. Fluconazole
D. Amphotericin B

8. In the same patient as question 7), the chest radiograph reveals a cavitary lesion, and sputum is sent for acid-fast bacilli smear microscopy along with a nucleic acid amplification test (NAAT-TB). In 48 hours, the microbiology lab calls with results of a positive NAAT. Which of the following medications is NOT part of the initial treatment of pulmonary *Mycobacterium tuberculosis*?

A. Ethambutol
B. Isoniazid
C. Clarithromycin
D. Pyrazinamide

9. The same patient as questions 7 and 8, is found to be HIV positive with a viral load of 88,000 copies/mL and an absolute CD4 count of 164. Which of the following medications is MOST appropriate for primary prevention of opportunistic infections?

A. Sulfamethoxazole-trimethoprim
B. Azithromycin
C. Dapsone
D. Atovaquone

Questions 10 to 12 pertain to the following case:

A 53-year-old woman with a history of hypertension and hyperlipidemia presents with sudden-onset headache and stupor. In the ED, she is minimally responsive to pain and has a flaccid left arm and increased tone in her lower extremities; she then requires intubation. Noncontrast head computed tomography (CT) is completed on admission and shown here.

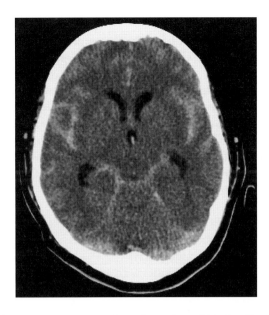

10. The patient is transferred to the ICU for further management and placement of an external ventricular drain (EVD). Which prophylactic antibiotic should be used before placing an EVD?

A. Cefazolin
B. Cefepime
C. Ciprofloxacin
D. Piperacillin-tazobactam

11. The same patient has now been hospitalized in the ICU for 3 days. Her EVD is still present, and in the intervening time she has required endotracheal intubation and mechanical ventilation because of a poor neurological exam. The chest radiograph is shown here. She has temperature of 38.4° C, white blood cell (WBC) count of 19 × 10³ cells/mm³, and purulent sputum. You decide to perform bronchoalveolar lavage (BAL) of the lung to assess for ventilator-associated pneumonia (VAP).

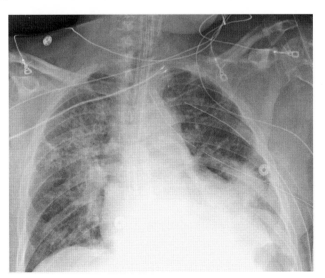

Which is the MOST likely causative pathogen of this patient's VAP?

A. Methicillin-resistant *Staphylococcus aureus* (MRSA)
B. *Pseudomonas aeruginosa*
C. *Streptococcus pneumoniae*
D. *Legionella pneumophila*

12. Which empiric antibiotic regimen is BEST for the likely causative pathogen of the patient's suspected VAP?

A. Ceftriaxone
B. Vancomycin
C. Piperacillin-tazobactam
D. Cefepime

Questions 13 and 14 pertain to the following case:

A 37-year-old man has a past medical history significant for quadriplegia since the age of 28 following injuries sustained in a motor vehicle collision. He has no known drug allergies. He reports foul odor from a sacral wound on dressing changes and overall feeling unwell. Vitals on admission include the following:

HR: 112 bpm
BP: 98/64 mm Hg
RR: 18 breaths/minute
Temperature: 38.7° C

Physical examination reveals a large foul-smelling sacral decubitus ulcer, and laboratory evaluation reveals WBC 18.7 × 10³ cells/mm³. Chart review discloses a history of extended-spectrum beta-lactamase (ESBL)-producing *Enterobacter aerogenes* and MRSA from the wound.

13. Which one of the following combination regimens is BEST to administer at this time?

A. Ceftriaxone and daptomycin
B. Cefepime
C. Piperacillin-tazobactam and vancomycin
D. Meropenem and daptomycin

14. The patient is taken to the surgery for operative debridement. Culture results on postoperative day 3 are reported here:

Acinetobacter baumannii		
Antibiotic	Minimum Inhibitory Concentration	Interpretation
Ampicillin-sulbactam	>32/16	R
Ceftriaxone	>64	R
Cefepime	>32	R

Gentamicin	>16	R
Levofloxacin	>8	R
Meropenem	4	I
Piperacillin-tazobactam	>128/4	R
Tobramycin	>16	R

Which one of the following is the BEST antibiotic strategy until additional susceptibility results are available?

A. Continue with meropenem
B. Change to amikacin
C. Add colistin to meropenem
D. Result is likely contamination

15. A 65-year-old woman admitted to the surgical ICU after being taken to an operating room emergently for partial bowel resection with primary anastomosis for mid to small bowel necrosis and perforation secondary to severe peripheral vascular disease. The surgical team reported significant peritoneal contamination with evidence of peritonitis. The patient received perioperative cefazolin and metronidazole. Which empiric antibiotic regimen would be MOST appropriate?

A. Piperacillin-tazobactam
B. Cefazolin
C. Ertapenem
D. Metronidazole

Question 16 and 17 pertain to the following case:

A 27-year-old 77-kg, 67-inch male presents to your hospital ED with headache, altered mental status, lethargy, and a temperature of 39° C. CT and magnetic resonance imaging (MRI) suggest encephalitis. Lumbar puncture (LP) is performed, and routine diagnostic lab tests are ordered on his cerebral spinal fluid (CSF). Complete blood count, basic metabolic panel, and blood cultures are pending.

16. What is the BEST regimen to initiate as empiric therapy?

A. Ceftriaxone and linezolid
B. Ceftriaxone, linezolid, and acyclovir
C. Ceftriaxone, vancomycin, and acyclovir
D. Cefepime, vancomycin, and acyclovir

17. The patient's CSF panel is as follows:

Opening pressure: 43 mm Hg
WBC count: 3500 cells/mm³ (24% neutrophils)

Protein: 178 mg/dL
Glucose: 62 mg/dL (serum glucose 100 mg/dL)
Red blood cell (RBC) count: 1000 cells/mm³

Bacterial antigen and CSF Gram stain were negative. Results of the remaining lab tests came back normal except for elevated serum WBC count of 14 × 10³ cells/ mm³. A CSF herpes simplex virus (HSV) polymerase chain reaction (PCR) test is positive, and blood cultures are negative. Which of the following is the BEST treatment regimen?

A. Oral (PO) acyclovir for 14 days
B. Intravenous (IV) acyclovir for 7 days
C. IV acyclovir for 14 days
D. Continue antibiotics with acyclovir

18. Following a business trip to Idaho, a middle-aged man with past medical history of obesity, type 2 diabetes (controlled with diet), and reflux disease presents with hyperglycemia, fever, confusion, abdominal pain, and rash. He takes pantoprazole daily; otherwise, his family denies any other chronic pharmacotherapy. On physical examination, a papule (shown here; image courtesy of Richard Jahan-Tigh, MD, MS) is noted on his right thigh.

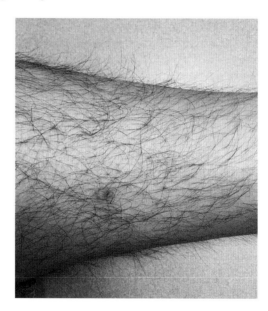

Which of the following is the MOST appropriate treatment?

A. Linezolid
B. Doxycycline
C. Amoxicillin
D. Discontinue pantoprazole

19. A 28-year-old female G_1P_{1001} is involved as a passenger in a motor vehicle collision with rollover. She is found to have a fractured humerus and left lung contusion and is admitted to the ICU for management. Abdominal CT shows no acute abnormalities, and FAST examination is negative. The bedside nurse reports that she complains of pruritis ani, abdominal pain, and nausea and had been intending to see her primary physician for her abdominal symptoms. Which of the following would be the MOST appropriate initial treatment?

A. Mebendazole
B. Ciprofloxacin
C. Cefazolin
D. Vancomycin

ANSWERS

1: Answer: D

Although the 2013 Pain, Sedation, Delirium guidelines recommend non–benzodiazepine-based sedation as the preferred type of sedation, this patient should not receive propofol or dexmedetomidine because she is in septic shock and both medications have a high incidence of hypotension and can increase vasopressor requirements. Hydromorphone is not appropriate because the patient is already receiving analgosedation, and her current BPS score is 3, which is indicative of no pain. Additionally, while hydromorphone may be used as a sedative agent, it is not a hypnotic agent, which may prevent a patient with pulmonary disease from tolerating mechanical ventilation. Additionally, because the duration of action of hydromorphone is 3 to 4 hours, the pharmacokinetics of such a drug lend it to accumulation. The BPS was first described in 2001 and includes a summative score of the following factors, with a total score range of 3 to 12:

ITEM	DESCRIPTION	SCORE
Facial expression	Relaxed	1
	Partially tightened (e.g., brow lowering)	2
	Fully tightened (e.g., eyelid closing)	3
	Grimacing	4
Upper limbs	No movement	1
	Partially bent	2
	Fully bent with finger flexion	3
	Permanently retracted	4
Compliance with ventilation	Tolerating movement	1
	Coughing but tolerating ventilation for most of the time	2
	Fighting ventilator	3
	Unable to control ventilation	4

Midazolam is a benzodiazepine, and benzodiazepine-based sedation, compared with non–benzodiazepine-based sedation, is associated with a shorter ICU length of stay and duration of mechanical ventilation. However, a landmark trial by Riker et al. failed to demonstrate a statistically significant increase in ICU length of stay when midazolam sedation was compared with dexmedetomidine sedation, but there was decrease in time to extubation. Midazolam remains an option for the acute treatment of agitation in mechanically ventilated patients given its clinical efficacy and hemodynamic profile. If a benzodiazepine is required, the smallest possible dose should be administered that will achieve the intended clinical outcome.

Midazolam has a benzepine ring that is commonly suspended in the preservative benzyl alcohol. In an acidic environment, the benzepine ring opens, facilitating solvency in water. As soon as parenteral midazolam encounters a neutral pH, the benzepine ring closes, and midazolam becomes lipid soluble. Parenteral midazolam is prepared with hydrochloric acid to achieve appropriate solubility. Benzyl alcohol toxicity has been associated with anion gap metabolic acidosis, but this is not frequently seen in adults receiving midazolam. The benzodiazepines diazepam and lorazepam, when administered as an IV infusion, may lead to an anion gap metabolic acidosis because they have significant quantities (50–80% volume) of propylene glycol as a diluent; propylene glycol toxicity is commonly manifested by seizures, renal failure, and central nervous system depression.

Keywords: Specialized areas; Pharmacology (indications, contraindications, and complications); Sedative-hypnotics

REFERENCES

Barr J, Fraser GL, Puntillo K et al. Clinical practice guidelines for the management of pain, agitation, and delirium in adult patients in the intensive care unit. *Crit Care Med.* 2013;41:263–306.

Fraser GL, Devlin JW, Worby CP et al. Benzodiazepine-based sedation for mechanically ventilated, critically ill adults: a systematic review and meta-analysis of randomized trials. *Crit Care Med* 2013;41:S30–S38.

Payen JF, Bru O, Bosson JL et al. Assessing pain in critically ill sedated patients by using a behavioral pain scale. *Crit Care Med* 2001;29(12):2258–2263.

Riker RR, Shehabi Y, Bokesch PM et al.; SEDCOM (Safety and Efficacy of Dexmedetomidine Compared with Midazolam) Study Group. Dexmedetomidine vs midazolam for sedation of critically ill patients: a randomized trial. *JAMA* 2009;301(5):489–499.

Shehab N, Lewis CL, Streetman DD, Donn SM. Exposure to the pharmaceutical excipients benzyl alcohol and propylene glycol among critically ill neonates. *Pediatr Crit Care Med* 2009;10(2):256–259.

2. ANSWER: D

Succinylcholine is a depolarizing paralytic that is used in single doses as part of rapid-sequence intubation or as intermittent administration. Additionally, succinylcholine may cause vagal stimulation and therefore lead to bradycardia, though infrequently. Rocuronium (aminosteroid), vecuronium (aminosteroid), and cisatracurium (benzylisoquinoline) are non-depolarizing paralytics that can be administered as continuous infusions. Vecuronium and rocuronium undergo renal or hepatic elimination and therefore are affected by acute renal and hepatic failure. Because this patient is in multiple-organ failure, cisatracurium would be the most appropriate paralytic agent because elimination is dependent on Hoffman elimination.

Chiari I malformation (CIM) is a source of significant morbidity in the ICU population, and while neuromuscular blockade administration (aminosteroid or benzylisoquinoline type) is a risk factor, there are no studies evaluating a difference in bolus versus infusion therapy for developing CIM. Other risk factors for developing CIM include hyperglycemia, corticosteroids, catecholamines, aminoglycoside antibiotics, parenteral nutrition, vasopressors, and advanced age.

Keywords: Specialized areas; Pharmacology (indications, contraindications, and complications); Neuromuscular blocking drugs

REFERENCES

Lacomis D, Petrella JT, Giuliani MJ. Causes of neuromuscular weakness in the intensive care unit: a study of ninety-two patients. *Muscle Nerve* 1998;21(5):610–617.

Murray M, DeBlock H, Erstad B et al. Clinical practice guidelines for sustained neuromuscular blockade in the adult critically ill patient. *Crit Care Med* 2016;44:2079–2103.

Papazian L, Forel JM, Gacouin A et al. Neuromuscular blockers in early acute respiratory distress syndrome. *N Engl J Med* 2010;363:1107–1116.

3. ANSWER: A

There is no definitive pharmacologic therapy for the treatment of ICU delirium, although it occurs in up to 30% of hospitalized patients and is associated with increased morbidity and mortality. Atypical antipsychotics have been evaluated in a few studies, but only one study comparing quetiapine to placebo showed a difference in the duration of delirium. The Society of Critical Care Medicine guidelines suggest that atypical antipsychotics may reduce the duration of delirium, but this is a recommendation with low or very low evidence. Despite weak evidence, atypical antipsychotics may be administered to patients with hyperactive delirium but should be avoided in patients with risk for significant adverse events (e.g., torsades de pointes).

Impaired cholinergic neurotransmission has been demonstrated to have an important role in the development of delirium, and serum anticholinergic activity has been found to be elevated in patients with delirium. Additionally, drugs with anticholinergic effects (e.g., glycopyrrolate) have been known to cause delirium, especially in elderly patients. Nonetheless, rivastigmine is not an appropriate therapy for the treatment of delirium because it has been demonstrated to trend toward a longer duration of delirium; in fact, the trial evaluating this application of rivastigmine was terminated early because of an association with higher mortality. Benzodiazepines should be avoided unless patients are experiencing alcohol or benzodiazepine withdrawal due to increased duration of mechanical ventilation and are associated with precipitating more delirium.

While there is no published evidence showing a benefit of haloperidol for the treatment of delirium above other pharmacologic agents, it is the most frequently prescribed neuroleptic agent in the ICU. Haloperidol must be used with caution because it has a variety of adverse effects, including dystonias, neuroleptic malignant syndrome, extrapyramidal effects, and the most worrisome—torsades de pointes. It should not be given to patients with electrocardiographic evidence of prolonged QT interval. QT interval daily measurements are recommended when haloperidol is initiated.

Keywords: Specialized areas; Pharmacology (indications, contraindications, and complications); Antipsychotics

REFERENCES

Barr J, Fraser GL, Puntillo K et al. Clinical practice guidelines for the management of pain, agitation, and delirium in adult patients in the intensive care unit. *Crit Care Med* 2013;41:263–306.

Devlin JW, Roberts RJ, Fong JJ et al. Efficacy and safety of quetiapine in critically ill patients with delirium: a prospective, multicenter, randomized, double-blind, placebo-controlled pilot study. *Crit Care Med* 2010;38:419–427.

van Ejik MM, Roes KC, Honing ML et al. Effect of rivastigmine as an adjunct to usual care with haloperidol on duration of delirium and mortality in critically ill patients: a multicenter, double-blind, placebo-controlled randomized trial. *Lancet* 2010;376:1829–1837.

4. Answer: D

Serotonin syndrome, seizures, and cardiac conduction abnormalities are serious adverse effects of selective serotonin reuptake inhibitor (SSRI) overdose; while rare, these clinical findings are more associate with venlafaxine or citalopram. More severe complications following SSRI overdose may include a constellation of symptoms and signs referred to as serotonin syndrome; this may follow SSRI or selective serotonin-norepinephrine reuptake inhibitor (SNRI) overdose. This disorder results from excessive stimulation of central and peripheral serotonin receptors and is depicted by a triad of altered mentation, autonomic dysfunction, and neuromuscular hyperactivity. Signs and symptoms range from mild to very severe and include delirium, diaphoresis, diarrhea, hyperthermia, tremor, hyperreflexia, muscular rigidity, and clonus. Laboratory findings are generally nonspecific, including findings such as elevated white blood cell count, creatine phosphokinase, and hepatic transaminases. Serotonin syndrome tends to develop within 6 hours of the poisoning event.

Therapy for SSRI (and incidentally SNRI) overdose is primarily supportive, with the first and most accessible therapy being the discontinuation of the offending drugs. Benzodiazepines are administered as first-line agents for agitation and muscle rigidity. Activated charcoal is effective only when administered within 1 hour of ingestion and is excluded as an option here given the timing of the patient's admission. Since the patient presented 6 hours after ingestion, he may actually be harmed because he is experiencing altered mental status and at increased risk for aspiration. Sodium bicarbonate should not be administered at this time because the patient is not experiencing QRS or QT prolongation. However, in the setting of tricyclic antidepressant (TCA) overdose, sodium bicarbonate may be useful in treating QRS or QT prolongation.

Cyproheptadine is administered as an adjunct to benzodiazepines for agitation and muscle rigidity, but a loading dose of 12 mg should be administered. Use of cyproheptadine, a serotonin receptor antagonist, is normally reserved for serotonin syndrome or severe cases of overdose. Given the rarity of its necessity for administration, there are limited data on the use of cyproheptadine.

Keywords: Specialized areas; Pharmacology (indications, contraindications, and complications); Antidepressants; SSRIs

Propafenone is a class 1C antiarrhythmic drug and primarily serves to block open sodium channels and slow conduction; it has a role, as dose flecainide, in treating widened QRS complex tachyarrhythmias because it slowly dissociates from the sodium receptor during diastole, thereby making it more effective at higher rates of tachycardia. In this case, because the patient experiencing TCA overdose, it would not be an appropriate therapy.

Hyperthermia is a manifestation of the anticholinergic effects of TCAs; therefore, magnesium is not the appropriate initial therapy. While it cannot be used to treat pyrexia, magnesium sulfate is commonly used to *facilitate* hypothermia. The proposed mechanism for supporting hypothermia is inhibition of shivering and increased vasodilation; additionally, improved post-hypothermia neurological outcomes after magnesium administration have been observed in clinical trials.

Keywords: Specialized areas; Pharmacology (indications, contraindications, and complications); Antidepressants; Tricyclic antidepressants

REFERENCES

Boyer EW, Shannon M. The serotonin syndrome. *N Engl J Med* 2005;352:1112–1120.
Reilly TH, Kirk MA. Atypical antipsychotics and newer antidepressants. *Emerg Med Clin North Am* 2007;25:477–497.
Sun-Edelstein C, Tepper SJ, Shapiro RE. Drug-induced serotonin syndrome: a review. *Expert Opin Drug Saf* 2008;7:587–596.

REFERENCES

Alapat PM, Zimmerman JL. *Chest* 2008;133:1006–1013.
Blackman K, Brown SG, Wilkes GJ. Plasma alkalinization for tricyclic antidepressant toxicity: a systematic review. *Emerg Med* 2001;13:204–210.
Pimentel L, Trommer L. Cyclic antidepressant overdoses. *Emerg Clin North Am* 2007;25:477–497.
Zweifler RM, Voorhees ME, Mahmood MA, Parnell M. Magnesium sulfate increases the rate of hypothermia via surface cooling and improves comfort. *Stroke* 2004;35(10):2331–2334.

5. ANSWER: B

Impaired cardiac conduction as a result of sodium channel blockade is a manifestation of TCA overdose. Sodium bicarbonate should be administered in patients with a QRS great than 100 or impaired cardiac conduction who present following TCA overdose. The sodium load can overcome the TCA blockade of the sodium channels by increasing the electrochemical gradient. In addition, alkalization of the blood may increase protein binding of the TCA, therefore decreasing the amount of free drug. Additionally, by causing drug ionization, the alkalization process may serve to reduce the affinity of TCAs for the myocardial sodium channel receptor. Finally, by increasing the serum sodium concentration, sodium channel blockade may be overcome.

The patient is currently not hypotensive or in shock; therefore, a bolus of IV fluids is not indicated at this time. Furthermore, sodium chloride will not serve to alkalinize the blood given its pH of 5.5 and would therefore inhibit the process described previously.

6. ANSWER: B

As a second-line agent, lithium use can result in many adverse effects, with the most common including nausea, tremor, thirst, polyuria, weight gain, loose stools, and cognitive impairment. Acute worsening of these symptoms may indicate lithium toxicity. Over the long term, lithium can adversely affect the kidneys and thyroid gland. Chronic lithium ingestion can cause resistance to antidiuretic hormone (ADH) by accumulating in the principal cells of the collecting duct. The accumulation interferes with the ability of ADH to increase water permeability, leading to nephrogenic diabetes insipidus. A potential mechanism for this is that lithium may increase expression of cyclo-oxyenase-2 and increase urinary prostaglandin excretion. Prostaglandin E_2 induces lysosomal degradation of aquaporin-2 water channels and decreases the ability to concentrate the urine. In addition, cardiac rhythm disturbances have been described; these almost always occur in patients with preexisting cardiac disease. By extension, hypernatremia would be the expected laboratory abnormality in this presentation.

Lithium is known to been associated with leukocytosis with a reversible 2×10^9/L increase in WBC count at the initiation of therapy. In this case, diabetes insipidus is more likely given the chronic nature of this patient's presentation. While lithium does not cause changes in platelet count, escitalopram (and SSRIs in general) has been shown to mildly decrease platelet count. Depression and antidepressants are thought to affect platelets because neurons and platelets share similar serotonin profiles, and changes in 5-HT2A receptor and the 5-HT transporter (5-HTT) of platelets can act as a surrogate biomarker to indicate depression. SSRIs have inhibitory effects on 5-HTT and serotonin receptors of platelets, thereby diminishing platelet aggregation. Because this patient has bipolar disorder, there is not an indication for SSRIs, making this answer a distractor.

Although checking serum chemistries is common when lithium therapy is initiated, it is not indicated after the patient is stabilized or after the first year of therapy. These labs are primarily used to assess creatinine and blood urea nitrogen. There are not expected potassium changes with lithium therapy.

Keywords: Specialized areas, Pharmacology (indications, contraindications, and complications); Antidepressants; Lithium

REFERENCES

Behl Tapan, Kotwani A, Kaur, I, Goel H. Mechanisms of prolonged lithium therapy-induced nephrogenic diabetes insipidus. *Eur J Pharmacol* 2015;755:27–33.

Lithium: a review of pharmacology, clinical uses, and toxicity. *Eur J Pharmacol* 2014;740:464–473.

Song HR, Jung YE, Wang HR et al. Platelet count alterations associated with escitalopram, venlafaxine and bupropion in depressive patients. *Psychiatry Clin Neurosci* 2012;66(5):457–459.

7. ANSWER: C

Oropharyngeal candidiasis with dysphagia is an indicator of esophageal candidiasis. Esophageal candidiasis should be treated with systemic therapy; therefore, nystatin is not an appropriate treatment option. Of note, because nystatin contains sucrose, its prolonged use can lead to dental caries. The treatment of choice for esophageal candidiasis is fluconazole. Fluconazole has an 80 to 90% effectiveness rate and was demonstrated to be superior to other azole derivatives by three randomized control trials. Echinocandins (caspofungin, micafungin, and anidulafungin) are associated with higher esophageal

disease relapse rates compared with fluconazole. As a class of antifungals, echinocandins are notable in that they were the first antifungals to target the cell wall. Amphotericin is an effective treatment for esophageal candidiasis but should be used as an alternative agent secondary to its potential for nephrotoxicity.

Keywords: Specialized areas; Pharmacology (indications, contraindications, and complications); Antimicrobials; Antifungal

REFERENCE

Pappas PG, Kaufman CA, Andes DR et al. Clinical practice guidelines for the management of candidiasis. *Clin Infect Dis* 2016;62:e1–e50.

8. ANSWER: C

The preferred regimen for tuberculosis that is not known to be drug resistant is 2 months of isoniazid, rifampin, pyrazinamide, and ethambutol followed by 4 months of isoniazid and rifampin. Clarithromycin is included in the treatment regimen for *Mycobacterium avium* complex but not *M. tuberculosis*.

Keywords: Specialized areas; Pharmacology (indications, contraindications, and complications); Antimicrobials; Antibiotics; tuberculosis

REFERENCES

Nahid P, Dorman, SE, Alipanah N et al. Official American Thoracic Society/Centers for Disease Control and Prevention/Infectious Diseases Society of America clinical practice guidelines: treatment of drug-susceptible tuberculosis. *CID* 2016;63:e147–e195.

Panel on Opportunistic Infections in HIV-Infected Adults and Adolescents. Guidelines for the prevention and treatment of opportunistic infections in HIV-infected adults and adolescents: recommendations from the Centers for Disease Control and Prevention, the National Institutes of Health, and the HIV Medicine Association of the Infectious Diseases Society of America. Available at http://aidsinfo.nih.gov/contentfiles/lvguidelines/adult_oi.pdf. Accessed December 10, 2017.

9. ANSWER: D

Atovaquone is the appropriate prophylactic agent to start because this patient is at increased risk for developing *Pneumocystis* pneumonia with a CD4 count of less than 200. Azithromycin is initiated for prophylaxis against *M. avium* complex when the absolute CD4 count is less than 50. Drugs such as dapsone and sulfamethoxazole increase the likelihood of cell hemolysis in patients with G6PD deficiency. Recall that G6PD is an important enzyme for maintaining red cell wall structural integrity. This is related to the fact that blood cells contain relatively high concentrations of reduced glutathione; glutathione functions as an intracellular reducing agent, thereby protecting the cell against oxidant injury. In patients with G6PD deficiency, acute hemolysis can occur with oxidant injury from medications, acute illnesses, and certain foods. Drugs that lead to hemolysis in this condition interact with hemoglobin and oxygen, leading to the formation of H_2O_2, among other oxidizing radicals, within RBCs. When these oxidants accumulate inside of these RBCs, hemoglobin and other proteins are oxidized because there is insufficient glutathione, leading to cell lysis. A comprehensive list of common medications that may lead to hemolysis in G6PD deficiency is lengthy and can be found at https://www.g6pd.org/en/G6PDDeficiency/SafeUnsafe/DaEvitare_ISS-it.

Antibiotics that are contraindicated in G6PD deficiency include dapsone, nitrofurantoin (and related drugs), and primaquine. Common antibiotics that have been considered unsafe by at least one source but *could be* safe at therapeutic doses based on an updated review of the literature include the following:

Antimalarials	Chloroquine, mepacrine, quinine
Fluoroquinolones	Ciprofloxacin, levofloxacin, ofloxacin
Sulfonamides	Co-trimoxazole, trimethoprim-sulfamethoxazole
Antimicrobials	Chloramphenicol, furazolidone, isoniazid, mepacrine

Therefore, administration of dapsone and sulfamethoxazole should be avoided in this patient because of his history of G6PD deficiency.

Keywords: Specialized areas; Pharmacology (indications, contraindications, and complications); Antimicrobials; Antibiotics; Other

REFERENCES

Panel on Opportunistic Infections in HIV-Infected Adults and Adolescents. Guidelines for the prevention and treatment of opportunistic infections in HIV-infected adults and adolescents: recommendations from the Centers for Disease Control and Prevention, the National Institutes of Health, and the HIV Medicine Association of the Infectious Diseases Society of America. Available at http://aidsinfo.nih.gov/contentfiles/lvguidelines/adult_oi.pdf. Accessed on December 10, 2017.

Youngster I, Arcavi L, Schechmaster R et al. Medications and glucose-6-phosphate dehydrogenase deficiency: an evidence based review. *Drug Saf* 2010;33:713–726.

10. ANSWER: A

This patient is presenting with subarachnoid hemorrhage, as evidenced by the CT scan presented, as well as hydrocephalus, as evidenced by the plan to place an EVD. Surgical site infections (SSIs) are a common cause of healthcare-associated infections. Depending on the type of procedure performed, the Centers for Disease Control and Prevention (CDC) established criteria that define surgical site infection as infection related to an operative procedure that arises at or near the surgical incision within 30 to 90 days of the procedure. EVDs are used as a method of diverting CSF out of the cranium. Soft tissue infections and ventriculitis are the most common ventriculostomy-related infections. Reported EVD infection rates range from 0 to 32%, but an average of about 10% or less is the general consensus for the underlying rate. Before placement of the EVD, it has been routine to initiate antibiotics. However, data regarding the use of prophylactic antibiotics throughout the duration of insertion of EVDs are inconclusive at present. Gram-positive organisms are classically associated with ventriculitis, as are some reported gram-negative bacteria, but these were probably related to a nosocomial colonization caused by prolonged hospital stay. Cefazolin is an appropriate choice for prevention of drain-related infections given its narrow-spectrum coverage of specific organisms.

Keywords: Specialized areas; Pharmacology (indications, contraindications, and complications); Antimicrobials; Antibiotics; Gram-negative organisms

REFERENCES

See question 12.

11. ANSWER: C

This patient has early-onset VAP. She does not have risk factors for infection with multidrug-resistant organisms (MDROs). VAP is defined as hospital-acquired pneumonia arising more than 48 hours after endotracheal intubation. It is further classified by the CDC as a ventilator-associated event and an infection-related ventilator-associated complication. VAP is usually caused by bacterial pathogens; the infection can be monomicrobial or polymicrobial in nature but is seldom caused by viral or fungal pathogens. The diagnosis of VAP is classified into two categories: early onset (less than 5 days from hospitalization) or late onset (5 days or more from hospitalization). Early-onset hospital-acquired pneumonia and VAP are usually community-associated organisms, including *Haemophilus influenzae*, methicillin-sensitive *S. aureus* (MSSA), *S. pneumoniae*, and enteric gram-negative bacilli. Atypical bacteria, such as *L. pneumophila*, do not commonly cause VAP, and it is not necessary to add antibiotic coverage for this class of organisms, although consideration should be given if there is a poor response to initial therapy. Late-onset VAP is often associated with MDRO infection. Patients with early-onset VAP and risk factors for MDRO should be managed similarly to patients with late-onset VAP (Box 7.1).

Keywords: Specialized areas; Pharmacology (indications, contraindications, and complications); Antimicrobials; Antimicrobial resistance

REFERENCES

See question 12.

12. ANSWER: A

Ceftriaxone is a reasonable agent for empiric management of early-onset VAP because it has activity against common pathogens. Broad-spectrum antibiotics, such as piperacillin-tazobactam and cefepime, would provide adequate coverage but would result in an unnecessary breadth of antibiotic exposure. In patients with suspected VAP, empiric antibiotic therapy should be initiated. To reduce the incidence of mortality, appropriate selection of antibiotic is critical. To decrease the likelihood of inappropriate therapy, empiric antibiotic selection should be based on multiple factors. First, timing of pneumonia from hospital admission can differentiate between early-onset and late-onset VAP because the pathogens involved in the disease

process are not the same. Regardless VAP onset, patients should be carefully evaluated for risk factors for MDROs. Despite current recommendations, it is strongly advised to select the antibiotic based on local antibiotic susceptibility patterns because of growing concern about antibiotic resistance. Antibiotic selection should include IV agents to achieve relevant lung concentrations related to pathogen minimum inhibitory concentration (MIC) and should be dosed optimally using evidence-based pharmacokinetic and pharmacodynamic principles.

Keywords: Specialized areas; Pharmacology (indications, contraindications, and complications); Antimicrobials; Antimicrobial resistance

REFERENCES

American Thoracic Society; Infectious Diseases Society of America. Guidelines for the management of adults with hospital-acquired, ventilator associated, and healthcare-associated pneumonia. *Am J Respir Crit Care Med* 2005;171:388–416.

Arabi Y, Memish ZA, Balkhy HH et al. Ventriculostomy-associated infections: incidence and risk factors. *Am J Infect Control* 2005;33(3):137–143.

Berríos-Torres SI, Umscheid CA, Bratzler DW et al. Centers for Disease Control and Prevention guideline for the prevention of surgical site infection, 2017. *JAMA Surg* 2017;152(8):784.

Blomstedt GC. Results of trimethoprim-sulfamethoxazole prophylaxis in ventriculostomy and shunting procedures. *J Neurosurg* 1985;62(5):694–697.

Dettenkofer M, Ebner W, Els T et al. Surveillance of nosocomial infections in a neurology intensive care unit. *J Neurol* 2001;248(11):959–64.

Dey M, Stadnik A, Riad F et al. Bleeding and infection with external ventricular drainage: a systematic review in comparison with adjudicated adverse events in the ongoing Clot Lysis Evaluating Accelerated Resolution of Intraventricular Hemorrhage Phase III (CLEAR-III IHV) trial. *Neurosurgery* 2015;76(3):291–300.

Klompas M, Branson R, Eichenwald EC et al. Strategies to prevent ventilator-associated pneumonia in acute care hospitals: 2014 update. *Infect Control Hosp Epidemiol* 2014;35:915–936.

Lyke KE, Obasanjo OO, Williams MA et al. Ventriculitis complicating use of intraventricular catheters in adult neurosurgical patients. *Clin Infect Dis* 2001;33(12):2028–2033.

Zabramski JM, Whiting D, Darouiche RO et al. Efficacy of antimicrobial-impregnated external ventricular drain catheters: a prospective, randomized, controlled trial. *J Neurosurg* 2003;98(4):725–730.

13. ANSWER: D

Because of the history of ESBL-producing Enterobacteriaceae, the drug of choice would be meropenem. Ceftriaxone, cefepime, and piperacillin-tazobactam would not be good choices to treat the ESBL-producing organism because of resistance and reports of clinical failure. Daptomycin and vancomycin both have activity against MRSA.

Keywords: Specialized areas; Pharmacology (indications, contraindications, and complications); Antimicrobials; Antibiotics; Gram-negative organisms

REFERENCES

See question 14.

14. ANSWER: C

The susceptibility panel reveals only intermediate susceptibility to meropenem; this alone is not a viable treatment option to avoid treatment failure. Treatment options for multidrug-resistant *Acinetobacter baumannii* are limited to tigecycline and polymyxins (i.e., colistin). Amikacin susceptibility is unknown in the case and therefore should not be included until further results are revealed.

Keywords: Specialized areas; Pharmacology (indications, contraindications, and complications); Antimicrobials; Antimicrobial resistance

REFERENCES

Kanj SS, Kanafani ZA. Current concepts in antimicrobial therapy against resistant gram-negative organisms: extended-spectrum beta-lactamase-producing Enterobacteriaceae, carbapenem-resistant Enterobacteriaceae, and multi-drug-resistant *Pseudomonas aeruginosa. Mayo Clin Proc* 2011;86:250–259.

Manchanda V, Sanchaita S, Singh NP. Multidrug resistant *Acinetobacter. J Glob Infect Dis* 2010;2:291–304.

Paterson DL, Bonomo RA. Extended-spectrum beta-lactamases: a clinical update. *Clin Micro Rev* 2005;18:657–686.

Pogue JM, Mann T, Barber KE et al. Carbapenem-resistant *Acinetobacter baumannii*: epidemiology, surveillance and management. *Expert Rev of Anti-infect Ther* 2013;11:383–393.

15. ANSWER: A

The patient presented with community acquired complicated intra-abdominal infection involving the middle small intestine. The common organisms involved with these complications include *Escherichia coli* and *Klebsiella* spp. A patient with severe disease should be broadly covered for presence of *P. aeruginosa* and enterococci. Piperacillin-tazobactam has empiric activity against these organisms. Anaerobic coverage is warranted if the distal small bowel and the large bowel are the sites of infection. This region is populated with anaerobic gram-negative and gram-positive organisms. Answers B and C do not have sufficiently broad coverage to include enterococci. and need for solely anaerobic coverage (with metronidazole) is not indicated in this case.

Keywords: Specialized areas; Pharmacology (indications, contraindications, and complications); Antimicrobials; Antibiotics,; Anaerobes

REFERENCES

Marshall JC, Innes M. Intensive care unit management of intra-abdominal infection. *Crit Care Med* 2003;31:2228–2237. (In-depth descriptive review of pathophysiology and management strategies of complicated intra-abdominal infection in critically ill patients.)

Solomkin JS, Mazuski JE, Bradley JS et al. Diagnosis and management of complicated intraabdominal infection in adults and children: guidelines by the Surgical Infection Society and the Infectious Diseases Society of America. *Clin Infect Dis* 2010;50:133–164.

16. ANSWER: C

While results are pending, empiric therapy for both bacterial and viral encephalitis should be initiated because of the MRI results. This patient is at risk for *Neisseria meningitidis* and *S. pneumoniae*. IV acyclovir should be started for management of the most likely cause of viral encephalitis, HSV. HSV-1 is the most common virus to cause sporadic encephalitis in the United State; it is responsible for about 90% of HSV encephalitis in adults and children; HSV-2 is the etiology for the other 10%. With a mortality rate of 70% when untreated, timely administration of acyclovir improves survival and outcomes, especially when introduced early in infection. Broad-spectrum antibiotics, such as linezolid and cefepime, would provide adequate coverage but would result in an unnecessary breadth of antibiotic exposure. Cefepime in particular would be reasonable for nosocomial infection, but not for community-acquired infection, which is implied in the stem.

Keywords: Specialized areas; Pharmacology (indications, contraindications, and complications); Antimicrobials; Antibiotics; Other

REFERENCES

See question 17.

17. ANSWER: C

HSV PCR, LP results, and radiologic evidence strongly confirm the diagnosis of HSV encephalitis. Because there is no strong indication of bacterial infection, antibiotics should be discontinued at this time. A 14-day course of acyclovir therapy is suggested in confirmed cased of HSV encephalitis. Dosing should be 10 mg/kg IV every 8 hours in the setting of good renal function. The patient should also be well hydrated while on acyclovir to prevent renal damage unless contraindicated.

Keywords: Specialized areas; Pharmacology (indications, contraindications, and complications); Antimicrobials; Antiviral

REFERENCES

Mailles A, Stahl JP. Infectious encephalitis in France: a national prospective study. *Clin Infect Dis* 2009;49:1838–1847.

Tunkel AR, Glaser CA, Bloch KC et al. The management of encephalitis: clinical practice guidelines by the Infectious Diseases Society of America. *Clin Infect Dis* 2008;47:303–327.

Tunkel AR, Hartman BJ, Kaplan SL et al. Practice guidelines for the management of bacterial meningitis. *Clin Infect Dis* 2004;39:1267–1284.

Whitley RJ, Kimberlin DW. Herpes simplex encephalitis: children and adolescents. *Semin Pediatr Infect Dis* 2005;16:17–23.

18. ANSWER: B

Doxycycline is an agent used for coverage of suspected spirochetal and rickettsial infection. Rickettsial infection is typically acquired from tick or mite bites and can be acquired anywhere in the United States, Canada, Mexico, Central America, or South America. Rocky Mountain spotted fever (RMSF) was first reported in Idaho and is the most common cause of rickettsial infection in the United States, with nearly 5000 cases reported in 2012. Linezolid and amoxicillin are distracters in this stem. The history of reflux disease with a chronic proton pump inhibitor (PPI) may appear to be related to the patient's complaint of rash, and PPIs are associated with a mild rash following chronic treatment. Normally, withdrawal of the PPI will result in resolution of the patient's rash within a few weeks, although this does not explain the patient's fever, confusion, or abdominal pain.

The image in the question of a lesion (erythema and perifollicular petechiae) on the left medial upper ankle/lower calf of a patient with tick-borne spotted fever caused by *Rickettsia parkeri*. The earliest rash of RMSF looks similarly subtle if the clinician is fortunate enough to see the rash before the patient begins to deteriorate clinically.

Keywords: Specialized areas; Pharmacology (indications, contraindications, and complications); Antimicrobials; Antibiotics; Spirochetal and rickettsial

REFERENCES

Biggs HM, Behravesh CB, Bradley KK et al. Diagnosis and management of tickborne rickettsial diseases: Rocky Mountain spotted fever and other spotted fever group rickettsioses, ehrlichioses, and anaplasmosis—United States. *MMWR Recomm Rep* 2016;65(2):1.

Tubiana S, Mikulski M, Becam J et al. Risk factors and predictors of severe leptospirosis in New Caledonia. *PLoS Negl Trop Dis* 2013;7(1):e1991.

Walker DH. Rickettsiae and rickettsial infections: the current state of knowledge. *Clin Infect Dis* 2007;45(Suppl 1):S39.

19. ANSWER: A

Although this patient has been admitted to the hospital with a trauma diagnosis, her workup to this point does not indicate an acute abdominal process. The complaint of anal itching in the setting of abdominal pain and nausea is consistent with a severe pinworm infection. The two most common nematode infections worldwide are *Enterobius vermicularis* (pinworm) and *Trichuris trichiura* (whipworm). Humans are the only natural host for *Enterobius*, and infection can occur in temperate and tropical climates. Enterobius is the most common helminthic infection in the United States and Western Europe, and it is believed that there are 40 million individuals infected in the United States. Trichuriasis occurs most commonly in tropical climates. The drug of choice for treating these infections is mebendazole. When mebendazole is given once initially and then again at the end of 2 weeks, the cure rate is nearly 100%. The "paddle test," in which a spatula or something similar with adhesive is applied to the perianal area and then placed against a slide that is then examined under a microscope, is a common and easy technique for diagnosis. This patient's presentation, consisting of nausea and abdominal pain, is particularly severe.

Keywords: Specialized areas; Pharmacology (indications, contraindications, and complications); Antimicrobials; Antiparasitic

REFERENCES

Centers for Disease Control and Prevention. Enterobiasis (*Enterobius vermicularis*). Available at www.dpd.cdc.gov/DPDx/HTML/Enterobiasis.htm. Accessed on March 3, 2018.

Moore TA, McCarthy JS. Enterobiasis. In: Guerrant R, Walker DH, Weller PF, eds. *Tropical infectious diseases: principles, pathogens and practice*, 3rd edition. Philadelphia: Saunders Elsevier; 2011, p. 788.

8.

ENDOCRINOLOGY

Navneet Kaur Grewal and George W. Williams

QUESTIONS

1. A 70-year-old male who was admitted 3 days ago for a left tibial fracture and pulmonary contusions following a motorcycle collision has a sodium level of 132 mg/L. He received massive transfusion in the operating room along with aggressive crystalloid resuscitation. He is being weaned on the ventilator and has no significant medical history. Which of the following most likely represents the pathophysiology behind his presentation?

    A. Hypotonic fluids
    B. Renal failure
    C. Syndrome of inappropriate secretion of antidiuretic hormone (SIADH)
    D. Malnutrition

2. A 40-year-old female is transported by helicopter to the hospital after being found in a ditch. The patient has a core body temperature of 34.5° C. Computed tomography (CT) demonstrates loss of gray-white differentiation. The patient's serum sodium is 187 mEq/L. Which of the following is the MOST appropriate next step in management?

    A. Desmopressin
    B. Warmed saline
    C. Hyperbaric oxygen
    D. Antibiotics

3. A 22-year-old female presents to the emergency department (ED) with nausea, vomiting, and abdominal pain. She says that she has had diabetes since she was 12 years old and has been very regular with her insulin regimen. She also states that to celebrate her 22nd birthday, she and her friend have been partying and binge-drinking beer for the past 3 days. Vital signs and labs include the following:

Heart rate (HR): 113 bpm
Blood pressure (BP): 95/65 mm Hg
Respiratory rate (RR): 22 breaths/min
Serum glucose: 800 mg/dL
Sodium: 127 mEq/L
Bicarbonate: 9 mEq/L
Urine: positive for ketones

The immediate next step in the management is:

    A. Check potassium level
    B. Give intravenous (IV) 0.45% normal saline at 250 mL/hour
    C. Administer regular IV insulin bolus of 0.1 U/kg followed by infusion
    D. Check serum osmolality

4. You suspect that a patient has adrenal insufficiency. Which of the following is the LEAST appropriate test to confirm the diagnosis in the ICU?

    A. Glucagon
    B. Prolonged adrenocorticotropic hormone (ACTH) stimulation
    C. Metyrapone
    D. Insulin-induced hypoglycemia

5. A middle-aged 95-kg male who fell from a ladder has been comatose since admission 4 days ago. The patient has no subarachnoid hemorrhage and was suspected to have diabetes insipidus due to polyuria and is treated with 200-mL D$_5$ water, but this treatment is discontinued. The patient's blood glucose is found to be 346, and an insulin infusion is initiated. The patient's serum sodium level remained below 145 mEq/L and continues to fall, now at 133 mEq/L. Which of the following is the MOST likely etiology of this presentation?

A. SIADH
B. Fluid overload
C. Cerebral salt wasting (CSW)
D. Hyperglycemia

6. Following a cerebral aneurysm clipping procedure, your patient has a hematocrit of 29% and is noted to have hyponatremia, mild hypotension, and elevated urine output on postoperative day 10. Which of the following is the MOST appropriate intervention?

A. Fludrocortisone
B. 2% saline
C. Packed Red Cells
D. "Triple H" therapy

7. A 32-year-old male with a past medical history significant for acromegaly status post–gamma-knife therapy 5 years ago presents with hypotension. He reports visual-field defects over the past year and has a borderline fever. Which of the following is the MOST likely diagnosis?

A. Septic shock
B. Pituitary apoplexy
C. Adrenal insufficiency
D. Hashimoto disease

8. A 52-year-old male is transported to the ED for worsening shortness of breath and palpitations for the past 2 days. While in the ED, the patient becomes agitated and delirious. The family reports that the patient recently lost his job and health insurance, has been very depressed, and has stopped taking his medications, which include atenolol, methimazole, and lisinopril. On examination, the patient is noted to have a thyroid mass. Vital signs include:

BP: 105/45 mm Hg
HR: 160 bpm
RR: 20 breaths/minute
SpO$_2$: 98% on room air

An electrocardiogram (ECG) performed in the ED is shown here in the following image.

The BEST immediate next step in the management is:

A. Electrical cardioversion
B. T$_3$, T$_4$, and thyroid stimulating hormone (TSH) levels
C. Propranolol, propylthiouracil (PTU), and hydrocortisone
D. Endotracheal intubation

9. A 75-year-old male is brought to the ED by emergency medical services after he was found unresponsive at home. According to the history obtained from family, the patient has been complaining of headaches and lethargy for the past 2 days and was found unresponsive this morning. The family also says that he recently finished a course of radioactive iodine treatment last week. His past medical history is significant for hypertension, heart failure, and a cerebral

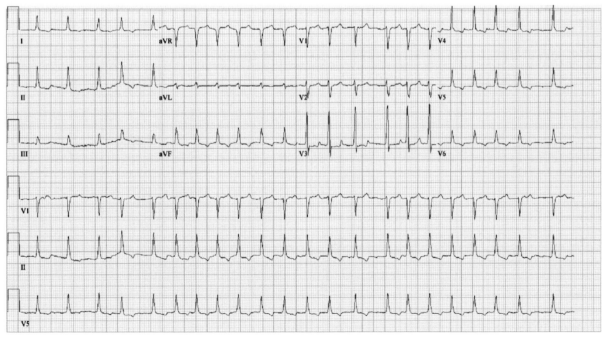

Figure Q8.1

aneurysm. The patient is intubated and transferred to the ICU with the following vital signs:

BP: 80/60 mm Hg
HR: 52 bpm
RR: 12 breaths/minute
Temperature: 35° C
Serum glucose: 72 mg/dL

Which of the following is the BEST next step in management?

A. Stat CT scan of the head
B. IV T_3, T_4, and hydrocortisone
C. T_3, T_4, and TSH levels
D. Transcranial Doppler ultrasound

ANSWERS

1. ANSWER: C

Assessment of hyponatremia is best achieved by determining volume status, with differentiation between hypovolemic and hypervolemic causes. No data are provided to indicate that the patient is hypovolemic; moreover, the patient received aggressive fluid resuscitation. Therefore, hypotonic fluids would not be appropriate, and renal failure is not likely. While malnutrition may lead to some electrolyte abnormalities following resumption of feeds, data supporting this are not provided in the stem. A patient on positive pressure ventilation and also in postoperative pain would be at increased risk for SIADH.

Keyword: SIADH

2. ANSWER: A

This patient is presenting with diabetes insipidus, which has resulted in severe hypernatremia. Desmopressin is the treatment of choice to temporarily correct this finding. Loss of gray-white differentiation is a finding consistent with severe anoxic brain injury. While hyperbaric oxygen administration would increase oxygen availability in the tissues, it would not serve to reverse this type of injury. Because the patient is hypothermic, brain death criteria are not met at this time; administration of warm fluids has been studied in the field and might be helpful. Administration of antibiotics at this time would not be indicated because there is no clear suspicion of infection. The authors recognize that a ditch is not an aseptic environment and that hypothermia could indicate sepsis, but this is not the MOST appropriate next step.

Keyword: Diabetes insipidus

REFERENCE

Haverkamp FJC, Giesbrecht GG, Tan ECTH. The prehospital management of hypothermia—an up-to-date overview. *Injury* 2018;49(2):149–164.

3. ANSWER: A

The first course of action when caring for a patient with diabetic ketoacidosis is to administer normal saline in order to expand the patient's depleted volume status. Half-normal saline is administered in the event of hypernatremia. Next, replacement of the patient's potassium deficit should occur, which must be measured in order to manage. If the potassium is more than 3.2 mEq/L, then an insulin infusion may be initiated. If potassium is less than 3.3, potassium should be administered before initiating an insulin infusion. Plasma osmolality would be expected to be elevated; it should not be addressed before potassium.

Keywords: Basic pathophysiology; Endocrine; Diabetes mellitus; Hyperglycemia, including diabetic ketoacidosis (DKA), nonketotic hyperglycemic coma (NKHC)

4. ANSWER: A

The prolonged ACTH stimulation test allows the clinician to differentiate between primary and secondary adrenal insufficiency. If the patient is experiencing primary adrenal insufficiency, then the nonfunctioning adrenal glands will never respond to the ACTH. If prolonged exposure to ACTH results in a response, this is more consistent with secondary (or tertiary) adrenal insufficiency. This test is not particularly useful in the ICU population. Metyrapone is an effective way to screen for adrenal insufficiency in postoperative pituitary patients. Metyrapone inhibits the final step of synthesis of cortisol; this results in stimulation of ACTH secretion due to a reduction in negative feedback from cortisol.

The insulin-induced hypoglycemia test is just what it sounds like and is only safe when a clinician is present for the test. When serum glucose drops to the goal of 35 mg/dL, cortisol levels are measured at 0, 30, and 45 minutes. The glucagon or growth hormone–releasing hexapeptide test has shown low sensitivity for diagnosing adrenal insufficiency.

Keyword: Adrenal insufficiency

REFERENCE

Alaioubi B, Mann K, Petersenn S. Diagnosis of adrenal insufficiency using the GHRP-6 Test: comparison with the insulin tolerance test in patients with hypothalamic-pituitary-adrenal disease. *Horm Metab Res* 2010;42(3):198–203.

5. ANSWER: C

Out of the choices provided, only CSW and SIADH would result in a true hyponatremia. Making the diagnoses in this case requires determining what is a distracting piece of information and what is pertinent for making a clinical decision. The brief administration of D_5 water would not reliably result in substantial sodium changes in a 95-kg male. It is important to be aware that severe hypoglycemia may result in pseudo-hyponatremia; this correction can be calculated by 2.4 × (serum glucose – 100). In this case, the correction could be no more than 5.9 mEq/L, which would not explain the patient's change in sodium.

The presence of polyuria is more consistent with CSW because SIADH would present with an oliguric clinical picture. Fluid overload would not be consistent with the clinical stem as presented because the volume of D_5 water administered is small compared with the patient's actual body weight.

Keyword: Cerebral salt wasting

REFERENCE

Hillier TA, Abbott RD, Barrett EJ. Hyponatremia: evaluating the correction factor for hyperglycemia. *Am J Med* 1999;106(4):399–403.

6. ANSWER: A

This patient clinically appears to be presenting with CSW syndrome. Recall that CSW is a hypovolemic hyponatremic lesion. It is commonly seen in aneurysmal subarachnoid hemorrhage; however, it can be seen in a variety of neurological conditions resulting in brain injury or following neurological surgery. Hypertonic saline (as well as normal saline) is commonly administered in this clinical presentation; however, determination of the cause of hyponatremia is of paramount importance. In particular, establishing the distinction between CSW and SIADH is important because SIADH is a hypervolemic lesion. Fludrocortisone facilitates both retention of volume and elevation of serum sodium, again through retention, and is therefore the correct choice.

Therefore, administering volume to such a patient could be clinically detrimental. As studies such as the TRICC trial have demonstrated, a gradual reduction in hematocrit can be expected in critically ill patients, especially after 7 days of admission. No transfusion threshold for aneurysmal subarachnoid hemorrhage has been established, although a hematocrit of more than 30% is not commonly suggested by current guidelines. Further discussion about "triple H" therapy is given in Chapter 1, but initiating such therapy, however debatable, in the absence of clinical symptoms or evidence of vasospasm during this admission would not be indicated.

Keywords: Management, endocrine; Management strategies, steroids (glucocorticoid and mineralocorticoid)

REFERENCE

Diringer MN, Bleck TP, Claude Hemphill J 3rd et al.; Neurocritical Care Society. Critical care management of patients following aneurysmal subarachnoid hemorrhage: recommendations from the Neurocritical Care Society's Multidisciplinary Consensus Conference. *Neurocrit Care* 2011;15(2):211–240.

7. ANSWER: C

This patient is presenting with panhypopituitarism due to having radiation therapy in the past. While gamma knife is intended to be a precise method of providing such treatment, frequently nearby tissues are affected, with more than 50% of patients presenting with endocrinologic deficiencies 4 years after such treatment; this frequency of adverse outcome is not consistent with the expected outcomes based on the design of stereotactic surgery at its outset. The types of endocrinopathies following stereotactic surgery can include the entire array of pituitary-related lesions such as TSH, ACTH, and follicle-stimulating hormone (FSH)/luteinizing hormone (LH) deficiencies.

Recall that pituitary apoplexy is a hemorrhage into the pituitary and is commonly characterized by headache along with visual-field deficits; the onset of visual-field defects is usually sudden. Imaging is needed to make the diagnosis, with magnetic resonance imaging being the most reliable modality.

Although the patient does demonstrate a mildly elevated temperature, there are no clinical data presented in the stem consistent with septic shock. Additionally, the patient's symptoms and presentation may be consistent with hypothyroidism; however, the information provided in the stem is more suggestive of a pituitary-oriented lesion in lieu of autoimmune thyroiditis.

Keywords: Critical illness diagnosis and management, endocrine; Diagnoses, adrenal, adrenal insufficiency; Diagnosis and management, endocrine; Diagnoses, pituitary

8. ANSWER: C

Beta-blockers are part of the first-line treatment of thyroid storm, with propranolol being a commonly chosen drug because it inhibits type 1 deiodinase, which can help reduce serum T_3 levels. Beta-blockers should be used with caution in the setting of heart failure. Thionamides (PTU, methimazole, or carbimazole) block thyroid hormone synthesis and should be part of any treatment paradigm for thyroid storm. Glucocorticoids inhibit conversion of T_4 to T_3 and can inhibit an underlying autoimmune process if it is applicable. The patient's atrial fibrillation and tachycardia are the result of the thyroid storm; additionally, because the atrial fibrillation is not unstable (hypotensive), no cardioversion is indicated. Obtaining thyroid hormone levels, while helpful, is not the most immediately pressing item of action. Because the patient is ventilating and oxygenating well, endotracheal intubation is not indicated.

Keywords: Basic pathophysiology, endocrine; Thyroid function abnormalities, hyperthyroidism, including thyroid storm

REFERENCE

Satoh T, Isozaki O, Suzuki A et al. 2016 Guidelines for the management of thyroid storm from the Japan Thyroid Association and Japan Endocrine Society, 1st edition. *Endocr J* 2016;63(12):1025–1064.

9. ANSWER: B

Myxedema coma is a highly morbid endocrine emergency with a mortality rate of 30 to 50%. Combined therapy with T_4 and T_3 is most efficacious for myxedema coma. Glucocorticoids are administered until adrenal insufficiency is ruled out. It is important to initiate treatment as soon as possible, thereby necessitating a bypass of laboratory confirmation when initially intervening.

Keywords: Basic pathophysiology, endocrine; Thyroid function abnormalities, hypothyroidism, including myxedema

REFERENCE

Kwaku MP, Burman KD. Myxedema coma. *J Intensive Care Med.* 2007;22(4):224–231.

9.

IMMUNOLOGY AND INFECTIOUS DISEASES

Joti Juneja Mucci

QUESTIONS

1. A 66-year-old male is admitted with photophobia, diffuse maculopapular rash, and diarrhea. His past medical history includes coronary artery disease, diabetes, chronic kidney disease, and end-stage liver disease (ESLD). He had a liver transplantation 3 weeks ago. His home medications are metoprolol, insulin, trimethoprim-sulfamethoxazole, prednisone, and mycophenolate mofetil (CellCept). His labs are shown here:

Sodium	134	Total bilirubin	7.2
Potassium	3.8	Aspartate aminotransferase	122
Chloride	108	Alanine aminotransferase	140
Bicarbonate	29	International normalized ratio (INR)	1.7
Blood urea nitrogen	67	Albumin	2.4
Creatinine	1.82		

Which of the following is MOST likely the cause of his symptoms?

 A. Trimethoprim-sulfamethoxazole
 B. Infection
 C. Mycophenolate mofetil
 D. Graft-versus-host disease (GVHD)

2. A 67-year-old male present to the intensive care unit (ICU) with diarrhea and abdominal pain, concerning for sepsis. He is tachycardic, febrile, and hypotensive. His past medical history includes hypertension, diabetes, congestive heart failure, and leukemia, for which he is status post–bone marrow transplantation several months ago. Which of the following medications is considered BEST first-line treatment for his likely diagnosis?

 A. Hydrocortisone
 B. Methylprednisolone
 C. Sirolimus
 D. Mycophenolate

3. A 65-year-old male patient presents to the hospital with a differential diagnosis of GVHD. Which of the following is LEAST likely to be a manifestation of acute GVHD?

 A. Maculopapular rash
 B. Voluminous diarrhea
 C. Abnormal liver function tests
 D. *Candida* esophagitis

4. A 36-year-old male presents to ICU with sepsis. He reports several weeks of fatigue, malaise, and night sweats. He denies any sick contacts but does admit to recently having unprotected sex. He is worked up for influenza and mononucleosis, and results are negative for both tests. Which of the following cell lines are affected by his likely diagnosis?

 A. Macrophages
 B. CD4$^+$ T cells
 C. Dendritic cells
 D. Neutrophils

5. A 50-year-old male was recently diagnosed with acute HIV-1. RNA levels on diagnosis were more than 10^7 copies/mL, while p24 antigens levels were higher than 100 pg/mL. Several weeks later, before any sort of treatment was initiated, plasma RNA levels are noted to have fallen precipitously by 2 to 3 logs. What is the primary reason for this?

 A. Proliferation of CD4$^+$ T cells
 B. Macrophage uptake of virus
 C. Emergence of CD8$^+$ cytotoxic T lymphocytes
 D. Emergence of B cells

6. A 39-year-old male is admitted with unresolving flu-like symptoms for the past few weeks including fever and chills. Infectious workup is completed and reveals acute HIV-1 infection. What is the CD4$^+$ threshold for when antiviral therapy should be initiated?

A. CD4$^+$ >350
B. CD4$^+$ <350
C. CD4$^+$ <200
D. CD4$^+$ <100

7. A 39-year-old male is admitted with nonresolving flu-like symptoms for the past few weeks including fevers, chills, fatigue, and myalgias. Past medical history includes hypertension and end-stage renal disease requiring intermittent hemodialysis. Infectious workup reveals acute HIV-1 infection. Which of the following combinations would be preferred in the initial treatment of acute HIV infection in this patient?

A. Abacavir-lamivudine plus dolutegravir
B. Tenofovir-emtricitabine plus raltegravir
C. Abacavir-lamivudine
D. Tenofovir-emtricitabine

8. A 43-year-old female is admitted to the ICU with respiratory failure. There is not much time to get a detailed history, and the patient is mildly obtunded. Her past medical history includes hypertension, for which she takes hydrochlorothiazide. You notice mild deformation of multiple joints along with poor neck extension. What lab test would be LEAST helpful in the diagnosis?

A. Complete blood count (CBC) with differential and platelet count
B. Rheumatoid factor (RF)
C. Anti–cyclic citrullinated peptide (anti-CCP) antibodies
D. Antinuclear antibody (ANA)

9. In rheumatoid arthritis (RA), the enzyme primarily responsible for the breakdown of cartilage, bone, and tendons is:

A. Glycosidase
B. Myeloperoxidase
C. Elastase
D. Metalloproteinase

10. Which of the following antibodies is MOST useful for diagnosis of mixed connective tissue disease (MCTD)?

A. ANA
B. Anti-U1 ribonuclear protein (RNP)

C. Anti-CCP antibodies
D. RF

11. A 42-year-old female is admitted to the ICU with concerns of sepsis several days after a tooth extraction. Her past medical history includes hypertension, obesity, type 2 diabetes, and a bicuspid aortic valve that was replaced 2 years ago. Which of the following prophylactic antibiotics is LEAST appropriate to prevent bacterial endocarditis?

A. Amoxicillin
B. Clindamycin
C. Meropenem
D. Cefazolin

12. Antimicrobial prophylaxis is suggested for patients with cardiac conditions that confer the highest risk for adverse outcome from endocarditis. Which of the following is the MOST clear indication for prophylaxis against endocarditis?

A. Vaginal delivery
B. Bronchoscopy with biopsy
C. Insertion of urinary catheter
D. Endoscopy

13. A 73-year-old female is admitted to the ICU in septic shock from a likely urinary infection. Her past medical history includes coronary artery disease, hypertension, obesity, and RA. Laboratory assessment reveals a significant neutropenia. Which of her medications is LEAST likely to be contributing to her neutropenia?

A. Methotrexate
B. Adalimumab (Humira)
C. Anakinra (Kineret)
D. Eliquis (Apixaban)

14. System lupus erythematosus is associated with which of the following immunologic abnormalities?

A. Decrease in circulating plasma cells
B. Autoantibodies forming immune complexes with antigens
C. Phagocytosis and clearing of immune complexes
D. Thrombocytosis

15. ANA testing is typically positive at some point during the course of the patient's disease. What other test is highly specific for systemic lupus erythematosus (SLE)?

A. Antiphospholipid antibodies
B. Anti-dsDNA antibodies
C. Anti-Ro/SSA
D. Anti-U1 RNP

16. A 63-year male with ESLD is admitted to the ICU for concerns of sepsis. His past medical history includes hypertension and alcoholic cirrhosis, which has been complicated by esophageal varices and ascites. He is febrile and complaining of abdominal pain. Paracentesis is performed and demonstrates a high neutrophil count (>250 cells/mm³); cultures are pending. Which of the following antibiotics is LEAST appropriate for prophylaxis in the future?

A. Trimethoprim-sulfamethoxazole
B. Ciprofloxacin
C. Norfloxacin
D. Ampicillin and gentamycin

17. A 22-year-old female college student presents with fever, myalgias, sore throat, and rash. She also has axillary and cervical lymphadenopathy. She denies any recent sick contacts. On further questioning, she admits to having unprotected sex occasionally with several men. Which is the best initial test to help diagnose acute HIV infection?

A. Combination antigen-antibody immunoassay
B. HIV viral load (reverse transcriptase polymerase chain reaction [RT-PCR] testing)
C. Western blot testing
D. Antibody-only HIV-1/HIV-2 differentiation immunoassay

ANSWERS

1. ANSWER: D

The most important diagnosis to rule out in this situation given the proximity to transplantation is GVHD. Acute GVHD occurs when the T cells of the donor recognize the presence of histocompatibility antigens in the host that differ from the donor cells. This antigen recognition is followed by amplification of the T cells. The proliferation of activated T cells leads to the production and secretion of a variety of cytokines, which are responsible for the inflammatory effects and tissue damage associated with GVHD. Much of the damage is caused by inflammatory cytokines such as interleukin (IL)-1, IL-2, tumor necrosis factor (TNF), and gamma-interferon. Liver dysfunction is commonly seen in patients with advanced GVHD, along with a diffuse maculopapular rash. Furthermore, interstitial pneumonitis, nephritis, and ocular manifestations such as photophobia and hemorrhagic conjunctivitis may be seen.

One of the first manifestations of acute GVHD is a maculopapular rash. Other symptoms can be nausea and emesis, abdominal cramps, diarrhea, and a rising bilirubin. Acute infection may lead to symptoms similar to GVHD (e.g., fever) but does not reliably demonstrate symptoms correlating with this disease. Of course, in the post-transplantation population, infection should remain on one differential diagnosis for the acute onset of symptoms. Risk factors for acute GVHD may include younger age, acute leukemia (when compared with other hematologic malignancies), and a graft from an unrelated donor.

Trimethoprim-sulfamethoxazole (commonly called Bactrim) may result in adverse reactions in less than 10% of the population, but this rate may be much higher in the HIV population. Common side effects include nausea, vomiting, and skin rash; adverse reactions may be treated by removing the drug in many instances. Bactrim is not associated with elevation in liver function assays or bilirubin.

While gastrointestinal (GI) symptoms such as diarrhea are commonly seen in patients receiving mycophenolate mofetil (up to 75% of patient), it is generally well managed with dosing adjustments; additionally, bone marrow suppression is common. Many of the symptoms that this patient exhibited, such as rash and photophobia, are not associated with administration of mycophenolate mofetil.

Keyword: Graft-versus-host disease

REFERENCES

Antin JH, Ferrara JL. Cytokine dysregulation and acute graft versus host disease. *Blood* 1992;80:2964.
Ferrara JL. Deeg HJ. Graft versus host disease. *N Engl J Med* 1991; 324:667.

Lee SE, Cho BS, Kim JH et al. Risk and prognostic factors for acute GVHD based on NIH consensus criteria. *Bone Marrow Transplant* 2013;48(4):587–592.

2. ANSWER: B

Methylprednisolone is considered frontline therapy for treatment of GVHD. The therapy for GVHD depends on the severity of symptoms and the organs involved. The goal of therapy is to suppress the donor T cells. T cells are also responsible for the immunologic effects of the transplant; hence, the aim is to balance the GVHD symptoms with the immunologic effect. Patients with severe manifestations are treated with systemic corticosteroids. Methylprednisolone differs from prednisone by addition of a 6-alpha-methyl group. This chemical group blocks the binding of this steroid to transcortin, the protein that transports steroids in plasma. Instead, methylprednisolone binds primarily to albumin. Because of this, there is a larger partition coefficient resulting in significantly greater penetration into certain tissues, especially pulmonary. The side effects of methylprednisolone may be dependent on the hosts' albumin levels.

Keyword: Graft-versus-host disease

REFERENCES

Dignan FL, Clark A, Amrolia P et al. Haemato-oncology Task Force of British Committee for Standards in Haematology, British Society for Blood and Marrow Transplantation: diagnosis and management of acute graft-versus-host disease. *Br J Haematol* 2012;158(1):30–45.
Martin PJ, Rizzo JD, Wingard JR, Ballen K et al. First- and second-line systemic treatment of acute graft-versus-host disease: recommendations of the American Society of Blood and Marrow Transplantation. *Biol Blood Marrow Transplant* 2012;18(8):1150–1163.
Oosteruis B, ten Berge IJ, Schellekens PT et al. Prednisolone concentration-effect relations in humans and the influence of plasma hydrocortisone. *J Pharmacol Exp Ther* 1986;239:919.

3. ANSWER: D

The skin, GI tract, and liver are the principal target organs in patients with acute GVHD. In most patients, the first and most common manifestation is a diffuse, maculopapular rash. The upper and lower GI tracts are also involved and may manifest as nausea, vomiting, diarrhea, and anorexia. Liver involvement may be suggested by abnormal liver function tests, with the earliest and most common findings of rising conjugated bilirubin and alkaline phosphatase.

Keywords: Immunosuppression; Graft-versus-host disease

REFERENCES

Aslanian H, Chander B, Robert M et al. Prospective evaluation of acute graft-versus-host disease. *Dig Dis Sci* 2012;57(3):720–725.

Jagasia M, Arora M, Flowers ME et al. Risk factors for acute GVHD and survival after hematopoietic cell transplantation. *Blood* 2012;119(1):296.

Ratanatharathorn V, Nash RA, Przepiorka D, et al. Phase III study comparing methotrexate and tacrolimus with methotrexate and cyclosporine for graft-versus-host disease prophylaxis after HLA-identical sibling bone marrow transplantation. *Blood* 1998;92:2303

4. ANSWER: D

HIV has several targets, including dendritic cells, macrophages, and CD4+ T cells. HIV-1 most often enters the host through the anogenital mucosa. The viral envelope protein, glycoprotein (GP)-120, binds to the CD4 molecule on dendritic cells. Interstitial dendritic cells are found in cervicovaginal epithelium as well as tonsillar and adenoidal tissue, which may serve as initial target cells in infection transmitted by genital-oral sex. Neutrophils as a group are least likely to be affected.

Keywords: HIV; AIDS

REFERENCES

Centlivre M, Sala M, Wain-Hobson S, Berkhout B. In HIV-1 pathogenesis the die is cast during primary infection. *AIDS* 2007;21(1):1.

Kahn JO, Walker BD. Acute human immunodeficiency virus type 1 infection. *N Engl J Med* 1998;339:33.

Nilsson J, Kinloch-de-Loes S, Granath A et al. Early immune activation in gut-associated and peripheral lymphoid tissue during acute HIV infection. *AIDS* 2007;21(5):565.

5. ANSWER: C

At the time of initial infection with HIV, patients have a large number of susceptible CD4+ T cells and no HIV-specific immune response. Viral replication is therefore rapid; plasma HIV RNA levels may climb to more than 10^7 copies/mL, and p24 antigen levels may exceed 100 pg/mL.

Concomitant with the evolution of HIV-specific immunity, primarily due to the emergence of virus-specific CD8+ cytotoxic T lymphocytes, plasma RNA levels fall precipitously by 2 to 3 logs, and symptoms of the acute syndrome resolve. In the absence of treatment, plasma HIV RNA levels will stabilize at an individual's given "set point" within 6 months of infection.

Keywords: HIV; CD4 counts

REFERENCES

Cooper DA, Tindall B, Wilson EJ et al. Characterization of T lymphocyte responses during primary infection with human immunodeficiency virus. *J Infect Dis* 1988;157(5):889.

Quinn TC. Acute primary HIV infection. *JAMA* 1997; 278:58.

Robb ML, Eller LA, Kibuuka H et al.; RV 217 Study Team. Prospective study of acute HIV-1 infection in adults in East Africa and Thailand. *N Engl J Med* 2016;374(22):2120.

6. ANSWER: B

There is high-quality evidence that initiating ART in patients with a CD4+ count of 350 cells/μL or greater results in a significant decline in the risk for AIDS-related morbidity and mortality. In addition, initiating ART *before* the CD4 count is less than 200 cells/μL also reduces mortality in HIV-infected individuals. The mortality benefit of initiating ART is less clear in patients with a CD4 count higher than 350 cells/μL. However, initiating ART in such patients reduces serious AIDS-related and non–AIDS-related complication.

Keywords: HIV; CD4 counts

REFERENCES

Kitahata MM, Gange SJ, Abraham AG et al. Effect of early versus deferred antiretroviral therapy for HIV on survival. *N Engl J Med* 2009;360:1815.

Lodi S, Phillips A, Touloumi G et al.; CASCADE Collaboration in EuroCoord. Time from human immunodeficiency virus seroconversion to reaching CD4+ cell count thresholds <200, <350, and <500 cells/mm³: assessment of need following changes in treatment guidelines. *Clin Infect Dis* 2011;53(8):817–825.

Minga AK, Lewden C, Gabillard D et al.; Agence Nationale de Recherches sur le Sida (ANRS) 1220 Primo-CI Study Group. CD4 cell eligibility thresholds: an analysis of the time to antiretroviral treatment in HIV-1 seroconverters. *AIDS* 2011;25(6):819.

Study Group on Death Rates at High CD4 Count in Antiretroviral Naive Patients; Lodwick RK, Sabin CA, Porter K et al. Death rates in HIV-positive antiretroviral-naive patients with CD4 count greater than 350 cells per microL in Europe and North America: a pooled cohort observational study. *Lancet* 2010;376:340.

7. ANSWER: A

The most effective ART regimens contain two different nucleoside reverse transcriptase inhibitors and one integrase strand transfer inhibitor.

Of these, the only combination that is safe given his renal function is abacavir-lamivudine and dolutegravir.

Tenofovir should be avoided in patients with glomerular filtration rate less than 30 mL/minute.

Keywords: HIV; Pharmacologic management

REFERENCES

Panel on Antiretroviral Guidelines for Adults and Adolescents. Guidelines for the use of antiretroviral agents in HIV-1-infected adults and adolescents. US Department of Health and Human Services. https://aidsinfo.nih.gov/contentfiles/adultandadolescentgl003093.pdf, Accessed May 8, 2018.

Sax PE, Tierney C, Collier AC et al.; AIDS Clinical Trials Group Study A5202 Team. Abacavir-lamivudine versus tenofovir-emtricitabine for initial HIV-1 therapy. *N Engl J Med* 2009;361(23):2230.

8. ANSWER: A

When initially evaluating a patient with suspected RA, both RF and anti-CCP antibody testing is useful. The results of both tests are informative because a positive result for either test increases overall diagnostic sensitivity, while the specificity is increased when both tests are positive. Despite this, both tests are negative on presentation in up to 50% of patients. A negative ANA helps exclude SLE and other systemic rheumatic diseases. The ANA may be positive in up to one third of patients with RA. However, in those patients with a positive ANA, anti-dsDNA and anti-Smith antibody testing should also be performed because these antibodies have high specificity for SLE. CBC with differential and platelet count is likely to be least contributory because it lacks the specificity in establishing a diagnosis.

Keywords: Rheumatoid arthritis; Laboratory diagnostic modalities

REFERENCES

Aletaha D, Neogi T, Silman AJ et al. 2010 Rheumatoid arthritis classification criteria: an American College of Rheumatology/European League Against Rheumatism collaborative initiative. *Arthritis Rheum* 2010;62(9):2569.

Nishimura K, Sugiyama D, Kogata Y et al. Meta-analysis: diagnostic accuracy of anti-cyclic citrullinated peptide antibody and rheumatoid factor for rheumatoid arthritis. *Ann Intern Med* 2007;146:797.

Whiting PF, Smidt N, Sterne JA et al. Systematic review: accuracy of anti-citrullinated Peptide antibodies for diagnosing rheumatoid arthritis. *Ann Intern Med* 2010;152(7):456.

9. ANSWER: D

The destruction of cartilage, bone, and tendons in RA is initiated largely by metalloproteinases. Stromelysin (metalloproteinase-3 [MMP-3]) is a protease that degrades cartilage proteoglycans, fibronectin, and type IV collagen in basement membrane and activates collagenase. Patients with homozygous polymorphism in the promoter region of the gene for MMP-3 have more rapid progression of erosive form of the disease than those without this genotype.

Keywords: Rheumatoid arthritis; Laboratory diagnostic modalities

REFERENCES

Constantin A, Lauwers-Cancès V, Navaux F et al. Stromelysin 1 (matrix metalloproteinase 3) and HLA-DRB1 gene polymorphisms: association with severity and progression of rheumatoid arthritis in a prospective study. *Arthritis Rheum* 2002;46:1754.

Jain A, Nanchahal J, Troeberg L et al. Production of cytokines, vascular endothelial growth factor, matrix metalloproteinases, and tissue inhibitor of metalloproteinases 1 by tenosynovium demonstrates its potential for tendon destruction in rheumatoid arthritis. *Arthritis Rheum* 2001;44(8):1754.

Liu M, Sun H, Wang X et al. Association of increased expression of macrophage elastase (matrix metalloproteinase 12) with rheumatoid arthritis. *Arthritis Rheum* 2004;50(10):3112.

10. ANSWER: B

The MCTDs are a group of diseases with an overlap syndrome associated with anti-U1 RNP antibodies that incorporates selected clinical features of SLE, systemic sclerosis (scleroderma), and polymyositis.

The original description of MCTD included circulating autoantibodies directed against ENA (an RNAse-sensitive extractable nuclear antigen), which has since been determined to be U1 RNP. The presence of this specific antibody remains a sine qua non for the diagnosis of MCTD.

Keywords: Mixed connective tissue disorders, laboratory diagnosis

REFERENCES

Bennett RM. Overlap syndromes. In: Firestein GS, Budd RC, Harris ED, et al., eds. *Textbook of rheumatology*, 8th edition. Philadelphia: Saunders; 2009. p. 1381.

Bennett RM, O'Connell DJ. Mixed connective tissue disease: a clinicopathologic study of 20 cases. *Semin Arthritis Rheum* 1980; 10:25.

Sharp GC, Irvin WS, Tan EM et al. Mixed connective tissue disease: an apparently distinct rheumatic disease syndrome associated with a specific antibody to an extractable nuclear antigen (ENA). *Am J Med* 1972; 52:148.

11. ANSWER: C

The presence of a bicuspid aortic valve by itself is not an indication for prophylaxis before procedures. Neither are mitral valve regurgitation with prolapse nor hypertrophic cardiomyopathy. However, this patient's valve has been replaced, which would be an indication for prophylaxis.

Prophylaxis is suggested in the following high-risk conditions:

- Prosthetic heart valves, including mechanical, bioprosthetic, and homograft valves (transcatheter-implanted as well as surgically implanted valves are included)
- Prosthetic material used for cardiac valve repair, such as annuloplasty rings and chords
- A prior history of infective endocarditis
- Unrepaired cyanotic congenital heart disease
- Repaired congenital heart disease with residual shunts or valvular regurgitation at the site or adjacent to the site of the prosthetic patch or prosthetic device
- Repaired congenital heart defects with catheter-based intervention involving an occlusion device or stent during the first 6 months after the procedure
- Valve regurgitation due to a structurally abnormal valve in a transplanted heart

Any of the antibiotics listed would be appropriate for prophylaxis during dental procedures except meropenem. The recommended regimen is to include an agent active against *Staphylococcus aureus* such as an anti-staphylococcal penicillin or cephalosporins.

Keywords: Endocarditis prophylaxis, antimicrobials

REFERENCE

Nishimura RA, Otto CM, Bonow RO et al. 2017 AHA/ACC focused update of the 2014 AHA/ACC guideline for the management of patients with valvular heart disease: a report of the American College of Cardiology/American Heart Association Task Force on Clinical Practice Guidelines. *J Am Coll Cardiol* 2017;70(2):252–289.

12. ANSWER: B

The other procedures are not an indication for prophylaxis against infective endocarditis.

The procedures associated with the highest risk for infection include:

- Dental procedures that involve manipulation of either gingival tissue or the periapical region of teeth or perforation of the oral mucosa; this includes routine dental cleaning
- Procedures of the respiratory tract that involve incision or biopsy of the respiratory mucosa
- GI or genitourinary (GU) procedures in patients with **ongoing** GI or GU tract **infection**
- Procedures on **infected** skin, skin structure, or musculoskeletal tissue

- Surgery to place prosthetic heart valves or prosthetic intravascular or intracardiac materials

Also see explanation for question 11.

Keyword: Endocarditis prophylaxis

REFERENCES

Durack DT. Prevention of infective endocarditis. *N Engl J Med* 1995; 332:38.
Nishimura RA, Otto CM, Bonow RO et al. 2017 AHA/ACC focused update of the 2014 AHA/ACC guideline for the management of patients with valvular heart disease: a report of the American College of Cardiology/American Heart Association Task Force on Clinical Practice Guidelines. J Am Coll Cardiol 2017;70(2):252–289.

13. ANSWER: D

Methotrexate reversibly inhibits dihydrofolate reductase and interferes with DNA synthesis, repair, and cellular replication. In addition to being used in rheumatoid arthritis, it is also used as an antineoplastic drug, It can cause significant neutropenia.

Adalimumab (Humira) is a recombinant, fully human anti-TNF monoclonal antibody.

A decrease in the number of peripheral blood neutrophils is common in patients who receive TNF-alpha inhibitors.

Anakinra (Kineret) is a recombinant human IL-1 receptor antagonist. It can also lead to neutropenia. Eliquis (Apixaban) is a antiplatelet agent, factor Xa inhibitor, has not been associated with neutropenia.

Keyword: Immunosuppression

REFERENCES

Andersohn F, Konzen C, Garbe E. Systematic review: agranulocytosis induced by nonchemotherapy drugs. *Ann Intern Med* 2007;146(9):657.
Vincent JL, Abraham E, Moore FA et al. *Textbook of critical care*, 6th edition. Philadelphia: Saunders; 2011.

14. ANSWER: B

The mediators of SLE are autoantibodies and the immune complexes they form with antigens; the autoantibodies are usually present for years before the first symptom of disease appears. Self-antigens that are recognized are presented primarily on cell surfaces, particularly by cells that are activated or undergoing apoptosis, where intracellular antigens access cell surfaces, where they can be recognized by the immune system.

Phagocytosis and clearing of immune complexes, of apoptotic cells, and of necrotic cell-derived material are defective in SLE, allowing persistence of antigen and immune complexes. B cells and plasma cells that make autoantibodies are more persistently activated and driven to maturation by B-cell–activating factor. Persistently activated helper T cells also make B-supporting cytokines such as IL-6 and IL-10. Mild thrombocytopenia is commonly seen, and rarely severe thrombocytopenia requiring treatment can occur.

Keywords: Systemic lupus erythematosus; pathophysiology

REFERENCES

Arbuckle MR, McClain MT, Rubertone MV et al. Development of autoantibodies before the clinical onset of systemic lupus erythematosus. *N Engl J Med* 2003;349:1526.

Graham KL, Utz PJ. Sources of autoantigens in systemic lupus erythematosus. *Curr Opin Rheumatol* 2005;17:513.

Mountz JD, Wu J, Cheng J, Zhou T. Autoimmune disease: a problem of defective apoptosis. *Arthritis Rheum* 1994;37:1415.

Muñoz LE, Janko C, Grossmayer GE et al. Remnants of secondarily necrotic cells fuel inflammation in systemic lupus erythematosus. *Arthritis Rheum* 2009;60:1733.

15. ANSWER: B

The ANA test is positive in virtually all patients with SLE at some time in the course of their disease. If the ANA is positive, one should test for more specific antibodies such as dsDNA, anti-Sm, Ro/SSA, La/SSB, and U1 RNP. In some labs, a positive ANA test by indirect immunofluorescence will automatically result in testing for such additional ANAs that are often present in patients with SLE.

- Anti-dsDNA and anti-Sm antibodies are very specific for SLE; anti-Sm antibodies lack sensitivity. Anti-dsDNA antibodies are seen in 70% of SLE patients; anti-Sm antibodies are seen in 30% of patients with SLE
- Anti-U1 RNP antibodies are present in 25% of SLE patients and are also seen in MCTD
- Anti-Ro/SSA antibodies are present in 30% of SLE patients
- Anti-La/SSB antibodies are present in 20% SLE patients
- Both Anti-RO/SSA and Anti-La/SSB are associated with Sjögren syndrome

Keywords: Systemic lupus erythematosus, laboratory diagnostics, serologies

REFERENCES

Benito-Garcia E, Schur PH, Lahita R; American College of Rheumatology Ad Hoc Committee on Immunologic Testing Guidelines. Guidelines for immunologic laboratory testing in the rheumatic diseases: anti-Sm and anti-RNP antibody tests. *Arthritis Rheum* 2004;51:1030.

Riemakasten G, Hiepe F. Autoantibodies. In: Wallace DJ, Hahn BH, eds. *Dubois' lupus erythematosus and related syndromes*, 8th edition. Philadelphia: Elsevier Saunders; 2013, p. 282.

16. ANSWER: D

Antibiotic prophylaxis to prevent spontaneous bacterial peritonitis (SBP) is recommended for patients at high risk for developing SBP and is associated with a decreased risk for bacterial infection and mortality.

Guidelines suggest that antibiotic prophylaxis be given to the following patients:

- Patients with cirrhosis and GI bleeding. Antibiotic prophylaxis in this setting has been shown to decrease mortality in randomized trials.
- Patients who have had one or more episodes of SBP. In such patients, recurrence rates of SBP within 1 year have been reported to be close to 70%.
- Patients with cirrhosis and ascites if the ascitic fluid protein is less than 1.5 g/dL (15 g/L) along with either impaired renal function or liver failure. Impaired renal function is defined as follows: creatinine ≥1.2 mg/dL (106 μmol/L), blood urea nitrogen ≥25 mg/dL (8.9 mmol/L), or serum sodium ≤130 mEq/L(130 mmol/L]). Liver failure is defined as Child-Pugh score ≥9 and bilirubin ≥3 mg/dL (51 μmol/L).

The antibiotics listed are useful for SBP prophylaxis in an outpatient setting where a patient is able to take them orally. The most commonly targeted microorganisms are *Escherichia coli* and *Klebsiella* species.

Ampicillin and gentamycin have been shown to be not as effective and associated with higher nephrotoxicity and higher superinfection rates and hence are the least appropriate choice.

Keywords: Prophylaxis for spontaneous bacterial peritonitis, antimicrobials

REFERENCES

American Association for the Study of Liver Disease. Practice guideline. Available at http://www.aasld.org/practiceguidelines/Documents/ascitesupdate2013.pdf.

Felisart J, Rimola A, Arroyo V et al. Cefotaxime is more effective than is ampicillin-tobramycin in cirrhotics with severe infections. *Hepatology* 1985;5(3):457.

Fernández J, Ruiz del Árbol L, Gómez C et al. Norfloxacin vs ceftriaxone in the prophylaxis of infections in patients with advanced cirrhosis and hemorrhage. *Gastroenterology* 2006;131:1049.

Runyon BA; AASLD. Introduction to the revised American Association for the Study of Liver Diseases Practice Guideline management of adult patients with ascites due to cirrhosis 2012. *Hepatology* 2013;57:1651.

Toto L, Rimola A, Ginès P et al. Recurrence of spontaneous bacterial peritonitis in cirrhosis: frequency and predictive factors. *Hepatology* 1988; 8:27.

17. ANSWER: A

In the United States, the recommended algorithm for screening involves an initial fourth-generation combined antigen-antibody immunoassay. If this is positive, it should be followed by a confirmatory antibody-only HIV-1/HIV-2 differentiation immunoassay, which should be followed by HIV viral testing if there is a discrepancy. In this algorithm, acute or early HIV is diagnosed when the initial immunoassay is reactive, the second immunoassay is nonreactive, and the viral test detects HIV RNA repeatedly or at a high level.

Some laboratories may still employ Western blot testing to confirm an initial reactive immunoassay. Detecting early HIV with this algorithm requires checking a viral RNA test if the Western blot is negative or indeterminate. In such cases, a reactive immunoassay followed by a negative or indeterminate Western blot followed by a positive viral RNA test is most likely indicative of early HIV infection. Thus, a reactive immunoassay followed by a negative or indeterminate Western blot should not be erroneously interpreted as a negative screening pattern for HIV without further testing.

Keywords: HIV testing, immunoassays

REFERENCE

Centers for Disease Control and Prevention (CDC). Detection of acute HIV infection in two evaluations of a new HIV diagnostic testing algorithm—United States, 2011–2013. *MMWR Morb Mortal Wkly Rep* 2013; 62:489. http://www.cdc.gov/hiv/pdf/HIVtestingAlgorithmRecommendation-Final.pdf.

10.

STATISTICS, ETHICS, AND MANAGEMENT

George W. Williams

QUESTIONS

1. A 62-year-old male is transferred to the intensive care unit (ICU) by helicopter transport because of a suspected stroke. His computed tomography (CT) scan is shown here, and cerebral angiography is pending.

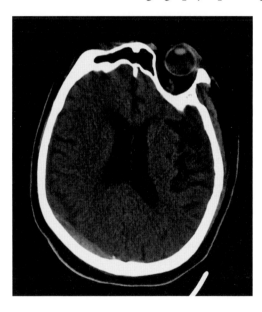

On the patient's admission to the ICU, your team discontinues the midazolam infusion and performs an examination. The patient is comatose and is noted to have a mildly hypothermic temperature of 36.0° C, is hypotensive requiring norepinephrine, demonstrates no brainstem reflexes, and has a serum creatinine of 2.71 and blood urea nitrogen (BUN) of 81. Which of the following is the BEST next step in determining brain death?

A. Intermittent hemodialysis
B. Apnea testing
C. Observation
D. Rewarming

2. During a medical staff meeting, the hospital CEO comments on the Hospital Consumer Assessment of Healthcare Providers and Systems (HCAHPS) scores for the ICU service being 45th percentile in the country. Which of the following MOST accurately describes the ramifications for the hospital administration?

A. Reduced payment the following year
B. Increased documentation requirements
C. Reduced ranking on a public website
D. Increased audit frequency

3. During morning rounds, your clinical pharmacist suggests that an aspirin drug should be administered to your patient based on a recent trial. In this trial, a linear regression was performed and demonstrated a positive correlation between aspirin administration and improved patient satisfaction scores, with an R^2 of 0.98. Which of the following BEST describes the R^2 value?

A. Probability of type 1 error
B. Precision of measured data
C. Variability in precision
D. Model accuracy

4. Following prolonged mechanical ventilation for acute respiratory distress syndrome (ARDS) management, a patient is being weaned off of sedation. The nurse reports that the patient is "CAM negative." Which of the following is the MOST appropriate next step in management.

A. Amantadine
B. Hospice consultation
C. Quetiapine
D. Spontaneous breathing trials

5. A 19-year-old male is declared brain dead following a motor vehicle collision in which he was an unhelmeted

operator of a motorcycle. Review of the patient's driver's license indicates that he is an organ donor, and over the following 24 hours, care consistent with preparation for organ donation is undertaken. When the patient's estranged wife first arrives on hospital day 3, she indicates that the patient would want to be "kept alive no matter what." Which of the following is the BEST description of what is appropriate for the intensivist to do in this case?

A. Proceed with organ donation
B. Negotiate with the family
C. Repeat brain death testing
D. Ethics consult

6. A quality improvement project assesses the rates of pneumonia when a new ventilator is used for critically in patients in a local hospital. A population of 108 patients are enrolled. Patients on ventilator A have a pneumonia rate of 9%, while patients on ventilator B have a pneumonia rate of 13%; a P value of 0.07 is given. The hospital administration concludes that there is no difference between the two ventilators. Which of the following BEST describes this conclusion?

A. Type 1 error
B. Bias
C. Underpowering
D. Confounding

7. A study for a new antibiotic enrolls 106 ICU patients to determine the likelihood of having green or purple urine following therapy. Which of the following statistical tests would be MOST appropriate to analyze this outcome?

A. Mann Whitney-U
B. Chi-squared
C. Wilcoxon rank sum
D. Student's t-test

8. A population of nine volunteers is studied to determine whether mini bronchoalveolar lavages (BAL) or tracheal aspirates are more frequently obtained after implementation of a new clinical protocol. Which of the following is the MOST appropriate test?

A. Fisher's exact
B. Bonferroni correction
C. Chi-squared
D. Analysis of variance (ANOVA)

9. Following an uneventful large bowel resection and nephrectomy, a patient without a past medical history of cardiac disease is admitted to the ICU for postoperative

monitoring. Overnight, the patient experiences hypotension and eventually cardiac arrest. On initial case review in the morning, there are no obvious errors made by the staff on call. Which of the following would be the MOST appropriate next step?

A. Medical examiners referral
B. Root cause analysis
C. Morbidity and mortality conference review
D. Medical staff office referral

10. A physician has been late to her shifts frequently over the past several weeks. On arrival to receive handoff for an evening shift, this physician is found by a colleague in the call room with signs of active cocaine use. There were no unstable patients or adverse outcomes from management decisions during the day, and the physician immediately removes herself from the call scheduled and volunteers to get treatment. Which of the following is the MOST appropriate entity to inform?

A. Hospital administration
B. Medical board
C. Risk management
D. National practitioner data bank

11. A 98-year-old female with an extensive past medical history and complex medical course is approached regarding initiating comfort care by the palliative care service. The patient indicates her desire to pursue comfort care, but the patient's daughter who is the medical power of attorney specifically denies permission to change goals of care. Which of the following is the MOST appropriate next step?

A. Ethics consult
B. Comfort care
C. Current goals of care
D. Meeting with all family members

12. A 98-year-old male with a past medical history significant for four-vessel coronary artery bypass graft (CABG), peripheral vascular disease, stage IV renal cell carcinoma, and hepatitis C is managed in your ICU for 23 days following a motor vehicle collision. The patient remains comatose and had a large left-sided ischemic stroke on day 4 of admission. Attempts to communicate with the family or change goals of care have resulted in threats to "sue the hospital if you try to kill my uncle." Which of the following is the MOST appropriate clinical plan of action?

A. Inform risk management
B. Ethics consult

C. Long-term acute care facility placement
D. "Soft" code status

C. Chi-squared
D. Relative risk

13. Hospital administrations requests you to lead a team reviewing retrospective data regarding central line–associated bloodstream infections (CLABSIs). The data provided include 1280 patients older than 10 years who had CLABSIs. You are asked to determine whether a new skin prep that the hospital gradually implemented over this time period reduced the CLABSI rate. Which of the following statistical techniques would be MOST appropriate?

    A. Student's t-test
    B. Odds ratio

14. You are caring for a patient who stopped taking his antirejection medications and now shows signs of renal transplant rejection. The transplant team notes that Medicare stops paying for antirejection drugs after 3 years. Which is the most effective way to change this policy?

    A. Call your congressman
    B. Participate in organized medicine
    C. Run for office
    D. Give money to a legislator

ANSWERS

1. ANSWER: C

This patient has a right parietal-occipital subdural hematoma (SDH). Given its size (<10-mm shift) and lack of other obvious pathology, this CT scan does not indicate a catastrophic brain injury. Because the patient has been receiving a midazolam infusion for an unclear amount of time, it would not be possible to confirm that the patient does not have residual sedation affecting his exam. Therefore, it would be most appropriate to consider this patient ineligible for brain death determination at this time. As such, apnea testing should not be performed at this time.

Uremic encephalopathy is noted to occur in the setting of stage IV or greater renal failure, and because we do not have enough data to determine the extent of this patient's renal disease, there is clearly the presence of an SDH. Intermittent hemodialysis is contraindicated in the setting of acute intracranial bleeding because the rapid shifts in urea could lead to worsening cerebral edema. Furthermore, traumatic brain injury patients are particularly sensitive to changes in cerebral perfusion pressure, which could occur as a result of intermittent hemodialysis, leading to increase use of continuous hemodialysis in traumatic brain injury patients. Of note, hemodialysis patients are at increased risk for presenting with subdural hematoma; additionally, no trauma history is present in 30 to 50% of patients with an SDH.

The lower limit of normal temperature is 36° C, or 96.8° F; in this case, the patient's temperature does not have an effect on the ability to determine brain death if desired. Rewarming would be appropriate if the patient were truly hypothermic.

Keywords: Specialized areas; ICU ethics; Brain death

REFERENCES

Wang IK, Lin CL, Wu YY et al. Subdural hematoma in patients with end-stage renal disease receiving hemodialysis. *Eur J Neurol* 2014;21(6):894–900.

Wijdicks EF, Varelas PN, Gronseth GS, Greer DM; American Academy of Neurology. Evidence-based guideline update: determining brain death in adults. Report of the Quality Standards Subcommittee of the American Academy of Neurology. *Neurology* 2010;74(23):1911–1918.

2. ANSWER: C

HCAHPS is a patient satisfaction survey that must be given to all patients admitted to an inpatient hospital service. This survey excludes psychiatric patients. The purpose of the survey is to assess patients' satisfaction with their inpatient hospital experience. Contrary to popular knowledge, this system was not established by the Affordable Care Act (or Obamacare), but was originally developed during the George W. Bush administration. If a hospital or physician has ratings lower than the 50th percentile, the hospital will be subject to a funding cut 2 years after the actual surveys were performed (i.e., poor survey results in 2015 will result in lower payment in 2017).

Because every program administered by Medicare must be revenue neutral, hospitals rating higher than the 50th percentile will receive a bonus funded by the cuts administered to the lower ranking hospitals. Wild documentation expectations may remain substantial in medical practice; there is no effect on this documentation requirement as a result of these surveys. Additionally, a lower ranking does not automatically result in an audit visit by Medicare.

HCAHPS scores and other key metrics for all hospitals are publicly available on a government-run website (https://www.healthcare.gov/). At this site, consumers can compare hospitals by name, region, and other parameters. A change the hospital's ranking by the HCAHPS system would be shown within weeks of the next reporting period. It should be noted that improved HCAHPS scores have not consistently correlated with patient outcomes in studies.

Keywords: Specialized areas; ICU management and organization; Outcome and performance measures (HCAHPS)

REFERENCES

Joseph B, Azim A, O'Keeffe T et al. American College of Surgeons level I trauma centers outcomes do not correlate with patients' perception of hospital experience. *J Trauma Acute Care Surg.* 2017;82(4):722–727.

Sacks GD, Lawson EH, Dawes AJ et al. Relationship between hospital performance on a patient satisfaction survey and surgical quality. *JAMA Surg* 2015;150(9):858–864.

3. ANSWER: D

Fundamentally, a linear regression is a graph of dependent and independent variables. The statistics software used attempts to plot a line that best matches the values given, and the "degree" of fitting the line can be described numerically. The standard format for a linear regression equation is:

$$Y = \beta° + \beta 1 \times + \varepsilon$$

where Y (the line) has an intercept ($\beta°$) with a slope ($\beta 1$) plus error term (ε). The regression (R^2) value represents the amount of variation in the *dependent* variable that is explained by the linear association with the independent variable by model. The generic graph generated in Figure 10.1 demonstrates

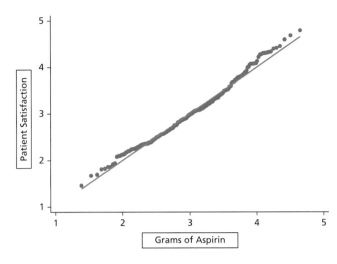

Figure 10.1 Sample of linear regression.
(Diagram produced by George Williams using Stata/IC 14.2 for Mac [64-bit Intel].)

values that correlate very closely. The threshold for considering an R^2 significant is generally agreed to be more than 0.8, although this is up to interpretation and varies by investigator. At its core, statistics is as much art as science; this concept leads to some variability as to numerical thresholds commonly used for technical concepts such as the R^2.

Keywords: Specialized areas; Biostatistics; Regression analysis

4. ANSWER: D

The Confusion Assessment Method for the ICU (CAM-ICU) score was originally published in the 1990s to serve as a screening tool for delirium by medical teams not staffed by psychiatrists. The CAM-ICU questionnaire is designed to be very simple, consisting of four elements: the first two elements are required and one of the latter two must be present to diagnose delirium. First published for clinical use in the ICU in 2001, the CAM-ICU tool has been widely adopted as a means for screening for delirium. It is important to remember that delirium is an independent risk factor for mortality in the ICU population. If a patient is CAM-ICU "positive," then the patient's examination is consistent with delirium (CAM-ICU has 100% sensitivity and 89% specificity for delirium when conducted by a physician).

There has been some research evaluating the role of neurostimulants such as amantadine for use in patients who have cognitive dysfunction manifested by lethargy in the ICU, with significant work being completed in the cardiac arrest, cardiac surgery, and traumatic brain injury populations. Because this patient is just completing a complicated clinical course and is following commands,

neurostimulants do not appear to be appropriate right now. Furthermore, because this patient is improving, consulting palliative care medicine would not be indicated.

In this case, because the patient is not showing clinical signs of delirium, there is no indication for antipsychotics such as Haldol or Seroquel.

Keywords: Specialized areas; ICU management and organization; Sedation, analgesia, delirium assessment (e.g. CAM, RASS)

REFERENCE

Ely EW, Margolin R, Francis J et al. Evaluation of delirium in critically ill patients: validation of the Confusion Assessment Method for the Intensive Care Unit (CAM-ICU). *Crit Care Med* 2001;29(7):1370–1379.

5. ANSWER: A

By indicating his wishes on his driver's license, this patient has completed a process called first-person authorization (FPA). Otherwise known as "donor designation," FPA allows an individual to choose to donate organs in a fashion that cannot be overridden by family members. Legislation enacting FPA has been passed in all 50 US states and the District of Columbia. This is, in part, because of the large number of patients awaiting a transplant at any given time. The number of patients awaiting organ transplantation increased by five-fold since 1990 to more than 100,000 in 2017; on the converse, the number of transplants increased two-fold from 15,000 to 34,000 over the same time span. FPA legislation was a nationwide effort to address this public health challenge, as are other efforts, such as donation after cardiac death (DCD).

Although it is clear that a situation like this would be emotionally charged and likely involve the patient experience and ethical support apparatus of a hospital, an ethics consult would not truly be helpful because the law is settled on this matter. Similarly, negotiation with the family would indicate that there are unclear legal grounds on which to carry out the patient's wishes, which is not true. Finally, repeated brain death testing is not indicated after the declaration of brain death has been made.

Keywords: Specialized areas; ICU ethics; Organ donation

REFERENCES

Choudhury RA, Prins K, Moore HB et al. Uncontrolled deceased cardiac donation: an unutilized source for organ transplantation in the United States. *Clin Transplant* 2018;33(3):e13474.

Traino HM, Siminoff LA. Attitudes and acceptance of First Person Authorization: a national comparison of donor and nondonor families. *J Trauma Acute Care Surg* 2013;74(1):294–300.

6. ANSWER: A

Although this scenario appears to be abstract, it reflects a frequently observed event in hospital administration. In determining whether results are statistically significant, it is important to understand what the role of a *P* value is. A *P* value is generally considered significant when less than 0.05; however, this designation is arbitrary in the field of medicine. When evaluating "significance," the clinician is essentially concluding if the result seen is likely by chance or not. The *P* value indicates the probability that the result occurred by chance, and in the field of medicine we have determined that a threshold of 5% or less is significant. This is analogous to running the exact same experiment 100 times and obtaining the result by chance 5% of the time.

Confounding is not relevant in this particular instance because we are not looking at other factors that could be affecting the outcome. Confounders for this project could include the presence of an immune deficiency or hypothermia, for example. Additionally, bias would be not applicable because this would occur in the setting of choosing patients for ventilator A versus ventilator B in a nonrandom fashion. There is no indication that this occurred in the stem. Finally, underpowering is an interesting phenomenon. If a *P* value is determined to be significant, then a study is not truly underpowered, although a larger population size is normally preferred in order to add validity to a study's results. Similarly, if a *P* value is not significant, underpowering may have occurred; however, the larger the population gets, the smaller is the detectable difference possible. If this ventilator study requires 100,000 patients in each arm in order to find a difference in the rate of pneumonia, that specific finding may not be clinically significant and not relevant for administrative consideration.

Importantly, type 1 error is incorrectly rejecting the null hypothesis, and type 2 error is incorrectly accepting the null hypothesis. In this case, the administrator is making a type 1 error.

Keywords: Specialized areas; Biostatistics; Type 1 and type 2 errors

7. ANSWER: C

Statistical tests are commonly employed in medical research, and their proper application is a key factor in properly interpreting the results gleaned from a project. In general, statistical tests should be organized based on the type of variables being analyzed. As such, it is important to recognize the three primary types of variables: continuous, categorical, and ordinal. Continuous variables include values that are heavily numerical with possible precision, such as weight or height. Categorical variables are values without an orderly organization, such as color or gender. Ordinal variables are still not continuous or categorical but may have continuous properties, such as a number scale that correlates with increasing risk or intensity. The American Society of Anesthesiologists (ASA) score is an excellent example of this in that an ASA 1 patient is certainly healthier than an ASA 2 patient, but there is no ASA 1.7 status.

In this case, the variable is a categorical variable (color), which would indicate use of a chi-squared test. A student's t-test is used to analyze continuous variables. When a nonparametrically distributed sample is obtained (i.e., the sample is skewed or not balanced), the Wilcoxon rank sum or Mann-Whitney U test is used. Because these tests are synonymous, there is no difference between answer choices A and C.

Keywords: Specialized areas; Biostatistics; Statistical tests; Nonparametric (e.g., Wilcoxon rank sum, Mann-Whitney U test, chi-squared test, Kaplan-Meier curve), Parametric (e.g.; t-test, ANOVA)

8. ANSWER: A

The question expounds on the concepts reviewed in question 7, with specific knowledge required for the application of categorical tests. A small population size ($> \sim 15$) cannot be appropriately studied with a chi-squared test. The Fisher's exact test was designed for a small population such as this (Figure 10.2).

The ANOVA is designed to compare means between multiple (three or more) groups at the same time. A Bonferroni correction specifically applies to hypothesis testing when multiple variables are tested against each other in different combinations. Take, for example, a group of six different variables in a study. Each of these variables is assigned a letter, A through F. If we compare group A to group B and the *P* value is 0.05, that specific value may be significant (type 1 error probability is 5%). However, as we compare the multiple groups in this data set, the probability of making a type 1 error when the overall set of combinations of this population is combined grows with each individual test. The goal of the Bonferroni correction is lower the individual p values needed for each test, so that the overall P value can remain statistically significant after all of the compounded type 1 error is accounted for.

Keywords: Specialized areas; Biostatistics; Statistical tests; Nonparametric (e.g., Wilcoxon rank sum, Mann-Whitney

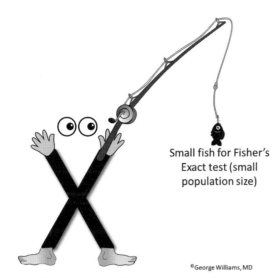

Small fish for Fisher's Exact test (small population size)

Full size X² for a normal population size

©George Williams, MD

Figure 10.2 Common categorical tests pneumonic.

U test, chi-squared test, Kaplan-Meier curve); Parametric (e.g., t-test, ANOVA)

9. ANSWER: B

In circumstances such as this, an RCA is an important part of the hospital's quality improvement process. Because this patient expired following a procedure in which mortality was not expected, further review is required. An RCA is a concept that was adapted from the business world to allow hospitals to function as highly reliable organizations by drilling down to the root of a systemic problem that may have contributed to an unexpected negative outcome. An RCA should not be part of a punitive process focused on an individual provider but should be focused on the system as a whole.

Because this case is an unexpected death, referral to the medical examiner's office is not necessarily required, although it could take place. Medical examiner referrals are generally reserved for patients who have died as a result of potentially criminal causes (e.g., gunshot wounds). Although this case will likely and should likely be reviewed in a departmental morbidity and mortality conference, such a conference is insufficient considering the magnitude of what has happened in this case. Finally, while medical staff office referral could be appropriate depending on the circumstances behind the event, it is not the paramount issue that should be considered by an administrative team running an ICU.

Keywords: Specialized areas; ICU management and organization; QA/QI (patient safety)

REFERENCE

Gershengorn HB, Kocher R, Factor P. Management strategies to effect change in intensive care units: lessons from the world of business. Part I. Targeting quality improvement initiatives. *Ann Am Thorac Soc.* 2014;11(2):264–269.

10. ANSWER: B

In most states, an individual is required to report an impaired physician, and if a person is knowledgeable of this requirement and does not report such a position, there could be legal consequences. Most laws provide immunity for the reporting individual, but each state is different. The National Practitioner Data Bank (NPDB) provides information about licensure status, professional conduct, and any malpractice claims against physicians; it does not serve as an appropriate reporting mechanism in circumstances such as this. Of note, admission into a treatment program is not reportable to the NPDB.

Although reporting to hospital administration or the risk management team may seem pertinent, such a report is not necessarily legally required and would not come before informing the medical board of a given state. The Americans with Disabilities Act (ADA), which was enacted in 1992, does provides protection for individuals who have substance abuse difficulty with alcohol specifically. Additionally, a person with alcoholism need not be in a treatment program in order to receive protection from the ADA. There is no disability protection for other illicit substances as are described in the stem.

Keywords: Specialized areas; ICU ethics; Impaired providers

REFERENCE

Bryson EO, Silverstein JH. Addiction and substance abuse in anesthesiology. *Anesthesiology* 2008;109(5):905–917.

11. ANSWER: B

Out of the four ethical principles—nonmaleficence, beneficence, and justice—the ethical principle of autonomy has been a pillar of the practice of medicine in the United States since the 1940s. Although this stem does not give us a great deal of information, it does indicate that the patient was able to communicate her wishes clearly. The presence of an extensive past medical history or being elderly does not prohibit patients from exercising their right of autonomy. As a result of this, the patient still has full authority to determine her goals of care. The person who is designated as the medical power of attorney cannot overrule a patient who is able to communicate his or her own wishes.

Therefore, an ethics consult on current goals of care would be inappropriate. Additionally, having more family members present would not be helpful because the patient would still determine her own plan care.

Keywords: Specialized areas; ICU ethics; Patient autonomy

REFERENCE

Rubin MA. The collaborative autonomy model of medical decision-making. *Neurocrit Care* 2014;20(2):311–318.

12. ANSWER: B

This clinical case describes a patient who is essentially moribund and for whom a goals of care discussion would be appropriate. Certain issues that are commonly seen in the ICU are raised, such as grief and resistance to electing for comfort care as a course of action. It remains important to consider the four principles of ethics when considering such cases: autonomy, justice, beneficence, and nonmaleficence. To properly assess whether this patient would desire to continue what appears to be futile care (autonomy), it would be necessary to have some perspective on the patient's wishes at baseline. As such, when considering how to answer such a question, it is important to evaluate the course of action that would facilitate assessing the patient's wishes.

Risk management, although certainly appropriate to include in this case, would not be the most appropriate service to engage at this time in dealing with the patient's clinical issue. Clearly, because this patient does not appear to have reasonable probability of ever leaving the hospital, it would seem inappropriate to refer the patient to a long-term acute care facility. While "soft" codes (allowing cardiopulmonary resuscitation for a few moments and then promptly declaring death) are described, they have been generally agreed to be inappropriate as a care plan because they do not allow for true disclosure of the medical plan of action. An ethics consult is the only realistic way to engage hospital administration for support while simultaneously evaluating the patient wishes.

Keywords: Specialized areas; ICU ethics; End-of-life, futility

REFERENCE

Neville TH, Wenger NS. The authors reply. *Crit Care Med* 2015;43(5):e152.

13. ANSWER: B

As a rule, odds ratios are most appropriate when patients are identified based on their outcome; prior exposure to an event (or agent) is then determined. The odds ratio is generally used when evaluating rare diseases (e.g., pseudohyperkalemia); therefore, one is more likely to see it used with large data sets (e.g., National Inpatient Sample). The risk ratio, or relative risk, is an applicable test for patients who are followed over time on the basis of an exposure in order to determine whether they have a specific outcome. Generally, relative risk is not applied to retrospective data sets.

Because these are retrospective data, the options of chi-squared and Student's t-test are distractors. Recall that these tests compare two groups for categorical and continuous variables, respectively.

Keywords: Specialized areas; Biostatistics; Odds ratio; Relative risk

REFERENCE

Meng QH1, Wagar EA. Pseudohyperkalemia: a new twist on an old phenomenon. *Crit Rev Clin Lab Sci* 2015;52(2):45–55.

14. ANSWER: B

The example given in this stem is reflective of an existing in common policy that Medicare enacted in 1995. This is a policy that is the result of a rule; rules are policies made by administration (executive branch) officials and do not require action from Congress. A rule in effect describes how a law should be carried out. For example, if Congress passed a law requiring all patients with sepsis to be given antibiotics, a rule by the executive branch to carry out that law could dictate what antibiotics should be given and at what doses and under what circumstances. This particular immunosuppressive drug rule is considered by many physicians to be poorly conceived because after spending tens of thousands of dollars on a transplantation, an individual would suddenly be in a position in which they cannot afford the very drugs needed to maintain the transplant. The fact that such a rule still exists is reflective of inadequate advocacy on the part of organized medicine; such inadequacy likely results from the general lack of physician knowledge of the importance of collective efforts in the political arena.

Running for office, while effective, is impractical for most people, although the authors do encourage physicians who are interested in participating in policymaking to run for office if they are able to do so. Participating in organized medicine is the single most effective way to communicate with rule-makers because large organizations have resources and staff who have relationships with the actual rule-making individuals. In particular, a political action committee is a financial vehicle (essentially a bank account) through which any group of people can contribute money for a collective cause; in this way, groups can participate in the political process and allow for the direct lobbying of individuals for a specific purpose. Finally, giving money directly to a politician is a very effective way to inject influence into the political process; however, in order to change a policy on this scale, a collective effort such as being involved in organized medicine would be necessary.

REFERENCES

Croft D, Jay SJ, Meslin EM et al. Perspective: is it time for advocacy training in medical education? *Acad Med*. 2012;87(9):1165–1170.

Medicare program; Medicare coverage of prescription drugs used in immunosuppressive therapy—HCFA. Final rule. *Fed Regist* 1995;60(32):8951–8955.

11.

PULMONOLOGY

Ted Lytle and Marc J. Popovich

QUESTIONS

The following case applies to questions 1 and 2:

You respond to a rapid response call for hypoxemia on a 24-year-old obese (body mass index [BMI] of 36) male who is 12 hours from repair of bilateral midshaft femoral fractures following a boating accident 36 hours ago. Additional past medical history includes obstructive sleep apnea (OSA), mild intermittent asthma, and alcohol abuse. He has an allergy to penicillin. Vital signs include temperature 38.5 ° C, heart rate (HR) 110 bpm, blood pressure (BP) 130/80 mm Hg, respiratory rate (RR) 30 breaths/minute, and pulse O_2 saturation 86% on room air. Physical exam shows clear lung auscultation bilaterally and no jugular venous distention. Current medications include acetaminophen, morphine sulfate, low-molecular-weight heparin, and cefazolin. The patient is placed on nasal oxygen and is sent for computed tomography (CT) lung scan, which shows bilateral ground-glass infiltrates. Because he remains persistently hypoxemic, the patient is transferred to the intensive care unit (ICU), where continuous positive pressure ventilation (PPV) by mask (continuous positive airway pressure [CPAP] 8, forced inspiratory oxygen [FiO_2] 0.5) is initiated, and O_2 saturations stabilize at 97%. Shortly thereafter, he becomes disoriented and belligerent, and a petechial rash is noted on his chest and neck. Arterial blood gas (ABG) analysis shows a PaO_2 of 50 and a PCO_2 of 40.

1. Which of the following is MOST helpful in establishing the patient's diagnosis?

    A. Complete blood count
    B. Liver function enzymes plus creatine phosphokinase
    C. CT of the head
    D. Pulmonary artery catheterization
    E. Fiberoptic bronchoscopy

2. Which of the following would be the MOST appropriate next step in management?

    A. Administer aerosolized albuterol by mask
    B. Administer intravenous (IV) epinephrine
    C. Begin IV heparin with bolus and infusion
    D. Initiate bilevel positive airway pressure
    E. Endotracheal intubation and mechanical ventilation

3. A 75-year-old male with hypertension, obesity, anxiety, and OSA undergoes urgent coronary artery bypass grafting with intra-aortic balloon bump placement following an ST-elevation myocardial infarction. He is extubated to mask CPAP on the second postoperative day. Two days later, he has diuresed, and the ICU team orders his mask CPAP and central line discontinued. The patient asks for his home lorazepam before line removal. Following line removal, he complains of dyspnea and develops hypoxia and tachycardia and then headache. BP is 90/50 mm Hg, and O_2 saturation is 88% on 2-L nasal cannula. Which of the following interventions is MOST appropriate?

    A. Give IV epinephrine 100 mcg
    B. Immediate intubation and mechanical ventilation
    C. Position patient left side down and put on high-flow oxygen
    D. Get transthoracic ultrasound
    E. Put patient back on CPAP and continue diuresis

The following case applies to questions 4 and 5:

A 30-year-old male with a history of prior IV drug abuse, alcohol use, and hepatitis C is transferred to your tertiary care IC from the emergency department (ED) after presenting with chest pain and dyspnea following a "wing-eating contest" 12 hours earlier, after which he vomited. He does not follow regularly with physicians and is on no medications. Physical exam shows an ill-appearing male with epigastric guarding. He is tachycardic and tachypneic, with a BP of 100/60 mm Hg. Urine appears concentrated. Initial laboratory evaluation includes a leukocytosis with left shift and a hemoglobin of 9.3 mg/dL. CT scan of the chest demonstrates distal esophageal perforation and left-sided pleural effusion.

4. Initial management should include:

A. Administration of red blood cells
B. Placement of a nasogastric tube
C. Thoracentesis of the left pleural space
D. Thoracic surgery consultation

5. Which of the following antimicrobials would be the BEST empiric choice?

A. Piperacillin-tazobactam
B. Vancomycin plus fluconazole
C. Meropenem plus fluconazole
D. Aztreonam

6. A 77-year-old male with a history of obesity, OSA (treated with home-use mask CPAP), diabetes mellitus, chronic renal failure with a baseline creatinine of 1.5 mg/dL, and post-traumatic stress disorder sustained a fall from horseback resulting in right anterior chest trauma. CT scan demonstrated fractures of ribs four through eight and moderate hemopneumothorax, for which a chest tube drain was placed. He received 4 mg of IV morphine sulfate and was admitted to the ICU with O$_2$ saturation of 90% on 2-L nasal cannula. He has notably severe right anterior chest discomfort. Physical exam demonstrates an obese male in a cervical collar, splinting, with paradoxical chest wall movement on the right as well as decreased breath sounds on the right base. The chest tube drain has an intermittent air leak. Repeat chest radiography shows the right lung moderately well expanded with elevated right hemidiaphragm.
The next BEST option for pain control is:

A. Enteral acetaminophen
B. IV morphine sulfate
C. IV ketamine
D. Intrapleural infusion of local anesthetic
E. Regional anesthesia

7. An obese 65-year-old male presents to the ICU postoperatively after urgent coronary artery bypass grafting. Intraoperative transesophageal echocardiography demonstrated low-normal biventricular function and mild-moderate tricuspid valve insufficiency. He arrives with an intra-aortic balloon pump, is orotracheally intubated with an 8.0 endotracheal tube, and has an orogastric tube.

Ten hours later, the patient self-extubates. He wakes up and is cooperative, in moderate discomfort with deep inspiration, and is intermittently dozing to sleep with snoring following IV fentanyl and associated modest desaturation to 85% and some associated bradycardia. He is kept supine because of the presence of the intra-aortic balloon pump. A chest radiograph shows mild elevation of hemidiaphragms and small bilateral pleural effusions. ABG shows a PaO$_2$ of 58 and a PCO$_2$ of 50.

Which of the following is the next management option?

A. Administer IV naloxone
B. Reintubate
C. Increase epinephrine infusion
D. Start noninvasive PPV and follow closely
E. Administer high-velocity nasal oxygen

For questions 8 to 14, match the ventilation mode with its description. Each description may be used once, more than once, or not at all.
Modes

8. Volume-controlled ventilation
9. Pressure-controlled ventilation
10. Pressure-controlled inverse ratio ventilation
11. Pressure support ventilation
12. Airway pressure release ventilation
13. Synchronized intermittent mandatory ventilation
14. Pressure-regulated volume control

Descriptions

A. Time triggered, pressure limited, time cycled
B. Flow triggered, pressure limited, flow cycled
C. Time triggered, flow limited, time cycled
D. Time triggered, pressure limited, volume cycled
E. Flow triggered, flow limited, time cycled

15. A 70-year-old female with a history of hypertension, diabetes mellitus, severe aortic stenosis, and severe coronary artery disease is admitted to a cardiology service and received diuretics for 2 days before undergoing primary median sternotomy, tissue aortic valve replacement, and coronary artery bypass grafting × 3, complicated by intraoperative bleeding and coagulopathy, postoperative respiratory failure, and need for inotropic support. On postoperative day 3, the patient develops increased sputum production and increased suctioning requirements of tracheal tube by respiratory therapy. Labs are notable for increased leukocytosis. A chest radiograph discloses a right perihilar infiltrate. Which of the following is the BEST option for management?

A. Increase diuresis
B. Bolus heparin and begin IV infusion

C. Start enteral levofloxacin
D. Start parenteral vancomycin and piperacillin-tazobactam

The following case applies to questions 16 and 17:
Following a weekend of significant alcohol consumption, a 27-year-old previously healthy male presents to the ED with epigastric pain and is subsequently diagnosed with severe acute pancreatitis. Given his moderately deranged hemodynamics and ongoing need for resuscitation, he is admitted to your ICU. He receives 5 L of crystalloid over the following 24 hours and develops increasing hypoxia and tachypnea with dyspnea. Chest radiograph the next day shows extensive bilateral alveolar opacities. He has minimal cough, no fever, and mild sputum production. Point-of-care ultrasound shows normal biventricular function.

16. Which of the following diagnoses BEST describes this patient?

A. Acute cardiogenic pulmonary edema
B. Acute bilateral pneumonia
C. Acute pulmonary embolism
D. Acute respiratory distress syndrome (ARDS)

17. The patient's tachypnea is primarily the result of:

A. Increased elastic work of breathing
B. Increased resistive work of breathing
C. Increased static compliance
D. Increased dynamic compliance

18. A 55-year-old male current smoker with hypertension, mild coronary artery disease, chronic alcohol abuse, compensated diastolic heart failure, anemia, and localized pancreatic cancer is recovering from an open pancreatectomy that was complicated by 1 L of blood loss, multiple small bowel enterotomies, and volume resuscitation of 4 L of crystalloid. He is extubated on postoperative day 1 and, following a day in the ICU, is transferred to step-down floor. He is not started on heparin prophylaxis because of intraoperative misadventures. The morning of day 2, he is transfused 1 unit of red blood cells for mild hypotension (90/60 mm Hg) and oliguria. During mobilization with physical therapy later that morning, he is noted to have increasing dyspnea, hypoxia, and tachycardia. On exam, the patient is in moderate distress with accessory muscle use and is febrile and tachypneic. There is

no jugular venous distention, his abdomen is tender, and there is +1 pitting edema in his lower extremities. Electrocardiogram shows sinus tachycardia. A chest radiograph is ordered and shows diffuse bilateral pulmonary infiltrates. Bedside transthoracic echocardiography shows left ventricular hypertrophy. Which of the following diagnoses is MOST likely?

A. Pulmonary embolism
B. Aspiration pneumonia
C. Transfusion-associated circulatory overload (TACO)
D. Transfusion-related acute lung injury (TRALI)
E. Myocardial infarction

The following case applies to questions 19 and 20:
A 68-year-old 50-kg, 5'0"-tall female with a medical history significant for tobacco abuse and chronic obstructive pulmonary disease (COPD) with bullous emphysematous changes on recent CT scan of the chest undergoes general endotracheal anesthesia and uncomplicated thyroidectomy for localized thyroid cancer. Because of postprocedural somnolence and hypercapnia, she is left intubated and transferred to your ICU, where she is placed on volume-controlled ventilation with RR of 16 breaths/minute, tidal volumes of 550 mL, PS of 8, positive end-expiratory pressure (PEEP) of 8, and FiO_2 of 50%. You are called to her bedside 30 minutes later because of desaturation and hypotension.

19. Which of the following is the BEST intervention?

A. Reduce the FiO_2
B. Reduce the PEEP
C. Reduce the respiratory rate
D. Reduce the tidal volume

20. After your intervention, the hypotension and desaturation improve, but shortly thereafter the patient is in extremis, writhing in bed, with a BP of 70/30 mm Hg, HR of 110 bpm, and jugular venous distention, and the ventilator peak pressure alarm is ringing. There are decreased breath sounds on the right. What is the initial management step?

A. Order a chest radiograph
B. Bolus propofol to achieve better ventilator synchrony
C. Administer epinephrine 100 mcg IV
D. Needle decompression on right side

ANSWERS

1. ANSWER: A

2. ANSWER: B

Fat embolism syndrome (FES) typically manifests 24 to 72 hours following an initial insult and is most commonly associated with long bone trauma and pelvic fracture. FES may also result from hardware manipulation during orthopedic procedures, soft tissue trauma (particular adipose tissue), cosmetic procedures, and rib fracture. Nontraumatic causes, including pancreatitis, infusion of lipid-containing agents, sickle cell crisis, and osteonecrosis, have been described. Early immobilization of fractures may decrease likelihood of fat embolism, as does surgical correction rather than simply traction.

The most common presenting symptoms are respiratory and may include tachypnea, dyspnea, and hypoxemia. Neurological deficits, including confusion or seizure, may develop, as may the characteristic petechial rash, although this is present on average about 30% of the time.

Chest radiograph is typically normal initially but may progress to bilateral pulmonary infiltrates if ARDS develops. CT scan may show bilateral ground-glass infiltrates. Respiratory insufficiency may progress to ARDS in perhaps as many as 50% of cases. Multiple-organ dysfunction may progress and is due to either mechanical obstruction of capillaries or production of toxic free fatty acids following hydrolysis of fat and cytokine production. Paradoxical arterial emboli may occur because of patent foramen ovale, pulmonary arteriovenous malformation, or pulmonary microvascular overload.

Up to two thirds of patients may have associated thrombocytopenia and anemia; thus, of the items listed in the first question, a complete blood count would be most likely to contribute to making the diagnosis. Liver enzyme tests and pulmonary artery catheterization are nonspecific modalities and typically are unnecessary steps in FES. Additionally, although bronchoscopy and lavage demonstrating fat droplets within alveolar macrophages have been reported as diagnostic, the neurological impairment is usually nonfocal; thus, CT is rarely helpful. Magnetic resonance imaging, however, may show a "star field" pattern of diffuse, punctate, hyperintense lesions on diffusion-weighted scans.

Treatment is supportive, and in this case the most appropriate choice for the second question would be intubation and mechanical ventilation, to include a lung protective strategy. IV heparin is not indicated for treatment of fat embolism. Aerosolized albuterol is not indicated because there is no evidence of an acute asthma exacerbation based on physical exam. Steroid therapy is controversial and implemented on a case-by-case basis. Bilevel positive airway pressure is not an ideal therapy in uncooperative patients or those with decreased mental status. There is no evidence of acute COPD exacerbation nor hypercapnia. Noninvasive PPV for acute lung injury and ARDS is controversial, and limited evidence exists. Epinephrine may be required if there is evidence of right ventricular failure or obstructive shock from emboli. In this case, there is none. Additionally, the rash described is not most consistent with allergic reaction to cefazolin, although cross-reactivity may occur in 2 to 7%, and in as many as 50% of those patients who have had an anaphylactic reaction to penicillin.

Keywords: Critical illness diagnosis and management, pulmonary; Diagnoses, embolic disorders, fat

REFERENCES

Akhtar S. Fat embolism. *Anesthesiol Clin* 2009;27:533.
Mellor A Soni N. Fat embolism. *Anesthesia* 2001;56:145.
Stein PD, Yaekoub AY, Matta F, Kleerekoper M. Fat embolism syndrome. *Am J Med Sci* 2008;336:472.

3. ANSWER: C

The timing of the respiratory symptoms in relation to line removal suggests venous air embolism. Venous air embolism may be encountered during surgical procedures, trauma, line placement or removal, or intravascular injection or may be due to barotrauma during PPV or rapid ascent by divers. Care must be taken during removal of a line from a patient not undergoing PPV such that positioning is at least supine (the patient should not be sitting up) and the insertion site is compressed and covered with an airtight seal—lest air be sucked in during inspiration. When suspected, assuming hemodynamic stability, the patient should be placed in left lateral decubitus position with head down, which brings the right ventricular outflow tract inferior to the right ventricle and inhibits further embolization. If a central line remains in place and the patient is in extremis, an attempt at withdrawing air through the central line may be made. It is estimated that as little as 50 mL of venous air can be fatal due to creation of an "air lock" and obstructive shock. Large bubbles of air are most associated with an air lock, whereas smaller bubbles enter the pulmonary capillary system, causing damage, vasoconstriction, and release of inflammatory mediators. If the patient is hemodynamically unstable, requiring inotropic or vasopressor support, and there is end-organ dysfunction, then hyperbaric oxygen therapy may be considered. Paradoxical air embolism may occur with overload of pulmonary capillary system or through a patent foramen ovale or pulmonary arteriovenous malformation. Small amounts of air (0.5–2 mL) can have devastating consequences in cerebral and coronary vasculature.

Neither epinephrine nor intubation is yet indicated given current clinical stability. Transthoracic ultrasonography is the first test of choice for diagnosing intracardiac air; however, this would follow immediate therapy to prevent additional complications. Indirect effects of air emboli may include capillary leak, which would be supportively treated with diuresis. However, in this case, given the scenario, this is not the best choice.

Keywords: Basic pathophysiology, pulmonary; Embolic disorders

REFERENCES

Muth CM, Shank ES. Gas embolism. *N Engl J Med* 2000;342:476.
Palmon SC, Moore LE, Lundberg J, Toung T. Venous air embolism: a review. *J Clin Anesthesiol* 1997;9:251.

4. ANSWER: D

5. ANSWER: C

Infections of the mediastinum may develop as a complication of cardiac surgery, may spread from odontogenic or retropharyngeal infections, or may result from primary penetrating trauma, hematogenous spread of infection, or esophageal perforation. General principles of therapy for mediastinitis include debridement and source control, early antibiotic therapy, restoration of luminal integrity (if applicable and possible), and appropriate monitoring and follow-up.

Any organism can cause mediastinitis. Typically, a single-agent beta-lactam with sufficient gram-negative coverage would suffice; however, because of this patient's substance abuse and chronic liver disease, the addition of antifungal coverage is warranted.

In cardiac postsurgical patients, mediastinitis would be a surgical site infection; thus, the most common organism is typically methicillin-sensitive *Staphylococcus aureus*. Risk factors for post–cardiac surgery mediastinitis include diabetes, obesity, tobacco use, peripheral arterial disease, prolonged procedure, emergency surgery, prior cardiac surgery, return to operating room, prolonged preoperative or postoperative ICU stay, preoperative intra-aortic balloon bump, and dialysis. Clinical presentation is typical for an infectious process with elevated white blood cell count, fever, pain, and radiographic findings of fluid collection. Sternal instability may occur. Treatment includes reopening and debridement as well as antimicrobial therapy.

Esophageal perforation and resultant mediastinitis may have devastating morbidity and high mortality rates if not treated promptly, with mortality doubling to 28% if treatment begins more than 24 hours after the initial event. Etiologies of perforation include iatrogenic (primarily during endoscopy), traumatic, ingestion of foreign body, and retching. Following the previous general principles, antimicrobial therapy should be started immediately, covering both aerobic and anaerobic organisms and possibly yeast (this may include immunosuppressed patients, those on antibiotic therapy before perforation, and those on long-term acid suppression, as well as patients who do not make clinical progress after initial therapy). Consultation with thoracic surgery should occur as an option for source control by chest tube placement, for possible luminal repair (either by stent or primarily), and if the patient deteriorates acutely and requires further surgical exploration. Clearly, leakage of esophageal contents into the mediastinum can initiate an inflammatory cascade leading to multiple-organ failure, and supportive care as needed must be provided.

There is no indication for blood transfusion in this case as initial management.

Keywords: Basic pathophysiology, pulmonary; Infection, mediastinitis

REFERENCES

Abu-Omar Y, Kocher GJ, Bosco P et al. European Association for Cardio-Thoracic Surgery expert consensus statement on the prevention and management of mediastinitis. *Eur J Cardiothorac Surg* 2017;51:10.
Brinster CJ, Singhal S, Lee L et al. Evolving options in the management of esophageal perforation. *Ann Thorac Surg* 2004;77:1475.
Vallböhmer D, Hölscher AH, Hölscher M et al. Options in the management of esophageal perforation: analysis over a 12-year period. *Dis Esophagus* 2010;23:185.

6. ANSWER: E

Paradoxical chest wall movement—inward motion of the chest during inspiration—is indicative of flail chest, which requires either double fractures of three or more contiguous ribs or a single fracture in multiple ribs along the same vertical line. Flail chest is most commonly caused by blunt force trauma.

Many strategies for pain control in patients with rib fractures exist, and there is no specific consensus. What is clear, however, is that patients with rib fractures are at risk for significant pulmonary complications related to severe pain with deep breaths and coughing, decreased respiratory work from mechanical dissociation, and possible lung contusion. Retained hemothorax and subsequent development of empyema may also complicate the hospital course, as can ongoing air leaks. More than 50% of patients with flail chest require mechanical ventilation, and the incidence of pneumonia in patients older than 65 years may be one in three. Having more than six rib fractures increases the risk for death.

The Eastern Association for the Surgery of Trauma (EAST) recommends an individual, tailored approach, including involvement of a dedicated pain service and use of regional anesthesia, particularly epidural analgesia, for patients with four or more rib fractures, those older than 65 years, and those who have significant cardiopulmonary disease or diabetes mellitus. Enteral acetaminophen, although ultimately a reasonable part of a multimodal approach, is likely insufficient, and given the current clinical status, the patient should be kept nothing by mouth (NPO) for possible intubation. IV morphine sulfate is not the best choice because of renal insufficiency, and IV ketamine is not the best choice because of the patient's history of post-traumatic stress disorder. Studies have shown ketamine to be a useful adjunct in trauma patients. There is no good evidence to support intrapleural local anesthesia.

Keywords: Basic pathophysiology, pulmonary; Chest trauma (e.g., pulmonary contusion, flail chest)

REFERENCES

Bulger EM, Edwards T, Klotz P, Jurkovich GJ. Epidural analgesia improves outcome after multiple rib fractures. *Surgery* 2004;136:426.

Dehghan N, de Mestral C, McKee MD et al. Flail chest injuries: a review of outcomes and treatment practices from the National Trauma Data Bank. *J Trauma Acute Care Surg* 2014; 76:462.

7. ANSWER: D

OSA results from the repetitive collapse of the upper airway during sleep, leading to apneas and hypopneas. Snoring, gasping, and sleep interruptions are common, as are fatigue and daytime sleepiness. OSA is more common in men with a BMI higher than 30 and narrowed oropharyngeal airways. Systemic and pulmonary hypertension, as well as nocturnal cardiac arrhythmias, may be present. Through screening tools such as STOP-Bang, which may predict a patient's predilection for OSA based on the presence of risk factors, the diagnosis is made by polysomnographic testing.

However, not infrequently, patients present postoperatively with either clinically undiagnosed OSA or unanticipated worsening of their known condition. The prevalence of OSA in surgical patients is estimated at 10%, but in certain high-risk surgical subspecialties, it may be as high as 70%. Strategies to reduce postoperative complications of OSA include upright positioning, judicious use of opioids, and close monitoring,

especially in the first 48 hours, when the majority of complications occur.

When obstruction is noted, the clinician may elect to use noninvasive PPV. CPAP may be used to maintain upper airway patency and improve oxygenation—particularly in an airway that has been manipulated and is at risk for swelling and crowding. Bilevel positive airway pressure may be an option in obese patients who cannot be perfectly positioned, those receiving opioid analgesia, and if hypercapnia is a primary concern. IV naloxone is not indicated given the patient's level of wakefulness and cooperativity, and neither is reintubation, assuming resolution of obstruction with noninvasive PPV. Bradycardia is likely related to desaturation, and thus increasing the epinephrine is not indicated. High-flow-velocity nasal oxygen may be an additional option; however, given the positioning constraints and intermittent sleeping with obstructive symptoms, this is not the best option.

Keywords: Basic pathophysiology, pulmonary; Respiratory failure; Sleep apnea, obstructive

REFERENCE

American Society of Anesthesiologists Task Force on Perioperative Management of patients with obstructive sleep apnea. Practice guidelines for the perioperative management of patients with obstructive sleep apnea: an updated report by the American Society of Anesthesiologists Task Force on Perioperative Management of patients with obstructive sleep apnea. *Anesthesiology* 2014;120:268.

8. ANSWER: C

9. ANSWER: A

10. ANSWER: A

11. ANSWER: B

12. ANSWER: B

13. ANSWER: E

14. ANSWER: D

Even though PPV has existed as a mainstay of patient management in anesthesia and critical care for more than 50 years, lung inflation still occurs by manipulation of either volume or pressure. The main differences in evolution of ventilation modes relates to improvement in synchronization of mandatory (i.e., determined by the clinician) breaths with the patient's own spontaneous efforts. As such, each mode of ventilation may be described in terms of three parameters: trigger, limit, and cycle.

The "trigger" is the parameter that initiates a positive pressure breath. If a rate is set, without provision for spontaneous effort, then the mode is described as "time triggered," whereas if the patient's effort determines the onset of the breath, it is either "pressure triggered" or "flow triggered." Controlled modes are typically described as time triggered (even though modern ventilators with controlled modes allow for the patient to initiate a breath, typically these modes are primarily used with the patient's efforts as a secondary concern).

The "limit" is the parameter held constant throughout the inspiratory portion of the respiratory cycle. Volume-based modes have traditionally held flow constant as the tidal volume is reached, whereas pressure-based modes hold pressure constant.

The "cycle" is the parameter that ends the positive pressure breath, allowing the patient to exhale. Again, if a rate and inspiration-to-expiration (I:E) ratio are set, then the mode is time cycled. Modes can also be volume cycled (a tidal volume is reached) or flow-cycled (patient's inspiratory flow is reduced below a threshold).

Pressure support ventilation is entirely a spontaneous mode, so the trigger and cycle are determined by the patient's respiratory efforts. In synchronized intermittent ventilation, a patient's spontaneous effort (trigger) will align with the mandatory breath, which will then time-cycle. Pressure-regulated volume control is a hybrid mode, which delivers a set tidal volume with a pressure-controlled breath pattern (pressure is limited, cycles when volume is reached).

Keywords: Critical illness diagnosis and management, pulmonary; Management strategies, ventilatory support

REFERENCE

Chiumello D, Pelosi P, Calvi E et al. Different modes of assisted ventilation in patients with acute respiratory failure. *Eur Respir J* 2002;202:925.

15. ANSWER: D

Patients are diagnosed with ventilator-associated pneumonia (VAP), a type of hospital-acquired pneumonia, when they have been intubated and mechanically ventilated for 48 hours or longer and develop progressive radiographic infiltrates and signs and symptoms of infection and positive respiratory cultures. VAP is a serious health issue, with an all-cause mortality rate of 20 to 50%. The differential diagnosis of VAP is broad and may include pulmonary embolism, pulmonary infarction, aspiration, ARDS, vasculitis, and drug reaction, among others. Multiple risk factors for the development of VAP have been identified, and practice guidelines exist for prevention. Strategies to reduce VAP include using noninvasive ventilation when possible, minimizing sedation, using mechanical ventilation weaning protocols, initiating early patient mobilization, elevating the head of the bed, minimizing pooled secretions above the tracheal tube cuff, and ensuring appropriate maintenance of ventilator circuits.

With clinical signs and symptoms of VAP present, cultures should be drawn before initiation of antimicrobial therapy, which is empiric until finalized cultures return. Empiric therapy for VAP needs to include coverage for *Staphylococcus aureus, Pseudomonas aeruginosa*, and other gram-negative organisms and should be started as soon as possible. The Infectious Diseases Society of America 2016 guidelines recommend treatment duration for VAP of 7 days. De-escalation after 48 to 72 hours if no cultures are positive is an important component of enhanced antibiotic stewardship.

For the case presented, the severity of illness and unclear MRSA resistance rates would suggest using broad-spectrum IV empiric therapy as opposed to enteral therapy. Although pulmonary embolism is in the differential diagnosis, the increasing sputum production and more gradual presentation suggest VAP.

Keywords: Critical illness diagnosis and management, pulmonary; Diagnoses, infection, pneumonia

REFERENCES

Bonten MJ. Healthcare epidemiology. Ventilator-associated pneumonia: preventing the inevitable. *Clin Infect Dis* 2011;52:115.

Erb CT, Patel B, Orr JE et al. Management of adults with hospital-acquired and ventilator-associated pneumonia. *Ann Am Thorac Soc* 2016;13:2258.

16. ANSWER: D

17. ANSWER: A

ARDS is a result of diffuse alveolar damage caused by more than 60 identified etiologies. It manifests clinically as increasing dyspnea and hypoxemia and radiographically shows diffuse bilateral pulmonary infiltrates. Through the release of inflammatory mediators, both pulmonary and systemic effects ensue, which may lead to significant short-term and long term multisystem morbidity as well as mortality rates estimated at 26 to 58%. Most patients who die will die from the inciting etiology of ARDS or complications during supportive therapy rather than from respiratory failure alone.

Tachypnea is a result of increased elastic work of breathing, which worsens with decreasing compliance. Increased compliance and resistive work of breathing are processes associated with obstructive diseases like emphysema.

Treatment for ARDS is supportive and includes appropriate, evidence-based approaches to sedation, protective lung ventilation, pain control, delirium monitoring and management, nutrition, judicious fluid management, glycemic control, stress ulcer and deep vein thrombosis prophylaxis, and early mobilization. Patients and families must be educated on short-, medium-, and long-term effects of ARDS and critical illness.

In the case presented, based on transthoracic echocardiography, there is no cardiogenic pulmonary edema, which is important to rule out in making the diagnosis of ARDS.

There is no convincing evidence for pulmonary embolism.

Acute bilateral pneumonia may present in a similar fashion and may progress to ARDS. However, in our scenario, the etiology of hypoxic respiratory failure is most consistent with ARDS secondary to ARDS.

Keywords: Basic pathophysiology, pulmonary; Respiratory failure, ARDS

REFERENCE

Bellani G, Laffey JG, Pham T et al. Epidemiology, patterns of care, and mortality for patients with acute respiratory distress syndrome in intensive care units in 50 countries. *JAMA* 2016;315:788.

18. ANSWER: D

TRALI is a potentially devastating consequence of blood component transfusion that most typically presents 1 to 2 hours after initiation transfusion. By definition, TRALI may present within 6 hours after transfusion. Most commonly, patients experience hypoxemia, pink frothy secretions, fever, and hypotension, and tachypnea and tachycardia may be present. The treatment for TRALI or possible TRALI includes discontinuation of transfusion, alerting the blood bank, and supportive care, which may include mechanical ventilation with a protective strategy. The

incidence of TRALI in critically ill patients may be as high as 5 to 8%, and the mortality rate associated with it may be as high as 35 to 58%. Blood components with high plasma volume are most implicated in TRALI; however, it has been described in all blood products. Recipient risk factors have been described as well and for this case include current smoking, positive fluid balance, and chronic alcohol abuse.

Although pulmonary embolism remains a possibility given the lack of anticoagulation in a postoperative patient, there is no jugular venous distention, and no right ventricular dysfunction is noted on transthoracic echocardiography. Diffuse bilateral pulmonary infiltrates are most consistent with acute lung injury. There is nothing to suggest aspiration in the case, nor are there electrocardiographic changes suggestive of myocardial infarction.

Keywords: Basic pathophysiology, pulmonary; Respiratory failure, TRALI

REFERENCES

Chapman CE, Stainsby D, Jones H et al. Ten years of hemovigilance reports of transfusion-related acute lung injury in the United Kingdom and the impact of preferential use of male donor plasma. *Transfusion* 2009;49:440.

Clifford L, Jia Q, Subramanian A et al. Risk factors and clinical outcomes associated with perioperative transfusion-associated circulatory overload. *Anesthesiology* 2017;126:409.

19. ANSWER: C

20. ANSWER: D

Primary pneumothorax develops in a person without underlying lung disease spontaneously, without antecedent event, whereas secondary spontaneous pneumothorax develops in the setting of underlying lung disease, such as COPD, malignancy, cystic fibrosis, and necrotizing pneumonia.

Patients with emphysema are at high risk for development of barotrauma without careful choice of ventilation management. In this case, the high respiratory rate leads to dynamic hyperinflation (auto-PEEP), which worsens the risk for barotrauma. Although the tidal volume is relatively high, the best maneuver is to reduce the respiratory rate to allow the patient more time to exhale. Although she responds initially, the stage had already been set for barotrauma.

Tension pneumothorax is an emergency and requires immediate intervention in the form of chest tube placement or needle decompression. If suspected, there is no indication to wait for chest film. Furthermore, in severe emphysema, it may be difficult to delineate the characteristic radiographic findings (pleural line may be difficult to distinguish from outline of large bullae). The hypotension and jugular venous distention suggest obstructive shock and a prearrest state.

A standard 14- or 16-gauge angiocatheter is introduced over the superior border of the third rib in the midclavicular line, and there should be a rush of air. After decompression and stabilization of hemodynamics ensue, preparations should be made for more definitive management (tube thoracostomy).

Keywords: Basic pathophysiology, pulmonary; Airway disruption; Pneumothorax, volutrauma

REFERENCES

Noppen M, De Keukeleire T. Pneumothorax. *Respiration* 2008;76:121.

Rouby JJ, Brochard L. Tidal recruitment and overinflation in acute respiratory distress syndrome: yin and yang. *Am J Respir Crit Care Med* 2007;175:104.

12.

CARDIOVASCULAR I
PHYSIOLOGY AND MANAGEMENT

Linda W. Young

QUESTIONS

1. A 65-year-old male presents to the emergency department (ED) after a syncopal episode. The patient states that over the past few months he felt "funny" and sometimes short of breath. There were no aggravating or alleviating activities. Vital signs are: blood pressure (BP) 109/68 mm Hg, heart rate (HR) 122 bpm, and respiratory rate (RR) 25 breaths/minute. In the ED, imaging and laboratory studies were performed and included: Na 139 mEq/L, K 4.4 mEq/L, Mg 2.1 mEq/L, creatinine 2.1 mg/dL, and brain natriuretic peptide (BNP) 68 pg/mL. You obtain a stat 12-lead electrocardiogram (ECG), shown here (image courtesy of George Williams, MD).

The MOST likely diagnosis is:

A. Atrial flutter
B. Ventricular tachycardia
C. Atrial fibrillation
D. Torsades de pointes

2. A 96-year-old female presents to the ED from a skilled nursing facility after being found unresponsive. On emergency medical services arrival, cardiopulmonary resuscitation (CPR) was initiated; no shockable rhythm was detected with automated external defibrillator (AED). The patient received 2 mg of epinephrine, was intubated, and had return of spontaneous circulation (ROSC) after 3 minutes. In the ED, the patient was

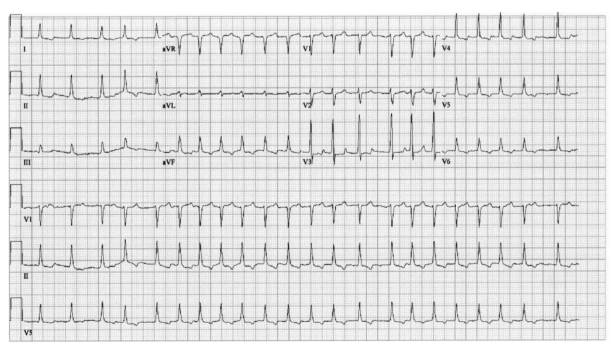

Figure Q1.1

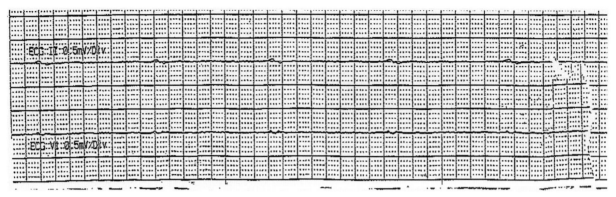

Figure Q2.1

placed on an epinephrine infusion and admitted to the intensive care unit (ICU). You are called to the patient's room immediately on admission to the ICU. You check the monitor, and the above rhythm is noted. You have ensured all ECG leads are connected, as shown here (image courtesy of George Williams, MD).

The MOST likely diagnosis is:

A. Pulseless electrical activity (PEA)
B. Supraventricular tachycardia (SVT)
C. Sinus bradycardia
D. Asystole

3. A 65-year-old male presents to the ED with chest pain on and off for 2 days, worsening since this morning. While in the ED, the patient is noted to be hemodynamically stable, awake, and responsive; however, during the discussion with the ED physician, he says he feels funny and is noted to suddenly become unresponsive. The rhythm shown here is noted on the monitors (image courtesy of George Williams, MD).

The MOST likely diagnosis is:

A. SVT
B. Ventricular fibrillation
C. Afib with rapid ventricular response
D. Rapid firing of a pacemaker

4. An otherwise healthy 76-year-old male was admitted to ICU after presenting to the ED by ambulance after feeling faint and "passing out." His wife reported that it lasted a few seconds and he returned to normal. The patient's past medical history is significant for hypercholesterolemia. Laboratory and imaging studies obtained in the ED were within normal limits. Computed tomography (CT) of the brain was normal. An ECG was

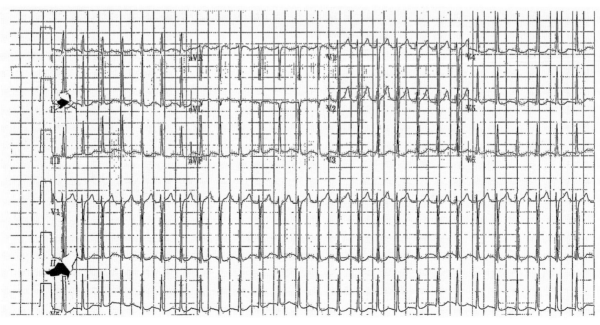

Figure Q3.1

obtained and is shown here (image courtesy of George Williams, MD). This rhythm represents:

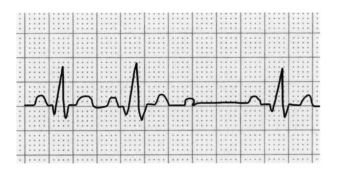

A. Wolff-Parkinson-White (WPW) syndrome
B. Sinus bradycardia
C. Normal sinus rhythm
D. Heart block

5. A 78-year-old male, admitted to the ICU 2 days ago with a diagnosis of acute renal failure, is hyperkalemic with a potassium level of 6.8 mEq/L. At the time of admission, a temporary dialysis catheter was placed, and emergent dialysis was initiated. Laboratory studies this morning showed Na 145 mEq/L, K 3.7 mEq/L, chloride 89 mEq/L, HCO_3 23 mEq/L, blood urea nitrogen (BUN) 22 mg/dL, creatinine 2.2 mg/dL, white blood cell (WBC) count $7 \times 10^3/\mu L$, hemoglobin (Hgb) 6 g/dL, hematocrit 18%, and platelet count $222 \times 10^3/\mu L$. You are called to the patient's room by the nurse intern, who reports that the patient is unresponsive. You report to the room, and the ECG is shown here (image courtesy of George Williams, MD).

You cannot palpate a pulse. The MOST likely rhythm is:

A. Second-degree heart block
B. Sinus bradycardia

C. PEA
D. Third-degree heart block

6. A patient presented to the ED with complaint of crushing substernal chest pain. A ST-elevation myocardial infarction (STEMI) alert was activated. Laboratory samples were drawn and results pending. The patient was diaphoretic and ECG revealed ST elevation in leads V_3 to V_5. The patient complained of pain and received morphine 2 mg, and was placed on a nitroglycerin infusion. Fifteen minutes later, the patient stated that he felt more comfortable. In the middle of the conversation, the patient suddenly became unresponsive, and the following rhythm was observed (image courtesy of Shaina M. Sheppard, MD):

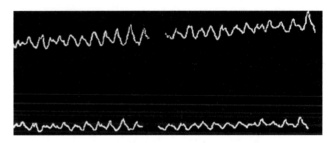

The MOST likely rhythm was:

A. Sinus tachycardia
B. SVT
C. Ventricular fibrillation
D. Atrial fibrillation

7. A 44-year-old male is admitted to the ICU for recurrent syncopal episodes. On evaluation, the patient reports that this is the third recurrence in 2 months, and it "runs in his family." He stated that it happened to his

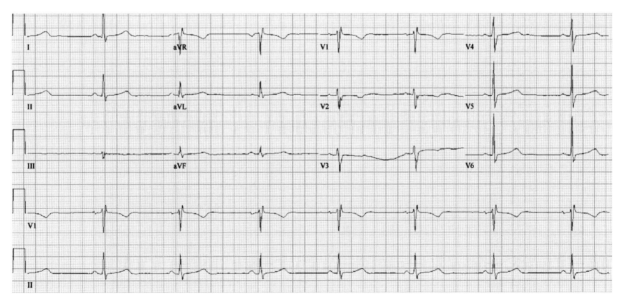

Figure Q5.1

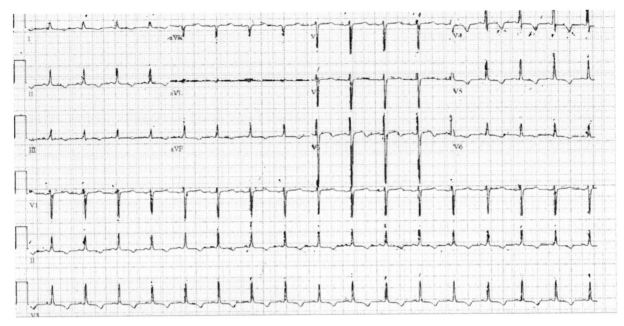

Figure Q7.1

father who is now deceased, and has also now occurred with his youngest brother. Initial workup of laboratory, imaging, and electroencephalography (EEG) studies are within normal limits. An ECG has been obtained and is shown here (image courtesy of George Williams, MD).

The MOST likely diagnosis is:

A. WPW syndrome
B. Brugada syndrome
C. Hypertrophic cardiomyopathy (HCM) or hypertrophic obstructive cardiomyopathy (HOCM)
D. Atrial fibrillation

8. A 22-year-old male patient presented to the ED after "passing out." CT of the brain without contrast was performed; results were normal. An ECG

was performed and is shown here (image courtesy of Francisco Fuentes, MD).

The MOST likely diagnosis is:

A. Atrial fibrillation
B. Third-degree heart block
C. WPW syndrome
D. Ventricular fibrillation

9. A 72-year-old male with a history of coronary artery disease presented to the ED with crushing substernal chest pain in leads V_3, V_4, V_5, and V_6. The patient emergently underwent coronary angiography with percutaneous coronary intervention (PCI). The patient was then transferred to ICU. The patient was ordered aspirin 81 mg daily to be continued, now with the

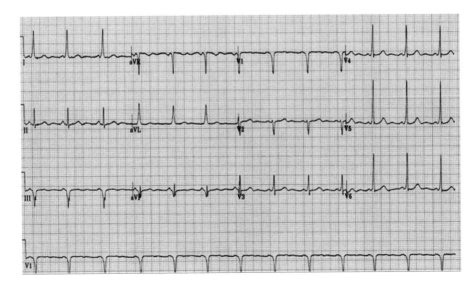

Figure Q8.1

drug-eluting stent placement. What is the BEST medication in addition to aspirin that is required post-PCI?

A. Dabigatran
B. Clopidogrel
C. Prasugrel
D. Ticagrelor

10. A 130-kg 30-year-old female presented to the ED with shortness of breath (SOB). She reported that she had been on a flight from California to New York City last summer and developed SOB at that time and went to the ED. She was told at that time that "she had a small blood clot in her lung and her left leg." She stated that she stayed in the hospital for 2 days and then was discharged home. She did not remember receiving any medications for her "blood clot in the lung" while in the hospital. She was instructed to follow up with her primary care physician for additional laboratory work and care, but never returned to her physician. The patient stated that she started having SOB 2 weeks ago and it is now worsening. The patient also reported pain in her right leg, now swollen. On physical examination, the patient's lungs are clear to auscultation, jugular venous distention is present, S_3 sounds are on auscultation, and she is normotensive with a positive Homan sign. A venous Doppler ultrasound of bilateral extremities reveals a right posterior tibial deep vein thrombosis (DVT). Laboratory results were within normal limits, with the exception of a D-dimer being slightly elevated. CT pulmonary angiogram is shown below.

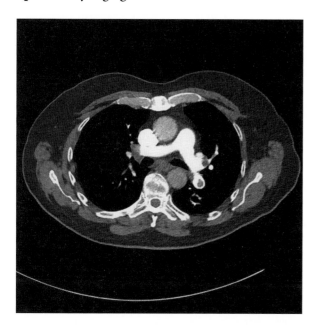

Echocardiography was performed and showed ejection fraction (EF) of 45 to 50%, slight right ventricular dysfunction, right ventricular hypertrophy, right atrial enlargement, and pulmonary arterial pressure (PAP) of 64 mm Hg. The MOST likely diagnosis is:

A. Bronchitis
B. Acute pulmonary embolus
C. Chronic thromboembolic pulmonary hypertension (CTEPH)
D. Acute right heart failure

11. A patient presented to the ED with a complaint of vomiting up blood overnight. The patient reported vomiting three times during the night and now complains also of nausea. The patient's medical history is significant for chronic atrial fibrillation, and controlled HR is 84 bpm. He takes a blood thinner but does not remember the name. The patient was recently diagnosed with a foot infection and has been on a 14-day course of antibiotics. He now complains of being progressively weaker throughout the day. Laboratory studies revealed Hgb of 6.8 g/dL and international normalized ratio (INR) of 5; basic metabolic panel is within normal limits. The patient is transferred to the ICU. The MOST likely drug responsible for the elevation of INR is:

A. Dabigatran
B. Aspirin
C. Warfarin
D. Clopidogrel

12. A 26-year-old 135-kg female was just admitted to the ICU with hypoxia. She had presented to the ED after returning from Europe on an 8-hour transatlantic flight where she had been attending a college seminar. The patient's past medical history is benign, and her home medications are birth control pills daily and occasionally ibuprofen, and she has no known drug allergies. Laboratory and imaging studies were performed. Basic metabolic panel and complete blood count were within normal limits. Chest radiograph revealed no abnormality. ECG results revealed sinus tachycardia. Arterial blood gas (ABG) analysis showed pH 7.39, CO_2 39 mm Hg, PO_2 88 mm Hg, HCO_3 21 mEq/L, and base excess 1 mEq/L on 5-L/minute nasal cannula. Vital signs included BP 126/54 mm Hg, HR 108 bpm, RR 28 breaths/minute, and O_2 saturation 95%. CT pulmonary angiography revealed subsegmental pulmonary emboli bilaterally. Echocardiography was obtained and revealed EF 68%, no right ventricular strain, PAP 21 mm Hg, and no regional wall motion abnormalities. Venous Doppler ultrasound showed nonocclusive thrombus in the left femoral vein. The BEST medication to initiate at this time is:

A. Plavix
B. Unfractionated heparin infusion and monitor partial thromboplastin time (PTT)
C. Aspirin 81 mg daily
D. Argatroban infusion

ANSWERS

1. ANSWER: C

Atrial fibrillation is one of the most common arrhythmias encountered in clinical practice. The prevalence increases with age, from 0.9% at 40 years to 5.9% in patients older than 65 years. It is characterized by disorganized atrial depolarization without effective contractions. Fibrillatory waves (f waves) usually generate an atrial rate greater than 350 bpm but are not able to produce coordinated atrial contractions or consistent P waves. Atrial fibrillation is distinguished from other forms of irregular narrow-complex tachycardia by the absence of P waves. The ventricular response to atrial fibrillation is usually 90 to 180 bpm. Risk factors include diseases that produce atrial distention or enlargement such as congestive heart failure, hypertension, coronary artery disease, chronic obstructive pulmonary disease, thyrotoxicosis, and alcohol abuse. Atrial fibrillation most commonly occurs following cardiac surgery, typically on postoperative day 2 or 3. The goals of management in atrial fibrillation are to reduce the risk for thromboembolism and to control symptoms. To avoid the risk of stroke in atrial fibrillation that lasts more than 48 hours, anticoagulation and transesophageal echocardiography should be performed before attempts of cardioversion to sinus rhythm.

Keyword: Cardiovascular atrial fibrillation

REFERENCES

Gillinov AM, Bagiella E, Moskowitz AJ et al. Rate control versus rhythm control for atrial fibrillation after cardiac surgery. *N Engl J Med* 2016;374:1911–1921.

January CT, Wann LS, Alpert JS et al. 2014 AHA/ACC/HRS guideline for the management of patients with atrial fibrillation: executive summary. A report of the American College of Cardiology/American Heart Association Task Force on practice guidelines and the Heart Rhythm Society. *J Am Coll Cardiol* 2014;64:2246–2280.

Roberts PR, Todd SR, eds. *Comprehensive critical care: adult.* Mount Prospect, IL: Society of Critical Care Medicine; 2012.

Shen WK, Sheldon RS, Benditt DG et al. 2017 ACC/AHA/HRS guideline for the evaluation and management of patients with syncope: a report of the American College of Cardiology/American Heart Association Task Force on Clinical Practice Guidelines and the Heart Rhythm Society. *J Am Coll Cardiol* 2017;70:e39–e110.

2. ANSWER: D

Asystole is the absence of mechanical and electrical cardiac activity. Per advanced cardiac life support (ACLS) guidelines, correct management is essential with regard to selection of vasoactive medication and CPR techniques. It is imperative that underlying possible causes be addressed simultaneously. See the cardiac arrest algorithm that follows.

Keyword: Cardiovascular asystole

REFERENCES

Donnino MW, Andersen LW, Berg KM et al. Temperature management after cardiac arrest: an advisory statement by the Advanced Life Support Task Force of the International Liaison Committee on Resuscitation and the American Heart Association Emergency Cardiovascular Care Committee and the Council on Cardiopulmonary, Critical Care, Perioperative and Resuscitation. *Circulation* 2015;132:2448–2456.

Kleinman ME, Brennan EE, Goldberger ZD et al. Part 5. Adult basic life support and cardiopulmonary resuscitation quality. Circulation 2015;132:S414–S435.

McCarthy JJ, Carr B, Sasson C et al. Out-of-hospital cardiac arrest resuscitation systems of care: a scientific statement from the American Heart Association. *Circulation* 2018;137:e645–e660.

Neumar RW, Shuster M, Callaway CW et al. Part 1. Executive summary: 2015 American Heart Association Guidelines update for cardiopulmonary resuscitation and emergency cardiovascular care. *Circulation* 2015;132:S315–S367.

Olasveengen TM, de Caen AR, Mancini ME et al. 2017 International consensus on cardiopulmonary resuscitation and emergency cardiovascular care science with treatment recommendations summary. *Resuscitation* 2017;121:201–214.

3. ANSWER: A

SVT is a common rhythm seen in the ED and ICU. The ECG shows tachycardia at a rate of 160 to 180 bpm with narrow QRS complexes. Also, the presence of atrial activity—P wave—is noted. BP is usually normal and sometimes low-normal owing to a decrease in filling time. SVT usually results from an orthodromic re-entrant mechanism, but it can sometimes originate from rapid discharges of atrial ectopic focus.

Paroxysmal supraventricular tachycardia (PSVT) also has narrow QRS complexes. The onset and termination of the event are abrupt, which is distinct from sinus tachycardia, which has a more gradual onset. There are five types of PSVT. One of the most common types is atrioventricular nodal re-entry tachycardia (AVNRT). The HR in AVNRT ranges from 140 to 250 bpm. The rhythm is regular. The atria are activated in a retrograde fashion, resulting in inverted P waves in leads II, III, and aVF. Retrograde conduction is rapid; thus, atrial and ventricular depolarizations are simultaneous, causing P waves to be obscured by QRS complexes; P waves may not be seen on the ECG or may appear at the terminal portion of QRS complexes. In approximately 76 to 90% of AVNRTs, antegrade conduction proceeds through the posterior "slow" AV nodal pathway and retrograde conduction through the anterior "fast" pathway; this is sometimes referred to as slow-fast AVNRT. In approximately one third of these cases, a positive deflection in leads aVR or V_1 (sometimes both) is seen, which initiates a right bundle branch block or pseudo-S waves. This

Adult Cardiac Arrest Algorithm

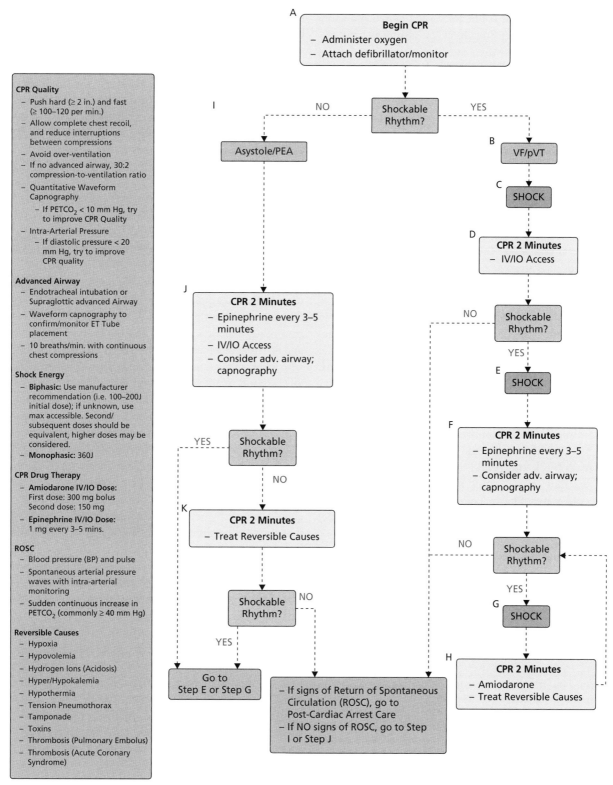

CPR Quality
- Push hard (≥ 2 in.) and fast (≥ 100–120 per min.)
- Allow complete chest recoil, and reduce interruptions between compressions
- Avoid over-ventilation
- If no advanced airway, 30:2 compression-to-ventilation ratio
- Quantitative Waveform Capnography
  - If PETCO₂ < 10 mm Hg, try to improve CPR Quality
- Intra-Arterial Pressure
  - If diastolic pressure < 20 mm Hg, try to improve CPR quality

Advanced Airway
- Endotracheal intubation or Supraglottic advanced Airway
- Waveform capnography to confirm/monitor ET Tube placement
- 10 breaths/min. with continuous chest compressions

Shock Energy
- **Biphasic:** Use manufacturer recommendation (i.e. 100–200J initial dose); if unknown, use max accessible. Second/subsequent doses should be equivalent, higher doses may be considered.
- **Monophasic:** 360J

CPR Drug Therapy
- **Amiodarone IV/IO Dose:**
  First dose: 300 mg bolus
  Second dose: 150 mg
- **Epinephrine IV/IO Dose:**
  1 mg every 3–5 mins.

ROSC
- Blood pressure (BP) and pulse
- Spontaneous arterial pressure waves with intra-arterial monitoring
- Sudden continuous increase in PETCO₂ (commonly ≥ 40 mm Hg)

Reversible Causes
- Hypoxia
- Hypovolemia
- Hydrogen Ions (Acidosis)
- Hyper/Hypokalemia
- Hypothermia
- Tension Pneumothorax
- Tamponade
- Toxins
- Thrombosis (Pulmonary Embolus)
- Thrombosis (Acute Coronary Syndrome)

Figure A2.1

represents a retrograde activation of the atria. Patients may present with symptoms of lightheadedness, palpitations, and near-syncope. Atrial contraction on a closed AV valve may produce neck pounding. Neck pounding is *virtually pathognomonic.*

Atrioventricular re-entry tachycardia (AVRT) involves an atrioventricular (AV) connection referred to as an accessory pathway. The cause is an incomplete separation of the atria and ventricles during fetal development. One of the most common accessory pathways is the Kent bundle located on the mitral or tricuspid annulus. The accessory pathways can conduct in both or either directions. AVRT normally proceeds antegrade, so the QRS complex is generally normal. A short RP interval with longer PR interval is typical. Both AVNRT and AVRT activate the annular atrial tissue first; P waves, if seen on the ECG, will be negative in the inferior leads. If upright P waves are seen in the inferior leads, it is atrial or sinus tachycardia.

If the direction through the AV node is antegrade conduction, it is known as orthodromic. The QRS complex is of normal width and follows the AV node–His Purkinje pathway. If antegrade conduction occurs through the accessory or bypass tract, it is called antidromic. Antidromic AVRT is identified on surface ECG with a short PR interval, a wider QRS, and delta waves. Delta waves are indicative of ventricular pre-excitation on the bypass tract. WPW syndrome is a form of ventricular pre-excitation. Recognition of antidromic AVRT is important because patients are at a higher risk for sudden cardiac death. Acute management for both AVNRT and AVRT termination includes vagal maneuvers like carotid sinus massage and focal immersion in cold water. Pharmacological interventions for AV blocking include adenosine, beta-blockers, calcium channel blockers, and digoxin.

Keyword: Cardiovascular SVT/tachyarrhythmias

REFERENCES

Link MS, Berkow LC, Kudenchuk PJ et al. Part 7. Adult advanced cardiovascular life support: 2015 American Heart Association guidelines update for cardiopulmonary resuscitation and emergency cardiovascular care. *Circulation* 2015;132:S444–S464.

Marino PL. *The ICU book*, 3rd edition. Philadelphia: Lippincott Williams & Wilkins; 2007, pp. 354–361.

Trohman RG. Supraventricular tachycardia: implications for the intensivist. *Crit Care Med* 2000;28:N129–N135.

Vincent JL, Abraham E, Moore FA et al. *Textbook of critical care*, 6th edition. Philadelphia: Churchill Livingstone; 2011, pp. 566–568.

4. ANSWER: D

Heart block presents as a conduction disturbance. The block can occur at the level of the AV node or below. Causes are multifactorial and include pharmacologic agents, myocardial injury or disease, metabolic disturbances, and trauma. Diseases involving endocrine, inflammatory, or infectious processes can also result in heart block. Heart block can also be neurally mediated.

First-degree AV block is defined as a PR interval greater than 0.20 second in adults. The QRS is usually narrow. The PR interval is fixed. It can be vagally mediated or medication induced. It may also represent AV nodal disease or progressive conduction defects. Patients usually do not have symptoms. It usually does not require any intervention. A pacemaker is required if first-degree AV block is accompanied with a bifascicular block (right bundle branch block and left anterior fascicular block) in the setting of myocardial ischemia.

Second-degree heart block has two types. Second-degree heart block (Mobitz type I), also known as Wenckebach, is defined as progressive prolongation of the PR interval and intermittent failure to conduct atrial impulse. The block in conduction is commonly within the AV node. In 90% of patients, the AV node is supplied by the right coronary artery. Patients diagnosed with an inferior wall myocardial infarction (MI) commonly experience Wenckebach. It is typically reversible, and no treatment is usually required. In patients with AV block who experience symptoms of hypoperfusion, patients usually respond to atropine. Second-degree heart block (Mobitz type II) originates in the His-Purkinje system below the level of the AV node. The His-Purkinje system in most patients is supplied by the left anterior descending coronary artery. The PR interval remains constant or fixed but inconsistent. If the conduction remains inconsistent, patients may have hemodynamic instability and thus may progress to complete AV block. Mobitz type II requires treatment. Underlying causes should be investigated because Mobitz type II can be reversed when caused by electrolyte derangements or enhanced vagal tone or when it occurs in patients after cardiac surgery or those with ischemic heart disease. Atropine is ineffective in the infranodal site of blockade, and a pacemaker is necessary.

Third-degree heart block is complete AV dissociation. This block can occur anywhere in the conduction system, including the AV node, bundle of His, or both bundle branches. The QRS can be narrow or wide. If the blockade is in the AV node, it will produce a narrow QRS complex with a junctional rhythm. The HR ranges from 40 to 60 bpm. However, if the infranodal block has a wide QRS greater than 0.10 second, it is usually symptomatic with hemodynamic instability because the HR ranges from 30 to 45 bpm. Third-degree heart block usually is seen 24 hours after MI. Patients who suffered an inferior wall MI may require temporary pacing. If complete heart block is due to an anterior MI, a permanent pacemaker is usually required. Treatment for third-degree heart block requires checking and correcting underlying causes and the use of immediate transcutaneous or transvenous pacemaker.

Keyword: Cardiovascular heart block

REFERENCES

Epstein AE, DiMarco JP, Ellenbogen KA et al. 2012 ACCF/AHA/HRS focused update incorporated into the ACCF/AHA/HRS 2008 guidelines for device-based therapy of cardiac rhythm abnormalities. *J Am Coll Cardiol* 2013;61:e6–e75.

John RM, Kumar S. Sinus node and atrial arrhythmias. *Circulation* 2016;133:1892–1900.

Kwok CS, Rashid M, Beynon R et al. Prolonged PR interval, first-degree heart block and adverse cardiovascular outcomes: a systematic review and meta-analysis. *Heart* 2016;102:672–680.

Shen WK, Sheldon RS, Benditt DG et al. 2017 ACC/AHA/HRS guideline for the evaluation and management of patients with syncope: a report of the American College of Cardiology/American Heart Association Task Force on Clinical Practice Guidelines and the Heart Rhythm Society. *J Am Coll Cardiol* 2017;70:e39–e110.

5. ANSWER: C

PEA, also known as electrical mechanical dissociation, is defined as an organized rhythm on surface ECG with no detectable pulse or HR. Evaluation of common causes includes recognition of the seven "H" and five "T" conditions:

SEVEN "H" CONDITIONS	FIVE "T" CONDITIONS
Hyperkalemia or hypokalemia	Tamponade
Hyperinflation (e.g., auto–positive end-expiratory pressure [auto-PEEP])	Trauma
Hypothermia	Tension pneumothorax
Hypoglycemia	Thrombosis (pulmonary or coronary)
Hydrogen ions (severe acidosis)	Toxic overdoses • Digoxin • Beta-blockers • Calcium channel blockers • Tricyclic antidepressants
Hypovolemia	-
Hypoxemia	-
	-

Evaluation by bedside echocardiography is recommended in the emergent situation. Focused cardiac ultrasound can provide immediate diagnosis to guide treatment protocols and decisions. Some of the goals of a focused cardiac ultrasound assessment include identification of pericardial effusion, marked right ventricular and left ventricular enlargement, evaluation of global systolic function, and intravascular volume assessment. One of the clinical indications for focused cardiac ultrasound is cardiac arrest and rapid diagnosis to guide treatment decisions. True PEA is the absence of ventricular contraction in the presence of electrical activity. Pseudo-PEA is the presence of ventricular contraction visualized on cardiac ultrasound in a patient without cardiac pulses.

Management of PEA includes identification of a wide versus a narrow QRS on initial ECG. If the QRS is narrow, it is a mechanical (right ventricle) issue. Examples include cardiac tamponade, tension pneumothorax, mechanical hyperinflation (auto-PEEP), pulmonary embolus, and acute MI (myocardial rupture). If the QRS is wide on ECG, it is a metabolic (left ventricle) problem; causes include severe hyperkalemia, sodium channel blocker toxicity, and acute MI (pump failure). Bedside echocardiography would reveal the left ventricle to be hypokinetic or akinetic, suggesting a true PEA.

Management of PEA after identification of QRS on ECG includes the following:

- If QRS is wide—utilization of pharmacologic management of severe hyperkalemia or sodium channel blocker toxicity with calcium chloride and sodium bicarbonate boluses
- If QRS is narrow—initiation of IV fluids wide open and identification of issues most efficiently by bedside echocardiograph, which helps to guide the use of pericardiocentesis for cardiac tamponade, needle decompensation for tension pneumothorax, ventilator management for mechanical hyperinflation (auto-PEEP), and thrombolysis for pulmonary embolism (PE).

Keyword: Cardiovascular pulseless electrical activity

REFERENCES

Labovitz AJ, Noble VE, Bierig M et al. Focused cardiac ultrasound in the emergent setting: a consensus statement of the American Society of Echocardiography and American College of Emergency Physicians. *J Am Soc Echocardiogr* 2010;23:1225–1230.

Littmann L, Bustin DJ, Haley MW. A simplified and structured teaching tool for the evaluation and management of pulseless electrical activity. *Med Princ Pract* 2014;23:1–6.

Mehta C, Brady W. Pulseless electrical activity in cardiac arrest: electrocardiographic presentations and management considerations based on the electrocardiogram. *Am J Emerg Med* 2012;30:236–239.

Neumar RW, Shuster M, Callaway CW et al. Part 1. Executive summary: 2015 American Heart Association guidelines update for cardiopulmonary resuscitation and emergency cardiovascular care. *Circulation* 2015;132:S315–S367.

Saarinen S, Nurmi J, Toivio T et al. Does appropriate treatment of the primary underlying cause of PEA during resuscitation improve patients' survival? *Resuscitation* 2012;83:819–822.

6. ANSWER: D

Ventricular fibrillation is a life-threatening emergency. It is the most common cause of sudden cardiac death. On ECG, it is an irregular, disorganized, rapid rhythm with 300 to 400 bpm, resulting in no cardiac output.

Etiology of ventricular fibrillation includes both cardiac and noncardiac causes. Noncardiac idiopathic ventricular fibrillation (IVF) can be caused by gene mutations of *DPP6, CALM1, RyR2,* and *IRX3.* Other causes of IVF include coronary artery disease, MI, coronary artery spasm, dilated cardiomyopathy, hypertrophic cardiomyopathy, arrhythmogenic right ventricular dysplasia/cardiomyopathy (ARVD/C), long QT syndrome, short QT syndrome, sudden cardiac death, and early repolarization syndrome.

The genetic mutations are caused by changes in the cardiac ion channels. Diagnosis other than ECG recognition includes basic metabolic profile, cardiac enzymes, electrolytes, thyroid panel, and toxicology screening. Imaging studies include echocardiography and chest radiography. In younger patients with minimal risk factors or no evidence of coronary artery disease, coronary CT or magnetic resonance angiography can be used as an alternative to coronary angiography. Treatment includes correction of electrolyte abnormalities and defibrillation per ACLS protocol.

Keyword: Cardiovascular ventricular fibrillation/ventricular tachycardia

REFERENCES

Brouwer TF, Walker RG, Chapman FW, Koster RW. Association between chest compression interruptions and clinical outcomes of ventricular fibrillation out-of-hospital cardiac arrest. *Circulation* 2015;132:1030–1037.

Link MS, Berkow LC, Kudenchuk PJ et al. Part 7. Adult advanced cardiovascular life support: 2015 American Heart Association guidelines update for cardiopulmonary resuscitation and emergency cardiovascular care. *Circulation* 2015;132:S444–S464.

Napolitano C, Priori SG, Bloise R. Catecholaminergic polymorphic ventricular tachycardia. *GeneReviews (Internet)* 2016 Oct 13. University of Washington, Seattle. PMID: 20301466.

Sapp JL, Wells GA, Parkash R et al. Ventricular tachycardia ablation versus escalation of antiarrhythmic drugs. *N Engl J Med* 2016;375:111–121.

Shen WK, Sheldon RS, Benditt DG et al. 2017 ACC/AHA/HRS guideline for the evaluation and management of patients with syncope: a report of the American College of Cardiology/American Heart Association Task Force on Clinical Practice Guidelines and the Heart Rhythm Society. *J Am Coll Cardiol* 2017;70:e39–e110.

Visser M, van der Heijden JF, Doevendans PA et al. Idiopathic ventricular fibrillation: the struggle for definition, diagnosis, and follow-up. *Circ Arrhythm Electrophysiol* 2016;9:e003817.

7. ANSWER: B

Brugada syndrome occurs during adulthood, with the average age of sudden death occurring at 40 years. ECG usually depicts ST-segment abnormalities in leads V_1 to V_3. This is a life-threatening or lethal rhythm and can result in sudden cardiac death. It is responsible for approximately 4% of all sudden cardiac deaths in patients worldwide and up to 20% in patients with structurally normal hearts. Other ECG findings or manifestations that can occur include first-degree AV block, an intraventricular conduction delay, right bundle branch block, and sick sinus syndrome.

Diagnosis includes routine testing to rule out other differentials, including thyroid-stimulating hormone, electrolytes, and basic metabolic panel as well as genetic testing for cardiac ion channel mutations. Single-gene testing for *SCN5A* accounts for 15 to 30% of cases. Imaging studies include chest radiography and echocardiography. Suspect Brugada syndrome in patients with recurrent syncope, history of polymorphic ventricular tachycardia, ventricular fibrillation, cardiac arrest, or family history of sudden cardiac death.

Management includes placement of an implantable cardioverter-defibrillator in patients with a history of cardiac arrest or syncope, isoproterenol for electrical storms, or quinidine 1 to 2 g daily. Patients should have an ECG every 1 to 2 years if they have been diagnosed with Brugada syndrome or have a family history of sudden cardiac death. Avoid class IA and class IC antiarrhythmics, elevated temperature (fever), antidepressants, and antipsychotics with mechanism of action that has sodium blockade effects.

Keywords: Other cardiac abnormalities, Brugada

REFERENCES

Bayés de Luna A, Brugada J, Baranchuk A, et al. Current electrocardiographic criteria for diagnosis of Brugada pattern: a consensus report. *J Electrocardiol* 2012;45:433–442.

Brugada R, Campuzano O, Sarquella-Brugada G et al. Brugada syndrome. *GeneReviews (Internet)* 2016 Nov 17. University of Washington, Seattle. PMID: 20301690.

Brugada R, Campuzano O, Sarquella-Brugada G et al. Brugada syndrome. *Methodist Debakey Cardiovasc J* 2014;10: 25–28.

Chung EH. Brugada ECG patterns in athletes. *J Electrocardiol* 2015;48:539–543.

8. ANSWER: C

Patients with WPW syndrome have a lifetime risk for sudden death. The risk can be eliminated by radiofrequency ablation of the accessory pathways.

WPW is a frequently encountered re-entrant arrhythmia that is characterized by a shortened PR interval less than 120 milliseconds, prolonged QRS greater than 120 milliseconds with an upsloping or "slurred" QRS complexes (delta waves), and occasional ST abnormalities. WPW is due to conduction abnormalities of the accessory pathways (bundle of Kent). The definitive treatment is radiofrequency ablation.

There are specific specialty markers that have been identified for sudden cardiac death. The markers include:

1. Anterograde effective refractory period of accessory pathway (APERP) of 240 to 250 milliseconds; if patient is taking isoproterenol, APERP <200 milliseconds
2. Shortest pre-excited RR interval (SPERRI) less than 250 milliseconds during or induced atrial fibrillation
3. Multiple accessory pathways
4. Ebstein anomaly
5. Familial WPW syndrome

The noninvasive parameters of a long refractory period of bypass tract (>250 milliseconds) include:

1. Intermittent pre-excitation
2. Disappearance of pre-excitation during exercise
3. Disappearance of pre-excitation during procainamide

The PACES/HRS consensus statement on the management of the symptom-free young patient with a WPW ECG pattern noted that SPERRI and APERP are important baseline parameters for risk stratification in patients with asymptomatic WPW.

Keywords: Other conduction abnormalities, WPW syndrome

REFERENCES

Cohen MI, Triedman JK, Cannon BC et al. PACES/HRS expert consensus statement on the management of the asymptomatic young patient with a Wolff-Parkinson-White (WPW, ventricular preexcitation) electrocardiographic pattern. *Heart Rhythm* 2012;9(6):1006–1024.

Finocchiaro G, Papadakis M, Behr ER et al. Sudden cardiac death in pre-excitation and Wolff-Parkinson-White. *J Am Coll Cardiol* 2017;69(12):1644–1645.

Obeyesekere MN, Leong-Sit P, Massel D et al. Risk of arrhythmia and sudden death in patients with asymptomatic preexcitation: a meta-analysis. *Circulation* 2012;125(19):2308–2315.

Page RL, Joglar JA, Caldwell MA et al. 2015 ACC/AHA/HRS Guideline for the management of adult patients with supraventricular tachycardia: a report of the American College of Cardiology/American Heart Association Task Force on Clinical Practice Guidelines and the Heart Rhythm Society. *J Am Coll Cardiol* 2016;67(13):e27–e115.

Pappone C, Vicedomini G, Manguso F et al. Risk of malignant arrhythmias in initially symptomatic patients with Wolff-Parkinson-White syndrome: results of a prospective long-term electrophysiological follow-up study. *Circulation* 2012;125(5):661–668.

Pappone C, Vicedomini G, Manguso F et al. The natural history of WPW syndrome. *Eur Heart J* 2015;17(Suppl):A8–A11.

9. ANSWER: B

The major determinants of arterial thrombus leading to acute coronary syndrome (ACS) are platelet adhesion, activation, and aggregation after plaque rupture. Antiplatelet therapy targets the pathways that lead to platelet activation and aggregation. Therapy is important for acute treatment and long-term secondary prevention of ischemic events in patients with ACS. Optimal treatment includes dual antiplatelet therapy with a combination of aspirin and either prasugrel or ticagrelor. Clopidogrel should be used when both prasugrel and ticagrelor are contraindicated.

Interventions include revascularization procedures for occlusive coronary stenosis that often relieve the anginal symptoms. However, these interventions have failed to reduce the risk for ACS and death. Statin medical treatment has been shown to prevent both first and recurrent ACS.

Platelets adhere to the vessel walls, which are sites of endothelial cell activation. This contributes to the development of chronic atherosclerotic lesions. As the lesions rupture, they trigger the acute onset of arterial thrombosis. Transient, repeated increases in the excretion of thromboxane metabolites have been seen and reported in patients with ACS. The episodic nature of platelet activation is consistent with the concept that coronary thrombosis is dynamic, in which repeated episodes of thrombus formation and fragmentation occur over a disrupted plaque. Treatment with either aspirin or streptokinase initiated within 24 hours after the onset of a suspected MI reduces the 5-week mortality rate by approximately 25%. The consistent finding of a 50% reduction in the risk for MI or death from vascular causes in patients with unstable angina who take aspirin shows the importance of thromboxane A_2 in platelet-mediated mechanism of the growth and stabilization of an intraluminal coronary thrombus. Evidence has repeatedly shown single antiplatelet agent is associated with 25% odds reduction in major adverse cardiovascular events, including MI. This includes patients with an acute or previous MI, acute or previous ischemic stroke, stable or unstable angina, and atrial fibrillation.

Initial antiplatelet or anticoagulant therapy in patients with definite or likely non–ST-elevation MI (NSTEMI)-ACS is recommended by the American College of Cardiology/American Heart Association taskforce (2014 guidelines), as follows:

- All patients with NSTEMI-ACS without contraindications should receive antiplatelet agent as soon as possible after presentation, followed by a maintenance dose (81–325 mg/day) continued indefinitely. For patients unable to take aspirin because of hypersensitivity or major gastrointestinal intolerance, a loading dose of clopidogrel, followed by a daily maintenance dose, should be administered.
- A P_2Y_{12} inhibitor (either clopidogrel or ticagrelor) should be given in addition to aspirin for up to 12 months to all patients with NSTEMI-ACS without contraindications who are treated with either an early invasive or ischemia-guided strategy.

- In patients with NSTEMI-ACS treated with early invasive strategies and dual antiplatelet therapy with intermediate- to high-risk features (i.e., positive troponins), a glycoprotein II_a/III_b inhibitor may be considered as part of the initial antiplatelet therapy. Preferred options include eptifibatide or tirofiban.

ASPIRIN (acetylsalicylic acid) inhibits platelet prostaglandin synthesis and the adenosine diphosphate (ADP)- and collagen-induced platelet release reaction. It permanently inactivates cyclo-oxygenase (COX) activity of prostaglandin H (PGH) synthase 1 and synthase 2, also known as COX-1 and COX-2, respectively. These isoenzymes catalyze the first committed step in prostanoid biosynthesis—the conversion of arachidonic acid to PGH_2. PGH_2 is an unstable biosynthetic intermediate and a substrate for several downstream isomerases that generate at least five different bioactive prostanoids to include thromboxane A_2 and prostacyclin (PGI_2). Although other mechanisms have been proposed, inhibitor of platelet COX-1 is sufficient to explain the antithrombotic effects of low-dose aspirin.

CLOPIDOGREL (thienopyridine ADP-receptor antagonist). Antagonist of P_2Y_{12}, one of the ADP receptors on platelets, clopidogrel is a prodrug that needs biotransformation to become active. It irreversibly inhibits the P_2Y_{12} receptor. Steady-state inhibition of platelet function is noted after 5 to 7 days of maintenance dosing. The recommended loading dose is 600 mg, and the maintenance dose is 75 mg daily. Clopidogrel has been shown to have a wide interindividual variability in inhibiting ADP-induced platelet function. The mechanisms of variability are multifactorial and include drug, environmental, and genetic interactions in addition to clinical features. Proton pump inhibitors (PPIs; i.e., omeprazole and esomeprazole, which are both substrates and inhibitors of CYP2C19) are associated with decreased inhibition of platelet aggregation by clopidogrel.

PRASUGREL (thienopyridine ADP-receptor antagonist) is also a prodrug that needs biotransformation to become active. It irreversibly inhibits the P_2Y_{12} receptor. The ischemic benefit of prasugrel compared with clopidogrel in patients with ACS undergoing PCI was particularly evident in those patients with diabetes. Prasugrel should not be used in patients who previously had a stroke or who have increased risk for bleeding—unless high-risk ischemic features are present. In the TRILOGY trial, prasugrel was not better than clopidogrel in reducing ischemic events in patients with NSTEMI who had not undergone revascularization.

TICAGRELOR is the first clinically available oral cyclopentyl triazolo-pyrimidine that inhibits P_2Y_{12} receptor and has low interindividual variability in antiplatelet response. Unlike thienopyridines, ticagrelor does not bind to the ADP-binding site and instead binds to a separate site

of the P_2Y_{12} receptor to inhibit G-protein activation and signaling. The recommended loading dose is 180 mg once, and the maintenance dose is 90 mg twice a day. Ticagrelor has a faster onset of action than clopidogrel, with inhibition of more than 40% of platelets in 30 minutes after dosing and with peak effect in 2 hours. Ticagrelor has a plasma half-life of 8 to 12 hours and reaches steady state after 2 to 3 days. With aspirin and thienopyridines, the effects can be offset with platelet transfusions, whereas thienopyridines need transfusion with a higher percentage of platelet mass. In contrast, because ticagrelor and its metabolites are likely to inhibit transfused platelets, studies suggest that platelet transfusion might not reverse the drug's properties.

	CLOPIDOGREL	PRASUGREL	TICAGRELOR
Prodrug	Yes	Yes	No
Percentage of active metabolite	15%	85%	90–100%
Onset of action	2–8 hours	30 minutes– 4 hours	30 minutes–4 hours
Offset of action	7–10 days	7–10 days	3–5 days
Interactions with CYP-targeted drugs	CYP2C19	No	CYP3A4 or CYP3A5
Drug class	Thienopyridine	Thienopyridine	Cyclopentyl triazolo-pyrimidine
P_2Y_{12} receptor blockade	Irreversible	Irreversible	Reversible

CILOSTAZOL inhibits phosphodiesterase III and increases levels of cyclic adenosine monophosphate, which leads to vasodilation, reduction of vascular smooth muscle proliferation, and inhibition of platelet aggregation. It is suggested for symptomatic management of peripheral vascular disease and has been used after PCI and for secondary prevention of noncardioembolic stroke or transient ischemic attack.

DIPYRIDAMOLE blocks the uptake of adenosine, which acts on the platelet A2 receptor to activate platelet adenylate cyclase, reducing platelet aggregation. It also inhibits phosphodiesterase. It is used for prevention of postoperative thromboembolic complications associated with cardiac valve replacement and for prevention of secondary stroke.

Keyword: Antiplatelet agents

REFERENCES

Amsterdam EA, Wenger NK, Brindis RG et al. 2014 AHA/ACC guideline for the management of patients with non-ST-elevation acute coronary syndromes. *J Am Coll Cardiol* 2014;64(24):e139–e228.

Davì G, Patrono C. Platelet activation and atherothrombosis. *N Engl J Med* 2007;357(24):2482–2494.

Libby P. Mechanisms of acute coronary syndromes and their implications for therapy. *N Engl J Med* 2013;368(21):2004–2013.

Patrono C, García Rodríguez LA, Landolfi R, Baigent C. Low-dose aspirin for the prevention of atherothrombosis. *N Engl J Med* 2005;353(22): 2373–2383.

10. ANSWER: C

CTEPH is a complication of acute PE. The diagnosis is associated with a history of acute venous thrombosis. The incidence is estimated to be 1 to 5%. DVT suspicion arises with clinical evaluation noted for a positive Homan sign. A positive Homan sign is not diagnostic of a DVT with a sensitivity ranging from 10 to 54%. Because it elicits concern to the provider, additional studies are obtained, including D-dimer or venous Doppler ultrasound. A D-dimer is a fibrin degradation product (protein) that is present in the blood after the blood clot has been degraded by fibrinolysis. A negative D-dimer usually can rule out thrombosis. It is useful for exclusion of thromboembolic conditions in patients with low probability. However, a positive D-dimer may indicate thrombosis, but other causes also must be investigated. Wells criteria for prediction of DVT are often used for risk assessment.

Wells Criteria

CLINICAL CHARACTERISTIC	SCORE
Active cancer (patient either receiving treatment for cancer within the previous 6 months or currently receiving palliative treatment)	1
Paralysis, paresis, or recent cast immobilization of the lower extremities	1
Recently bedridden for >3 days, or major surgery within the previous 12 weeks requiring general or regional anesthesia	1
Localized tenderness along the destination of the deep venous system	1
Entire leg swelling	1
Calf swelling at least 3 cm larger than that of the asymptomatic side (measured 10 cm below the tibial tuberosity)	1
Pitting edema confined to the symptomatic leg	1
Collateral superficial veins (nonvaricose)	1
Previously documented DVT	1
Alternative diagnosis at least as likely as DVT	–2

Wells Scoring System for DVT

PROBABILITY	POINT(S)
Low	–2 to 0
Moderate	1 to 2
High	3 to 8

CTEPH is associated with high morbidity and mortality. The etiology of development of CTEPH in patients after acute PE is unknown. Hypercoagulable states have been identified in some patients. Factor VIII elevated levels (>230 IU/dL) were more common among patients with CTEPH than control groups in some studies and continued to be elevated after thromboendarterectomy. Other prothrombotic states associated with CTEPH include antiphospholipid antibody and activated protein C and protein S deficiency However, less than 1% patients with CTEPH have deficiencies of antithrombin, protein C, or protein S.

Evaluation includes echocardiography, which shows an increased pulmonary artery systolic pressure, right atrial enlargement, and right ventricular hypertrophy with a decrease in systolic function. Pulmonary function tests show a decrease in diffusing capacity for carbon monoxide (DL_{CO}). A mild obstructive or restrictive defect may be seen. Chest radiography may reveal areas of hypoperfusion or hyperperfusion. Pulmonary hypertension may show an enlargement of the main pulmonary arteries, asymmetry in size of central pulmonary arteries, right atrial enlargement, or right ventricular enlargement.

When pulmonary hypertension is suspected or diagnosed, CTEPH must always be a consideration. Ventilation-perfusion (V/Q) scanning is the first imaging study performed. CTEPH can have segmental or larger mismatched V/Q defects. Patients with a diagnosis of CTEPH confirmed by V/Q scan should undergo a right heart catheterization and pulmonary angiography to confirm pulmonary hypertension, assess severity of pulmonary hypertension, and provide information regarding surgical access.

The diagnosis of CTEPH includes both pulmonary hypertension (PAP ≥25 mm Hg at rest, without elevated pulmonary artery occlusion pressure (i.e., ≤15 mmHg) and thromboembolic occlusion of the proximal or distal pulmonary vasculature as the presumed cause of the pulmonary hypertension.

Treatment of CTEPH includes medical and surgical entities. Surgical treatment includes pulmonary thromboendarterectomy and percutaneous pulmonary balloon angioplasty.

Keyword: Pulmonary hypertension

REFERENCES

Lang IM, Pesavento R, Bonderman D, Yuan JX. Risk factors and basic mechanisms of chronic thromboembolic pulmonary hypertension: a current understanding. *Eur Respir J* 2013;41(2):462–468.

Modi S, Deisler R, Gozel K et al. Wells criteria for DVT is a reliable clinical tool to assess the risk of deep venous thrombosis in trauma patients. *World J Emerg Surg* 2016;11:24.

Nosher JL, Patel A, Jagpal S et al. Endovascular treatment of pulmonary embolism: selective review of available techniques. *World J Radiol* 2017;9(12):426–437.

Preston IR, Roberts KE, Miller DP et al. Effect of warfarin treatment on survival of patients with pulmonary arterial hypertension (PAH) in the Registry to Evaluate Early and Long-Term PAH Disease Management (REVEAL). *Circulation* 2015;132(25):2403–2411.

Wells PS, Anderson DR, Rodger M et al. Evaluation of D-dimer in the diagnosis of suspected deep-vein thrombosis. *N Engl J Med* 2003;349:1227–1235.

11. ANSWER: C

Warfarin is a vitamin K antagonist and one of the most commonly used oral anticoagulants. The mechanism of action is antagonism of vitamin K causing disruption of formation of clotting proteins is vitamin K dependent, which include factors II, VII, IX, and X and proteins C and S. The half-life of warfarin is 40 hours, and complete anticoagulant effects occur 48 tot 72 hours after its administration. Activation and metabolism of this drug occur through enzymes including CYP2C9, CYP1A2, and CYP3A4. Reversal of anticoagulation effects of warfarin can be achieved by administration of vitamin K or infusion of clotting factors. Warfarin has a very narrow therapeutic index and requires routine blood testing to determine appropriate dose for the anticoagulant effect. The variability in patient response is multifactorial. It includes consumption of foods that contain vitamin K, which decreases warfarin's anticoagulation effect. On the other hand, depletion of vitamin K reserves (i.e., antibiotics given to a patient that inhibit intestinal flora production of vitamin K) potentiates its action. Also, inducers or inhibitors of certain CYP enzymes affect the properties of warfarin through altered metabolism. An example is the enhanced effect when amiodarone is coadministered. This is attributed to CYP2C9 inhibition. Drugs also involving CYP1A2 and CYP3A4 can affect the anticoagulation ability of warfarin. Vitamin K antagonists have a narrow therapeutic index, and blood monitoring is required.

Alternatives to warfarin are non–vitamin K oral antagonists, known as novel oral anticoagulants (NOACs), and include dabigatran, which targets factor IIa, and rivaroxaban, apixaban, and edoxaban, which target factor Xa. NOACs do not need blood monitoring and have a faster onset and offset of action. Chronic kidney disease affects half-life of drugs as well as plasma concentrations because of variable renal clearance.

Keyword: Warfarin

REFERENCES

Almutairi AR, Zhou L, Gellad WF et al. Effectiveness and safety of non-vitamin k antagonist oral anticoagulants for atrial fibrillation and venous thromboembolism: a systematic review and meta-analyses. *Clin Ther* 2017;39(7):1456–1478.

Cuker A, Siegal DM, Crowther MA, Garcia DA. Laboratory measurement of the anticoagulant activity of the non-vitamin K oral anticoagulants. *J Am Coll Cardiol* 2014;64(11):1128–1139.

Mega JL, Simon T. Pharmacology of antithrombotic drugs: an assessment of oral antiplatelet and anticoagulant treatments. *Lancet* 2015;386(9990):281–291.

12. ANSWER: B

Ischemic stroke causes 2.9 million deaths and results in 3.4 million years lived with a disability worldwide. Unfractionated heparin, low-molecular-weight heparin (LMWH), and heparinoids may decrease the risk for recurrence of an ischemic stroke, DVT, and PE. However, heparin and heparinoids also increase the risk for intracranial and extracranial hemorrhage.

Unfractionated heparin is a sulfated polysaccharide. It causes an anticoagulant effect by inactivating thrombin (factor IIa) and activated factor Xa through an antithrombin-dependent mechanism. For inhibition of thrombin, heparin binds reversibly to both the coagulation enzyme and antithrombin. However, binding the coagulation enzyme is not necessary for inhibition of factor Xa. It is a naturally occurring anticoagulant released from mast cells. Unfractionated heparin differs from LMWH in that the molecular weight of LMWH is 4.5 kDa, whereas that of unfractionated heparin is 15 kDa. Unfractionated heparin requires continuous infusions; activated partial prothrombin time (aPTT) monitoring is required when it is used. Unfractionated heparin also has a higher risk for bleeding and osteoporosis with long-term use.

LMWHs include enoxaparin, dalteparin, nadroparin, and tinzaparin.

Clinical considerations include the following:

- Increased bleeding in patients with clotting disorders, severe hypertension, and patients who have had recent surgery

	DABIGATRAN	RIVAROXABAN	APIXABAN	EDOXABAN
Factor target	IIa (thrombin)	Xa	Xa	Xa
Prodrug	Yes	No	No	No
Hours to C_{max}	1–3	2–4	3–4	1–2
Half-life (hours)	12–17	5–13	9–14	10–14
Liver metabolism	No	Yes (elimination)	Yes (elimination; minor CYP3A4 contribution)	Minimal
Absorption with H_2-blocker/PPI	12–30%	No effect	No effect	No effect

Table A11.1

- Patients with renal disease can experience accumulation of LMWHs or fondaparinux. Unfractionated heparin can be used without risk, or lower dosing of LMWH is preferred.
- Protamine sulfate can be used to reverse the effects of unfractionated heparin but has only a limited antidote effect on Lovenox.

Keywords: Heparin, heparinoids, LMWH

REFERENCES

Bath PW, Iddenden R, Bath FJ. Low-molecular-weight heparins and heparinoids in acute ischemic stroke: a meta-analysis of randomized controlled trials. *Stroke* 2018;31:1770–1778.

Lansberg MG, O'Donnell MJ, Khatri P et al. Antithrombotic and thrombolytic therapy for ischemic stroke: antithrombotic therapy and prevention of thrombosis, 9th edition. American College of Chest Physicians Evidence-Based Clinical Practice Guidelines. *Chest* 2012;141:e601S-e636S.

Mendez AA, Samaniego EA, Sheth SA et al. Update in the early management and reperfusion strategies of patients with acute ischemic stroke. *Crit Care Res Pract* 2018 ;2018:9168731.

Powers WJ, Rabinstein AA, Ackerson T et al. 2018 Guidelines for the early management of patients with acute ischemic stroke: a guideline for healthcare professionals from the American Heart Association/American Stroke Association. *Stroke* 2018;49:e46–e99.

Whiteley WN, Adams HP Jr, Bath PM et al. Targeted use of heparin, heparinoids, or low-molecular-weight heparin to improve outcome after acute ischaemic stroke: an individual patient data meta-analysis of randomised controlled trials. *Lancet Neurol* 2013;12(6):539–545.

13.

CARDIOVASCULAR II
MECHANICAL SUPPORT AND RESUSCITATION

John C. Klick

QUESTIONS

1. A 23-year-old male with a history of Wolff-Parkinson-White (WPW) syndrome arrives from the operating room to the surgical intensive care unit (ICU) after an open reduction and internal fixation (ORIF) procedure of an open femur fracture sustained during a motorcycle collision. He has bilateral lung contusions, and the anesthesiologist has opted to not attempt extubation. The patient is sedated and paralyzed on mechanical ventilation. His access includes two 16-gauge peripheral intravenous (IV) catheters and a radial arterial line. Shortly after arrival, he becomes tachycardic and hypotensive. A 12-lead electrocardiogram (ECG) reveals a wide-complex irregular tachycardia at a rate of approximately 165 bpm. His blood pressure (BP) is now 68/42 mm Hg. Which of the following is the most appropriate next step in the patient's management?

    A. Administer IV amiodarone
    B. Electrical cardioversion
    C. Diltiazem infusion
    D. Emergency radiofrequency ablation

2. A 68-year-old female with a history of atrial fibrillation has fallen and struck her head. She takes warfarin on a daily basis to prevent thromboembolism. Her Glasgow Coma Scale (GCS) score is 10, she is intubated, and head computed tomography (CT) shows a large subdural hematoma with mass effect. The neurosurgeons wish to take her emergently to the operating room for evacuation of the subdural hematoma but are concerned about her international normalized ratio (INR) of 3.2. What is the most effective way to reverse the effects of her warfarin?

    A. IV protamine administration
    B. Administration of fresh frozen plasma (FFP)

    C. Administration of a four-factor prothrombin complex concentrate (PCC)
    D. IV administration of vitamin K

3. A 21-year-old otherwise healthy woman presents to the emergency department (ED) complaining of increasing dyspnea on exertion for the past 2 to 3 days. She describes having an upper respiratory tract infection 3 weeks prior. Chest radiography reveals mild cardiac enlargement, and a subsequent transthoracic echocardiogram (TTE) shows a small circumferential pericardial effusion. She is discharged home with ibuprofen for presumed postviral pericarditis. Two days, later she is found unconscious in her bathroom. An ECG shows diffuse ST-segment elevation throughout the precordial leads. Cardiac catheterization reveals normal coronary arteries. She arrives at your tertiary care center intubated and sedated. Heart rate (HR) is 125 bpm, and BP is 66/32 mm Hg. Physical exam reveals an S3 gallop and diffuse pulmonary crackles. A stat TTE reveals a left ventricular ejection fraction (LVEF) of 10 to 15% with global hypokinesis and a small pericardial effusion. Inotropic support is initiated with dobutamine. Her white blood cell count is $31.2 \times 10^9/L$, and her troponin T level is 0.9 ng/mL. Creatinine is now 3.2, and her lactate is elevated at 3.5. Emergent right heart catheterization was performed with endomyocardial biopsy. The biopsy specimen reveals active lymphocytic myocarditis. Despite escalating inotropic support, she becomes anuric, and her lactate continues to climb. Which is the next most appropriate step in her management?

    A. Addition of IV phenylephrine
    B. Emergent sternotomy and surgical placement of an implantable left ventricular assist device (LVAD)
    C. Aggressive diuresis
    D. Percutaneous cannulation and initiation of venoarterial (VA) extracorporeal membrane oxygenation (ECMO)

4. A 72-year-old male with diabetes mellitus, hypertension, hyperlipidemia, atrial fibrillation, a 3.9 cm abdominal aortic aneurysm (AAA), peripheral arterial disease and chronic kidney disease presents with a non-ST segment elevation myocardial infarction (NSTEMI). His TTE shows an LVEF of 35%, mild mitral stenosis, moderate tricuspid regurgitation, mild pulmonary hypertension and moderate to severe aortic insufficiency. Cardiac catheterization reveals severe 3-vessel coronary artery disease and a CABG/AVR is planned for the following day. That night he develops severe substernal chest discomfort. Which of his following conditions precludes the use of an intra-aortic balloon pump (IABP)?

A. Chronic kidney disease
B. Moderate to severe aortic insufficiency
C. Mitral stenosis
D. Pulmonary hypertension

5. A 64-year-old male with a history of diabetes, hypertension, and new-onset end-stage renal disease presents to your ICU with hypoxemia, fever, and a widened pulse pressure. He is dialyzed through a tunneled hemodialysis catheter while waiting for his arteriovenous (AV) fistula to mature. His workup reveals pulmonary edema, and a TTE reveals severe aortic insufficiency (AI). Blood cultures reveal methicillin-resistant *Staphylococcus aureus*. A transesophageal echocardiogram (TEE) reveals vegetations on the mitral and aortic valves with an aortic root abscess and severe AI. Because of the patient's worsening hemodynamics and pulmonary edema, he is scheduled for urgent surgery. Postoperatively, he arrives in the ICU intubated, sedated, and on norepinephrine and vasopressin drips in sinus rhythm. Hemodynamics gradually improve, and vasopressor doses are decreased over the next 4 hours. Suddenly, the patient becomes bradycardic with HR of 34. ECG reveals a junctional escape rhythm. What is the next most appropriate step in the patient's management?

A. Start an infusion of isoproterenol
B. Bolus IV calcium chloride
C. Emergent placement of a transvenous pacing wire
D. Start an infusion of epinephrine

6. A 68-year-old morbidly obese woman with no known history of cardiovascular disease is 4 weeks postop from a left total knee replacement. She was found on the floor at home. Her BP on arrival to your ICU is 71/43 mm Hg, HR is 125 bpm, and O$_2$ saturation is 83% on a 100% non-rebreather mask. A central venous line was placed in the ED, and the central venous pressure (CVP) reads 38 mm Hg. You perform an immediate goal-directed TTE and see a hyperdynamic, underfilled left ventricle (LV) and a dilated hypokinetic right ventricle (RV) with

interventricular septal shift during systole. An image from a TTE is shown here (image copyright George Williams, MD, FASA, FCCP.)

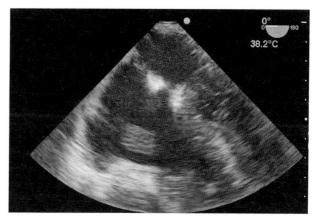

Based on these imaging results, what is the next MOST appropriate step in this patient's management?

A. Cardiopulmonary resuscitation (CPR)
B. Heparin infusion
C. Milrinone
D. IV thrombolytics

7. A 30-year-old male with a history of nonischemic cardiomyopathy is 9 months status post orthotopic heart transplantation (OHT). He had a Heartmate II LVAD for 2 years before his transplantation. He is admitted to the ICU after presenting with worsening renal function, shortness of breath, tachycardia to 125 bpm, and hypotension. A chest radiograph is shown here (image courtesy of George Williams, MD, FASA, FCCP). A pulmonary artery catheter is placed and reveals:

Cardiac output: 2.5 L/minute
Pulmonary capillary wedge pressure (PCWP): 23 mm Hg
CVP: 16 mm Hg
Systemic vascular resistance (SVR): 1300 dynes/sec/cm^5

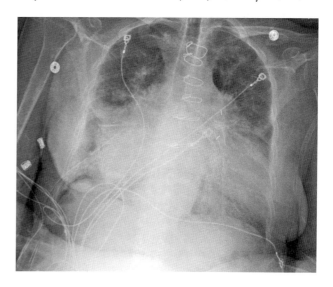

Which of the following is the MOST appropriate next step in this patient's management?

A. Administration of sodium nitroprusside
B. Beta-blockade
C. Placement of an IABP
D. Initiation of inotropic support

8. A 24-year-old man presents to your ICU after a syncopal episode preceded by hemoptysis. He is profoundly cyanotic despite being on a 100% non-rebreather oxygen mask. He reports being dizzy and severely fatigued. On exam, you notice a loud systolic murmur, abdominal swelling, and prominent clubbing of his fingertips. When asked about other medical problems, he states that he was told many years ago that he has a "hole in his heart" but has had no follow-up. An ECG from the ED shows severe right-axis deviation and P pulmonale. His hematocrit was 60% when checked in the ED. You perform a bedside TTE and note that the patient has severe RV hypertrophy and a large ventricular septal defect (VSD). You estimate the pulmonary arterial systolic pressures at about 115 mm Hg through continuous wave Doppler across the regurgitant tricuspid valve jet. What is the BEST description of this patient's diagnosis?

A. Pulmonary arterial hypertension (PAH)
B. Tetralogy of Fallot
C. Eisenmenger syndrome
D. Ebstein anomaly

9. The same 24-year-old patient with the VSD and Eisenmenger syndrome becomes acutely hypotensive; he also remains hypoxemic. Stat TTE shows an underfilled LV and shift of the interventricular septum into the LV during systole. Which of the following is the MOST appropriate treatment option at this point?

A. Emergent cardiac surgical consultation for emergent closure of the VSD
B. Inhaled nitric oxide (iNO)
C. IV epinephrine
D. Emergent ECMO

10. You are called emergently to the bedside of a 75-year-old man with a history of severe emphysema who was admitted to the ICU for treatment of a severe chronic obstructive pulmonary disease (COPD) exacerbation. He was using biphasic positive airway pressure (BiPAP) by face mask and is found to be hypotensive, with bulging neck vessels and a rapid narrow complex rhythm, and loses his pulse. As your team starts CPR and prepares to intubate the patient, you call for the echocardiography machine and perform a rapid subxiphoid image, on which you note a hyperdynamic LV with a compressed RV and no obvious pericardial fluid collection. During the pulse check pause of chest compressions, you rapidly scan the anterior chest. You note that the pleural line does not appear to move on the right. What should be your NEXT action in the resuscitation of this patient?

A. Loading dose of amiodarone
B. IV sodium bicarbonate
C. Fluid bolus
D. Needle decompression of the right chest

11. A 58-year-old man is admitted directly from the operating room where he has just undergone a redo sternotomy, aortic valve replacement, and replacement of the ascending aorta for a bicuspid valve. Ten years earlier, he had undergone a previous coronary artery bypass graft (CABG) × 4. During the first 2 hours in the ICU, he puts out about 300 mL of sanguinous fluid from his chest tubes every hour. His INR is 1.4, fibrinogen 220, platelet count 310. You order a thromboelastogram (TEG) to help determine whether there are any ongoing coagulation abnormalities. The K time, angle, and maximum amplitude are all within normal limits, but the R time is prolonged on the nonheparinase sample (normal R time is 6 minutes). Based on these TEG results, what is the MOST appropriate treatment to stop this patient's bleeding?

A. Allogeneic platelets
B. Allogeneic FFP
C. Protamine
D. Activated factor VII

12. A 69-year-old female was admitted to the ICU with acute shortness of breath. A pulmonary embolism protocol CT showed a large pulmonary embolism. A duplex ultrasound showed a large thrombus in the right superficial femoral vein. Several hours later, she becomes acutely hemodynamically unstable. Bedside echocardiography shows acute RV dysfunction with visible clot in the right atrium. IV recombinant tissue plasminogen activator (rTPA) is administered with improvement in RV function. However, she shortly becomes acutely dysarthric and hemiplegic. A stat noncontrast head CT shows an intracranial hemorrhage (ICH). Which of the following is the MOST appropriate next step in the management of this patient?

A. Emergent craniotomy for hematoma evacuation
B. IV vitamin K
C. IV epsilon–aminocaproic acid
D. Recombinant factor VIIa

13. A 65-year-old woman with severe COPD and previous replacement of her aortic valve with a mechanical prosthesis is recovering in the ICU 4 days after a CABG. Because of her severe lung disease, she is difficult to wean from mechanical ventilation and is extubated on postoperative day 3. Previous cardiac catheterization revealed 80% left main coronary artery occlusion and 75% right coronary artery (RCA) disease. An IABP was placed at the time of catheterization, and she was sent to the ICU on an IV heparin drip. She is on an unfractionated heparin drip until her Coumadin is therapeutic again. You note that her platelet count has dropped precipitously from 277,000/μL to 77,000/μ: over the past 24 hours. She has also developed new-onset left calf tenderness, and her pulses have been become diminished in the left leg with associated erythematous skin nodules as well. A platelet factor 4 (PF4)/heparin antigen assay comes back positive; serotonin release assay (SRA) is pending. What is the MOST appropriate next step in management of this patient?

A. IV bivalirudin
B. Warfarin
C. Referral to vascular surgery for urgent thrombectomy
D. Autologous platelets

14. A 64-year-old man with a history of congestive heart failure is in your ICU 1 day after an emergent exploratory laparotomy. During the exploratory laparotomy, a perforated diverticulum was found with fecal spillage, and the patient underwent colonic resection and diverting colostomy. He remains intubated and sedated but is hemodynamically unstable, requiring escalating doses of IV norepinephrine. The patient's CVP is 10 mm Hg, his urine output has fallen over the past 2 hours, and his creatinine has started to increase. Which of the following is the MOST appropriate next move in the management of this patient?

A. Continuous renal replacement therapy
B. Bedside TTE
C. IV dobutamine
D. IV methylene blue

15. A 74-year-old male with a history of a previous myocardial infarction (MI), COPD, type 2 diabetes, congestive heart failure, and chronic kidney disease arrives in your ICU, extubated, after a redo femoral-popliteal bypass graft. His native LVEF is 40%. A preoperative nuclear stress test had been positive, and subsequent cardiac catheterization had shown diffuse coronary artery disease with no intervenable lesions. His intraoperative course was relatively uneventful. Over the next 6 hours, he becomes progressively short of breath with bedside

monitor findings shown here (image courtesy of George Williams, MD, FASA, FCCP):

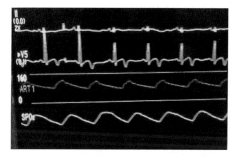

He remains in sinus rhythm with a HR of 95 bpm. What is the MOST appropriate next step in his medical management?

A. Beta-blockade
B. Oral aspirin
C. IV heparin
D. IV furosemide

16. You are called emergently to the postanesthesia care unit (PACU) where you find a 64-year-old male undergoing CPR and intubation. He is immediately postop from a radical prostatectomy and had been stable in the PACU for about 1 hour when he acutely went into ventricular fibrillation. He was loaded with amiodarone twice without any resolution of his arrhythmia. The PACU resident relays that the patient has a history of coronary artery disease and underwent percutaneous coronary intervention (PCI) with placement of a drug-eluting stent (DES) to his proximal left anterior descending coronary artery approximately 2 months ago. He had been on aspirin and ticagrelor after the PCI, but his urologist had instructed him to stop both agents for concern of bleeding during his procedure. Based on this presentation and history, what is the next MOST appropriate action to treat this patient?

A. Immediate thoracotomy and open cardiac massage
B. Load with IV procainamide
C. High-dose epinephrine infusion
D. Immediate consultation with interventional cardiologist and transfer to cardiac catheterization lab

17. A 55-year-old male with a history of refractory hypertension presents to the ED complaining of a headache. His BP is 276/135 mm Hg, and he is admitted to your ICU for management of hypertensive urgency. On admission, the patient begins to complain of severe chest pain that he says radiates to his back. A stat ECG shows ST depressions in leads II, III, and aVF. Bedside TTE demonstrates severe AI, a small pericardial effusion, hypokinesis of the RV and inferior LV wall, and

the appearance of a flap in the ascending aorta. Based on this presentation, what is the MOST appropriate next step in management?

A. Activate the cardiac catheterization lab
B. IV heparin
C. Consult CT surgery for emergent surgical intervention
D. Stat CT scan

18. The same patient from the previous question has arrived back in your ICU after his emergency surgery for his Stanford type A aortic dissection. He is intubated, on low-dose norepinephrine, and still producing urine after a prolonged cardiopulmonary bypass run and 39 minutes of deep hypothermic circulatory arrest. The surgeon replaced the entire aortic root, ascending aorta, and arch, as well as the aortic valve while reimplanting the coronary arteries. The innominate artery was involved, and the surgeon "bioglued" the layers of the innominate together to reimplant the innominate into the arch graft. The patient received multiple units of blood products in the operating room. The anesthesiologist tells you that TEE showed the dissection flap going over the arch and well below the diaphragm.

Over the course of the next 4 hours, the patient becomes increasingly hemodynamically unstable, requiring escalating doses of norepinephrine. He is not volume responsive, and you note that his lactate is steadily rising while he becomes increasingly acidotic. You note on exam that his abdomen is becoming increasingly distended.

Based on this presentation, what is your MOST concerning diagnosis in your differential?

A. Acute kidney injury
B. Rhabdomyolysis
C. Acute mesenteric ischemia
D. Acute cholecystitis

19. A 62-year-old male with a history of ischemic cardiomyopathy and progressive symptomatic heart failure is admitted to the ICU following implantation of a Heartmate II LVAD. He has had a previous sternotomy for CABG, and the surgeon notes that there were extensive adhesions. The blood loss was substantial, and the patient received multiple blood products in the operating room. The patient is intubated, is sedated, and has a pulmonary artery catheter in place. He is on a low-dose milrinone infusion for RV systolic dysfunction and has high chest tube output. The Heartmate II's revolutions per minute (RPMs) are set at 8400. While transfusing to correct his coagulopathy, you are called to the bedside for acute hypotension. You note that the pulsatility index has dropped, the displayed power has surged, and the CVP has increased from 11 to 24. You immediately perform a bedside TTE and note that the interventricular septum has shifted into the LV and there is now minimal LV fill. The MOST appropriate acute management of this patient is which of the following?

A. Reduce device RPMs, then slowly volume-load before increasing RPMs again
B. Initiate high-dose epinephrine drip
C. Start inhaled nitric oxide (iNO)
D. Give 80 mg IV furosemide

20. A 58-year-old woman arrives in your ICU from the operating room after a complex mitral valve repair for severe mitral regurgitation secondary to a Barlow valve. She is intubated on mechanical ventilation, has a pulmonary artery catheter, and is on a low-dose epinephrine infusion following an uneventful case. Over the next 2 hours, she becomes increasingly tachycardic, hypotensive, and oliguric. Her pulmonary arterial pressures have increased dramatically, and you note prominent V waves on the pulmonary artery pressure trace. The CVP has increased as well. Bedside TTE echocardiography shows a hyperdynamic underfilled LV with a significant posteriorly directed mitral regurgitation jet and systolic anterior motion (SAM) of the mitral valve, with obstruction of the LV outflow tract by the anterior mitral leaflet. Based on this information, which of the following options is the MOST appropriate action to treat this patient?

A. Increase the epinephrine infusion
B. Stat page the CT surgeon to go back to the operating room emergently
C. Stop the epinephrine infusion and administer 1 L of lactated Ringer's solution
D. IV milrinone infusion

ANSWERS

1. ANSWER: B

This patient is hemodynamically unstable with a wide-complex tachycardia. First-line treatment should be direct current cardioversion. This patient has a history of WPW syndrome and went into atrial fibrillation secondary to the high sympathetic tone associated with his traumatic injury and response to surgery.

WPW syndrome refers to the combination of supraventricular arrhythmias and an ECG pattern of pre-excitation. It occurs when there is an antegrade conducting accessory pathway along with one or more types of supraventricular arrhythmias. An accessory pathway is an anomalous pathway that connects the atria and ventricles, bypassing the normal AV node and His-Purkinje system. The pre-excitation pattern on a 12-lead ECG is due to the presence of this antegrade conducting accessory pathway and consists of a short PR interval, a widened QRS complex, and a delta wave, which is a slow upstroke of the QRS complex.

WPW syndrome most commonly presents in infancy and often resolves within the first year of life. Persistence of the WPW ECG pattern is associated with continued episodes of supraventricular tachycardia in 78% of patients. Atrial fibrillation may lead to sudden cardiac death due to the rapid ventricular response.

Digoxin or calcium channel blockers should not be used in patients with WPW syndrome because of the potential for facilitating conduction down the accessory pathway while blocking the AV node.

Chronically, these patients are usually treated with drugs that increase the refractory period of the accessory pathway, such as procainamide, propafenone, flecainide, disopyramide, ibutilide, and amiodarone. Electrophysiology consultation should be obtained. This patient may be a candidate for catheter ablation of the accessory pathway, which is successful in approximately 95% of cases.

Keywords: Cardiovascular; Rhythm disturbances; Atrial fibrillation; Other conduction abnormalities; ECG; Supraventricular tachyarrhythmias; Ventricular tachycardia/fibrillation

REFERENCES

Calkins H. Wolff Parkinson White syndrome: diagnosis and treatment. Available at www.clinicaladvisor.com.

Link MS. Evaluation and initial treatment of supraventricular tachycardia. *N Engl J Med* 2012;367(15): 1438–1448.

Mittnacht A, Riech D, Rhee AJ, Kaplan JA. Cardiac disease. In: Fleisher L et al. *Anesthesia and uncommon diseases*, 6th edition. Elsevier, Saunders: Philadelphia, PA: 2012, Chapter 2, page 28–74.

Zipes D, Jalife J, et al. *Cardiac electrophysiology: from cell to bedside*, 6th edition. Elsevier, Saunders: Philadelphia, PA: 2013.

2. ANSWER: C

This patient is systemically anticoagulated with warfarin as prophylaxis against thromboembolism due to her atrial fibrillation. An INR of 3.2 puts her into the supratherapeutic range. Warfarin inhibits the hepatic synthesis of vitamin K–dependent coagulation factors (II, VII, IX, X, as well as proteins C and S). Warfarin is hepatically metabolized and has a half-life of 20 to 60 hours. As a general rule, it should be stopped 5 days before elective surgery or neuraxial blockade.

Administration of vitamin K will decrease the time for the effects of warfarin to abate but will not reverse the effects rapidly enough for any kind of urgent interventional procedure. Administration of FFP will acutely reverse the anticoagulant effects of warfarin. Unfortunately, warfarin has a longer half-life than FFP. Administration of a four-factor PCC will rapidly and effectively reverse the anticoagulant effects of warfarin. It has been demonstrated to reverse the INR quicker with a lower red cell transfusion requirement and fewer adverse events than FFP.

Protamine given intravenously will rapidly reverse the effects of unfractionated heparin. Protamine will also partially reverse (60–70%) the anticoagulant effects of low-molecular-weight heparin. It will have no effect on the anticoagulant effects of warfarin.

Keywords: Anticoagulants and antithrombotics; Heparin, unfractionated, LMWH; Warfarin; Atrial fibrillation

REFERENCES

Hanley JP. Warfarin reversal. *J Clin Pathol* 2004;57:1132–1139.

Hickey M, Gatien M, Taljaard M et al. Outcomes of urgent warfarin reversal with frozen plasma versus prothrombin complex concentrate in the emergency department. *Circulation* 2013;128:360–364.

Klick J, Avery E. Anesthetic considerations for the patient with anemia and coagulation disorders. In: Longnecker DE, Brown DL, Newman MF, Zapol WM, eds. *Anesthesiology*, 2nd edition. New York: McGraw-Hill; 2012, pp. 196–217.

Lankiewicz MW, Hays J, Friedman KD, Blatt PM. Urgent reversal of warfarin anticoagulation with prothrombin complex concentrate. *Blood* 2004;104:2723.

Pesa N, Klick JC. Coagulopathies in the ICU. Society of Critical Care Anesthesiologists ICU Resident's Guide 2017. Society of Critical Care Anesthesiologists. Available at: www.socca.org.

3. ANSWER: D

This patient presents in cardiogenic shock from severely impaired LV systolic dysfunction due to viral myocarditis. Viruses may enter cardiac myocytes and macrophages through specific receptors, inciting a cytotoxic effect in the myocardium. The clinical spectrum of viral cardiomyopathy ranges from fulminant to acute to chronic. Most patients recover, but a subset may progress to a chronic dilated cardiomyopathy. In acute viral myocarditis, troponins may be elevated, and ECG may show ST elevation, mimicking an acute MI.

Echocardiography is an essential tool in the diagnostic workup to establish the LV function and to rule out other causes of heart failure such as amyloid or valvular disease. Classic findings include global hypokinesis with or without pericardial effusion.

Because patients generally present days to weeks after the initial viral infection, there is little role for antiviral therapy. There also appears to be little role for immunosuppressive therapy in acute viral myocarditis of less than 6 months' duration. Several studies suggest that patients with fulminant myocarditis who present with hemodynamic compromise have better outcomes than those with acute nonfulminant myocarditis, provided they are managed aggressively.

This patient is young and previously healthy. The onset of her myocarditis is fulminant, leading to cardiogenic shock. Despite aggressive use of inotropic therapy, she continues to show evidence of worsening end-organ function. Appropriate aggressive management of her condition would be to initiate mechanical circulatory support with VA ECMO. IV phenylephrine is purely a vasoconstrictor (sympathomimetic) and would have little role in the management of purely cardiogenic shock. Diuresis may help relieve the pulmonary congestion but would do little to address the fundamental cause of the patient's shock. The surgical placement of an implantable LVAD would not be the most expeditious means of initiating mechanical circulatory support for someone with cardiogenic shock who is already showing severe end-organ injury. An implantable LVAD may be considered once end-organ function has been stabilized with a more temporary means of circulatory support.

Keywords: Infectious, myocarditis, pericarditis; Myocardial function/dysfunction—left ventricular; ECG, imaging, cardiac ultrasound (TTE); Vasoactive or modulating drugs, inotropes; Circulatory support systems, left or right ventricular assist device, ECMO

REFERENCES

Asaumi Y, Yasuda S, Morii I et al. Favourable clinical outcome in patients with cardiogenic shock due to fulminant myocarditis supported by percutaneous extracorporeal membrane oxygenation. *Eur Heart J* 2005;26:2185–2192.

Nakamura T, Ishida K, Taniguchi Y et al. Prognosis of patients with fulminant myocarditis managed by peripheral venoarterial extracorporeal membranous oxygenation support: a retrospective single-center study. *J Intens Care* 2015;3:5

Schultz JC, Hiliard AA, Cooper LT, Rihal CS. Diagnosis and treatment of viral myocarditis. *Mayo Clin Proc* 2009;84(11):1001–1009.

4. ANSWER: B

IABPs are the most widely used form of mechanical circulatory assistance. The primary goal of its use is to increase myocardial oxygen supply and decrease myocardial oxygen consumption. The device is generally percutaneously placed through the femoral artery, with the tip sitting in the descending aorta just below the left subclavian artery. However, the device may also be inserted through the subclavian, axillary, brachial, or iliac arteries. Surgical approaches through a transthoracic or translumbar approach have also been described.

Counterpulsation refers to inflation of the balloon in diastole and deflation in early systole. Balloon inflation leads to an increase in coronary artery blood flow. Balloon deflation before opening of the aortic valve decreases the afterload against which the LV must pump. The magnitude of these effects is dependent on the balloon volume, the HR, and the aortic compliance.

Renal blood flow may increase up to 25% with a properly positioned and functioning IABP, so chronic kidney disease is not a contraindication to its use. Mitral stenosis and pulmonary hypertension are also not contraindications. In fact, use of the IABP may have favorable effects on RV function.

Absolute contraindications to the use of an IABP include aortic regurgitation, aortic dissection, chronic end-stage heart disease with no anticipation of recovery, and the presence of aortic stent grafts. Use of an IABP will worsen the magnitude of aortic regurgitation due to the diastolic inflation; therefore, this patient's aortic regurgitation makes him a noncandidate. Additionally, this patient's aortic aneurysm is a relative contraindication to placement of an IABP because the increased risk of aortic rupture. Severe peripheral arterial disease involving the aorta and femoral vessels is also a relative contraindication to placement of an IABP.

The most commonly used triggers for an IABP are the ECG waveform or the systemic arterial pressure waveform. Balloon inflation in diastole corresponds to the middle of the T wave on ECG. Deflation at the onset of LV systole corresponds to the peak of the R wave. Cardiac arrhythmias (such as atrial fibrillation in this patient) may result in erratic balloon inflation.

Proper timing of inflation and deflation may be observed on the arterial waveform display on the device console. The balloon should inflate just after aortic valve closure, which corresponds to the dicrotic notch on the arterial waveform. It should deflate immediately before the opening of the aortic valve, which corresponds to the point just before the upstroke of the arterial pressure waveform.

Keywords: Circulatory support systems, intraaortic balloon pump, left or right ventricular assist device; Peripheral vascular disease; Aneurysm, abdominal; Rhythm disturbances, atrial fibrillation; Myocardial dysfunction, left ventricular, right ventricular

REFERENCE

Krishna M, Zacharowski K. Principles of intra-aortic balloon pump counterpulsation. continuing education in anaesthesia. *Crit Care Pain* 2009;9(1):24–28.

5. ANSWER: C

Disruption of AV nodal conduction is a known complication of an aortic root abscess secondary to valvular endocarditis. It is also a recognized complication of surgical replacement of the aortic or mitral valve. Loss of conduction through the AV node results in third-degree heart block with resultant severe bradycardia. A junctional escape rhythm emerges with a low ventricular rate. Treatment involves emergent placement of a temporary transvenous ventricular pacing wire. Patients often have temporary epicardial pacing wires placed at the time of open heart surgery, and these may be used to provide temporary maintenance of an adequate ventricular rate. If the patient's hemodynamics deteriorate with the bradycardia, temporary transthoracic pacing may be used until a transvenous wire is placed. This is quite uncomfortable for patients, necessitating judicious use of sedation. IV atropine works by improving conduction through the AV node by reducing vagal tone. If the site of block is at the AV node, it may improve the ventricular rate but is clearly not the mainstay of treatment. Isoproterenol may be used as a temporary measure only to accelerate the ventricular escape rhythm, but it is associated with a high failure rate. Epinephrine has limited utility in the setting of a complete heart block. Calcium chloride has no therapeutic role in this setting.

Keywords: Infectious, endocarditis; Heart block, junctional or nodal rhythm; Imaging, cardiac ultrasound (TTE, TEE); Circulatory support systems, pacemakers/defibrillators

REFERENCES/FURTHER READING

Budzikowski AS et al. Third-degree atrioventricular block treatment and management. Available at www.emedicine.medscape.com.
Wang K, Gobel F, Gleason DF, Edwards JE. Complete heart block complicating bacterial endocarditis. *Circulation* 1972;XLVI:939–947.

6. ANSWER: D

This patient is experiencing an acute pulmonary embolism with acute RV failure. The hyperdynamic underfilled LV and evidence of RV pressure overload are supportive of the diagnosis, while the visualization of thrombus in this setting allows you to make the diagnosis. This patient is in imminent danger of cardiovascular collapse. Hemodynamically unstable patients with acute pulmonary embolism are predicted to have a more than 60% mortality rate without aggressive treatment. Thrombolysis should be initiated immediately in the absence of major contraindications. Major contraindications include intracranial disease, uncontrolled hypertension, and recent major surgery or trauma (within the past 3 weeks). The patient will require a minimum of 3 months of long-term anticoagulation if she survives. IV milrinone might help support the RV function but is not a definitive treatment. Milrinone, like inamrinone, is a phosphodiesterase inhibitor that increases cardiac contractility by reducing breakdown of cyclic adenosine monophosphate. Milrinone still increases cardiac output when beta-blockers have been administered and can be used in glucagon-resistant beta-blocker toxicity. IV heparin will be needed but is not the immediate potentially life-saving therapy of choice.

Keywords: Myocardial function/dysfunction, right ventricular; Imaging, cardiac ultrasound (TTE, TEE); Anticoagulants and antithrombotics, heparin, thrombolytics; Shock states, obstructive; hemodynamic monitoring, CVP

REFERENCES

Cohen R, Loarte P, Navarro V, Mirrer B. Echocardiographic findings in pulmonary embolism: an important guide for the management of the patient. *World J Cardiovasc Dis* 2012;2:161–164.
Giancarlo A, Bacattini C. Acute pulmonary embolism. *N Engl J Med* 2010;363:266–274.
Goldhaber SZ, Elliott CG. Acute pulmonary embolism: part I. *Circulation* 2003;108:2726–2729.
Rochefoucauld F. Pharmacological drug overdoses. In: Marino PL, ed. *The ICU book*, 4th edition. Philadelphia: Wolters Kluwer Health/Lippincott Williams & Wilkins; 2014; p. 972.

7. ANSWER: D

This patient is in cardiogenic shock secondary to severe LV systolic dysfunction. Inotropic support is the first-line therapy for patients in acute cardiogenic shock secondary to LV systolic dysfunction. The concern in this patient is that the LV dysfunction is secondary to rejection of the transplanted organ. Allograft rejection can be divided into four categories: (1) hyperacute rejection occurring minutes to hours after transplantation and mediated by preformed antibodies to ABO blood group, human leukocyte antigen (HLA), or endothelial antigens; (2) acute cellular rejection, occurring any time after transplantation and mediated by cellular immune mechanisms; (3) acute antibody-mediated rejection, occurring days to weeks after transplantation and caused by cell lysis secondary to antibody formation against donor HLA or endothelial antigens; and (4) chronic rejection, occurring months to years after transplantation and manifesting as coronary allograft vasculopathy.

Maintenance immunosuppression for OHT recipients consists of steroids tapered over the first year, a calcineurin inhibitor such as tacrolimus, and mycophenolate mofetil. Endomyocardial biopsies are performed frequently during the first 6 to 12 months to monitor for rejection.

Long-term complications also include infection, malignancy, and drug-induced complications from chronic immunosuppression, such as diabetes mellitus, kidney disease, hypertension, and obesity.

Acute cell-mediated rejection is primarily a host T-lymphocyte response against the allograft tissue. Most commonly, this occurs between 6 and 12 months after transplantation. Most cases are asymptomatic without allograft dysfunction.

Antibody-mediated rejection is diagnosed by the presence of antibody-mediated injury on endomyocardial biopsy. Risk factors include pregnancy, previous transplantation, blood transfusions, and use of ventricular assist devices. Treatment depends on clinical presentation and the degree of cardiac dysfunction but mostly involves IV corticosteroids and antithymocyte globulin. Patients in cardiogenic shock, such as this young man, may require plasmapheresis, IV immune globulin, heparin, and possibly mechanical support. Long-term management of antibody-mediated rejection may leave the patient with a low ejection fraction, restrictive physiology, and accelerated coronary artery disease. Rituximab, bortezomib, photopheresis, and possible redo transplantation are other options.

Keywords: Cardiac transplantation, rejection, complications; Vasoactive or modulating drugs, inotropes, chronotropes, lusitropes

REFERENCES

Alba AC, Bain E, Ng N et al. Complications after heart transplantation: hope for the best, but prepare for the worst. *Int J Transplant Res Med* 2016;2(2):022.

Maleszewski JJ. Heart transplant rejection pathology. Available at http://emedicine.medscape.com/article/1612493-overview.

Pajaro OE, Jaroszewski DE, Scott RL et al. Antibody-mediated rejection in heart transplantation: case presentation with a review of current international guidelines. *J Transplant* 2011;2011:351950.

Singh D, Taylor DO. Advances in the understanding and management of heart transplantation. *F1000Prime Reports* 2015;7:52.

Tonsho M, Ahmed Z, Alessandrini A, Madsen JC. Heart transplantation: challenges facing the field. *Cold Spring Harb Perspect Med* 2014;4:a015636.

8. ANSWER: C

This patient is suffering the sequelae of a long-standing uncorrected left-to-right intracardiac shunt. The uncorrected VSD has resulted in severe pulmonary hypertension, to the point at which right-sided pressure exceeds systemic pressures, reversing the shunt to right to left. This phenomenon is known as Eisenmenger syndrome. A telltale sign of a right-to-left shunt is the lack of improvement in O_2 saturation with the administration of oxygen. Arrhythmias or hypotension of any cause can lead to rapid deterioration.

PAH refers to conditions resulting in pressures within the pulmonary arteries that are due to vascular abnormalities in the pulmonary arterioles themselves. Of note, idiopathic and genetically induced PAH usually cannot be clinically distinguished. Other causes of PAH include congenital heart disease, portal hypertension, and drugs such as cocaine or amphetamines.

Tetralogy of Fallot is a congenital cardiac abnormality consisting of four findings: an aorta that overrides the RV outflow tract, RV outflow obstruction, a large subaortic VSD, and hypertrophy of the RV.

Ebstein anomaly is a congenital cardiac abnormality marked by inferior displacement of the tricuspid valve into the RV, resulting in atrialization of the RV. The result is a small hypocontractile RV. The posterior and septal leaflets of the RV are often very small with a large anterior leaflet. The condition is frequently associated with an atrial septal defect and accessory AV conduction pathways.

Keywords: Congenital heart disease in adults; Eisenmenger syndrome; Tetralogy of Fallot; ECG, cardiac ultrasound; myocardial function/dysfunction, right ventricular; Rhythm disturbances

REFERENCES

El-Chami MF. Eisenmenger syndrome workup. Available at www.emedicine.medscape.com.

Krasuski RA. Congenital heart disease in the adult. Cleveland Clinic Center for Continuing Education. August 2010. https://teachmemedicine.org/cleveland-clinic-congenital-heart-disease-in-the-adult/

Oechslin E, Mebus S, Schulze-Neick I et al. The adult patient with Eisenmenger syndrome: a medical update. Part III: specific management and surgical aspects. *Curr Cardiol Rev* 2010:6;363–372.

9. ANSWER: B

This patient is in trouble. Eisenmenger syndrome represents the end stages of an uncorrected left-to-right shunt. By this point, the patient's pulmonary hypertension is relatively fixed, and there is no benefit to surgical closure of the VSD. For surgical correction to be beneficial, it must be done early in the course of the disease.

Limited data show improved hemodynamics for patients with Eisenmenger syndrome who are placed on pulmonary vasodilators. Inhaled nitric oxide may drop the pulmonary vascular resistance enough to prevent the pressure overload of the RV. If it works, it might decrease the degree of right-to-left shunt and improve systemic oxygenation. Lack of response to a short-acting selective inhaled pulmonary vasodilator such as iNO is a bad prognostic sign. It implies that the pulmonary vascular resistance is fixed and the patient is running out of therapeutic options.

Heart-lung transplantation and bilateral lung transplantation remain therapeutic options for patients with Eisenmenger syndrome who are not candidates for repair of the underlying cardiac defect.

IV epinephrine would increase the pulmonary vascular resistance and potentially increase the right-to-left shunt.

ECMO would do nothing to correct the underlying pathophysiology. The only potential role for ECMO would be as a bridge to urgent transplantation.

Keywords: Congenital heart disease in adults; Eisenmenger syndrome; Myocardial function/dysfunction, right ventricular; Cardiovascular management strategies; Vasoactive or modulating drugs

REFERENCES

El-Chami MF. Eisenmenger syndrome workup. Available at www.emedicine.medscape.com.

Franklin WJ, Patel MD. An approach to pulmonary arterial hypertension in the adult patient with congenital heart disease-expert analysis. June 12, 2013. Available at www.acc.org.

Krasuski RA. Congenital heart disease in the adult. Cleveland Clinic Center for Continuing Education. August 2010. https://teachmemedicine.org/cleveland-clinic-congenital-heart-disease-in-the-adult/

Oechslin E, Mebus S, Schulze-Neick I et al. The adult patient with Eisenmenger syndrome: a medical update. Part III: specific management and surgical aspects. *Curr Cardiol Rev* 2010:6;363–372.

10. ANSWER: D

This patient has experienced a tension pneumothorax, most likely from rupture of an emphysematous bleb when positive pressure ventilation was employed. The intrathoracic pressure buildup caused limitation of venous return and the subsequent pulseless electrical activity (PEA) arrest. Needle decompression will decompress the pressure buildup in the right chest, allowing restoration of venous return. Needle decompression is an emergent procedure and would need to be followed by tube thoracostomy.

Causes of PEA can be divided into mechanical and metabolic issues. Most often, mechanical issues are manifested with a narrow QRS ECG pattern. These include cardiac tamponade, tension pneumothorax, mechanical hyperinflation, and pulmonary embolism. Metabolic issues tend to manifest a wide-complex QRS on the ECG. These include severe hyperkalemia, metabolic acidosis, and sodium

channel blocker toxicity. The clinical scenario can help guide the clinician toward the most likely etiology, as in this patient with severe COPD who was using positive pressure ventilation.

The use of bedside ultrasound can be invaluable in the management of PEA. Cardiac ultrasound can distinguish between true PEA with a severely hypokinetic or akinetic LV and "pseudo-PEA" in which the LV is actually hyperdynamic but the pulse cannot be felt. Pseudo-PEA is associated with a much better prognosis. Thoracic ultrasound can also be used to diagnose a pneumothorax, as in this case.

For patients with narrow-complex PEA from a suspected mechanical etiology, aggressive fluid resuscitation should be initiated while bedside ultrasound is used. Based on these results, needle decompression, pericardiocentesis, adjustment of ventilation, or thrombolytic therapy may be warranted. For wide-complex PEA, IV calcium chloride and sodium bicarbonate should be administered if the clinical scenario suggests hyperkalemia or sodium channel blocker toxicity.

Keywords: Rhythm disturbances; Pulseless electrical activity (PEA); Myocardial function/dysfunction; Shock states, cardiogenic; Imaging, cardiac ultrasound

REFERENCES

Beun L, Yersin B, Osterwalder J, Carron PN. Pulseless Electrical Activity Cardiac Arrest: Time to Amend the Mnemonic "4H&4T"? Swiss Med Wkly. 2015;145: w14178.

Chardoli M, Rabiee H, Sharif-Alhoseini M et al. Echocardiography integrated ACLS protocol versus conventional cardiopulmonary resuscitation in patients with pulseless electrical activity cardiac arrest. *Chinese J Traumatol* 2012;15(5):284–287.

Littman L, Bustin DJ, Haley MW. A simplified and structured teaching tool for the evaluation and management of pulseless electrical activity. *Med Princ Pract* 2014;23: 1–6.

11. ANSWER: C

In contrast to standard tests of coagulation, TEG measures the mechanical properties of the developing clot, along with the maximal clot strength and clot lysis (image copyright George Williams, MD, FASA, FCCP). It provides a measure of whole blood coagulation. Use of TEG has led to a reduction in the administration of blood products in cardiac surgery.

Using kaolin-activated sample cups, the parameters assessed include the R time, the K time, the alpha angle, and the maximum amplitude. The R time represents the start of the test until initial fibrin formation. K time represents the time taken to achieve a certain level of clot strength. The angle measures the speed at which fibrin buildup and cross-linking take place. The maximum amplitude represents the

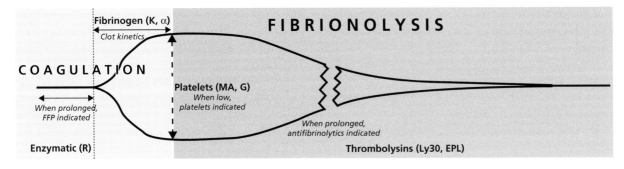

Figure A11.1

ultimate strength of the fibrin clot and reflects the dynamic properties of fibrin and platelet bonding through glycoprotein IIb/IIIa. This correlates to platelet function.

During and after cardiac surgery, two samples are typically run, one with a heparinase enzyme, one without heparinase. Heparinase is an enzyme that cleaves heparin. By comparing the R times of the heparinase and nonheparinase samples, the clinician can get a sense of the effect of residual heparin on the R time. In this case, the normal R time on the heparinase sample but prolonged R time on the nonheparinase sample indicates that residual heparin is the cause of the ongoing bleeding. Administration of protamine will reverse the effects of the residual heparin.

Keywords: Anticoagulants and antithrombotics, heparin, heparinoids

REFERENCE

Sharma AD, Al-Achi A, Seccombe JF et al. Does incorporation of thromboelastography improve bleeding prediction following adult cardiac surgery? *Blood Coagul Fibrinolysis* 2014;25(6):561–570.

Spiess BD, Wall MH, Gillies BS et al. A comparison of thromboelastography with heparinase or protamine sulfate added in-vitro during heparinized cardiopulmonary bypass. *Thromb Haemost* 1997;78(2): 820–826.

Thakur M, Ahmed AB. A review of thromboelastography. Int J Periop Ultrasound Appl Technol 2012;1(1):25–29.

12. ANSWER: C

The use of thrombolytic agents can be life-saving for the treatment of massive pulmonary embolism causing hemodynamic instability. However, hemorrhagic complications are a concern. Symptomatic ICH is the most feared complication and is associated with up to a 50% mortality rate. BP control (<180/105 mm Hg) after treatment and avoiding use of anticoagulant and antiplatelet agents in the first 24 hours after treatment may reduce the potential for ICH.

IV rTPA causes local thrombolysis by converting plasminogen into plasmin, which then degrades fibrin into fibrin split products. It is very short acting, with approximately 50% cleared within 5 minutes and 80% within 10 minutes. Clearance is through the liver with urinary excretion. Despite the rapid clearance, the prothrombin and activated partial thromboplastin (aPTT) times may be prolonged for more than 24 hours, along with reductions in the fibrinogen levels. The reduction in fibrinogen appears to correlate best with the degree of thrombolysis. The occurrence of ICH after IV administration of rTPA may be related not just to the coagulopathy but also to disruption of the blood-brain barrier.

Emergent craniotomy for hematoma evacuation is not the first-line treatment. The acute coagulopathy severely limits the ability to achieve surgical hemostasis.

Vitamin K promotes hepatic synthesis of factors II, VII, IX, X, along with proteins C and S. It takes several hours for the liver to synthesize those factors. In thrombolytic-related bleeding, the main mechanism of the coagulopathy is not related to factor deficiency but to reduction in fibrinogen. Thus, vitamin K is not useful in the acute reversal of this coagulopathy.

Recombinant factor VIIa is a vitamin K–dependent glycoprotein that activates the extrinsic coagulation cascade, promoting the formation of thrombin, which in turn converts fibrinogen to fibrin. It is not routinely recommended because of lack of demonstrated clinical benefit and increased risk for thrombotic events.

Epsilon–aminocaproic acid inhibits fibrinolysis by blocking the conversion of plasminogen to plasmin. It also directly inhibits the proteolytic activity of plasmin, leading to clot stabilization. It has a short half-life (roughly 2 hours) and exhibits peak action about 3 hours after administration. It has been shown not only to inhibit fibrinolysis but also to increase fibrinogen levels that are reduced in thrombolytic-related ICH. There is a potential risk for increased thrombotic events, although meta-analyses do not support the concern. Epsilon–aminocaproic acid should be used in combination with cryoprecipitate or fibrinogen concentrates and platelet transfusion.

Keywords: Shock states, obstructive; Imaging, CT, cardiac ultrasound; Anticoagulants and antithrombotics, antifibrinolytics, thrombolytics

REFERENCES

Martin C, Sobolewshi K, Bridgeman P, Boutsikaris D. Systemic thrombolysis for pulmonary embolism: a review. *P&T* 2016;41(12):770–775.

Shadi Y, Eisenberger A, Willey JZ. Symptomatic intracerebral hemorrhage in acute ischemic stroke after thrombolysis with intravenous recombinant tissue plasminogen activator: a review of natural history and treatment. *JAMA Neurol* 2014;71(9):1181–1185.

Tengborn L. Fibrinolytic inhibitors in the management of bleeding disorders. *Treatment of Hemophilia* 2012;42.

13. ANSWER: A

Despite not having the SRA results back, there is adequate clinical reason to suspect that this patient is developing heparin-induced thrombocytopenia (HIT). HIT is an immune-mediated, prothrombotic complication that occurs with unfractionated heparin and low-molecular-weight heparin, although to a lesser degree. It is caused by the interaction of heparin with a specific platelet protein, PF4. Clinically, there are two types of HIT. HIT type I is a benign non–immune-mediated sequestration of platelets in the spleen and occurs in 1 to 2% of patients who receive heparin. HIT type II is an immune-mediated syndrome caused by an antibody to the PF4/heparin complex. HIT type II is the clinically concerning entity that occurs in 0.1 to 0.2% of patients who receive heparin. It is associated with an increase in thrombotic episodes. The immunoglobulin G antibodies to the heparin/PF4 complex result in platelet activation, which may lead to overt arterial thrombosis, often referred to as the "white clot syndrome."

Typical onset of HIT occurs 5 to 10 days after initiation of heparin. Thrombocytopenia is the first sign in most cases, manifested by a platelet count below 150,00/μL or more than a 50% drop from baseline. Platelet counts usually fall to values between 40,00 and 80,000/μL. About 30 to 70% of cases will have thrombotic complications. Deep vein thrombosis and pulmonary embolism are the most common, followed by MI, arterial occlusive lower limb ischemia, mesenteric venous or arterial occlusion, and skin necrosis.

Enzyme-linked immunosorbent assay (ELISA) is most commonly test used to detect HIT antibodies. The test is very sensitive but is not very specific. SRA is a functional test that is very specific but takes longer to perform and is often a send-out test.

If there is a strong clinical suspicion of HIT, all heparin must be stopped. This technically includes even the use of any heparin-bonded catheters. Platelet transfusions are not indicated because of the risk for subsequent platelet activation and increased risk for thrombosis. Alternative anticoagulation should be started immediately without waiting for confirmatory testing if the clinical suspicion is high. Alternative anticoagulants include direct thrombin inhibitors such as bivalirudin and argatroban, and factor Xa inhibitors such as danaparoid.

Bivalirudin is an IV direct thrombin inhibitor. It has a 25-minute half-life, but the half-life increases to 4 hours in patients with renal failure on dialysis. Bivalirudin can be monitored by aPTT or the activated clotting time.

Vitamin K antagonist therapy is contraindicated in patients with HIT because of the increased risk for thrombosis in the presence of thrombocytopenia. Use of warfarin may induce lower limb venous gangrene or severe skin necrosis.

Vascular surgical consultation is not indicated in the presence of HIT, especially when alternative anticoagulation has not been tried.

Keywords: Anticoagulants and antithrombotics, thrombin inhibitors, heparin

REFERENCES

Cuker A, Crowther MA. 2013 Clinical practice guideline on the evaluation and management of adults with suspected heparin-induced thrombocytopenia (HIT). American Society of Hematology. Available at www.hematology.org.

Konstantinides S. *Management of acute pulmonary embolism.* Totowa, NJ: Humana; 2007.

Sakr Y. Heparin-induced thrombocytopenia in the ICU: an overview. *Crit Care* 2011;15:211.

14. ANSWER: B

This patient is in shock. Clinically, he is in septic shock, as evidenced by the perforated viscus with fecal soilage. Sepsis most often leads to a low systemic vascular resistance state, for which norepinephrine would be an appropriate drug. However, there are a number of confounding variables here. We do not know what this patient's intravascular volume status is. CVP is notoriously unreliable as a measure of intravascular volume status. It is dependent on too many variables (e.g., positive intrathoracic pressure from a ventilator, the patient's native cardiac compliance) to be used as a reliable measure of intravascular volume status. In addition, we do not know what this patient's native cardiac function is. The reader is informed that he has a history of congestive heart failure, which may indicate that the patient has impaired LV systolic function at baseline. Sepsis itself may lead to impairment of LV function and impairment of RV systolic function. With this patient's renal function getting worse, it is entirely possible that he is hypovolemic or else that his native cardiac output is too low because of poor LV contractility. Poor LV contractility would indicate the need to add inotropic support into the pharmacological therapy.

Bedside TTE will allow you to assess not only the patient's native biventricular contractility but also the patient's intravascular volume status. It will permit you to assess valvular function and rule out any hemodynamically significant valvulopathy such as aortic stenosis.

Using Doppler technology, direct calculations of the patient's cardiac output and stroke volume are easily obtained. A passive leg raise maneuver may then be performed to assess whether there is a significant (>12%) increase in the patient's stroke volume, which would be a clear indicator that the patient should still be volume responsive.

Keywords: Hemodynamic monitoring, cardiac output monitoring, CVP; Shock states, cardiogenic, distributive, hypovolemic, arterial pressure; Myocardial function/dysfunction, left ventricular

REFERENCES

Angus DC, Van der Poll T. Severe sepsis and septic shock. *N Engl J Med* 2013;369:840–851.

Hunter JD, Doddi M. Sepsis and the heart. *Br J Anaesth* 2010;104(1):3–11.

Mercado P, Maizel J, Beyls C et al. Transthoracic echocardiography: an accurate and precise method for estimating cardiac output in the critically ill patient. *Crit Care* 2017;21(136):1–8.

Vieillard-Baron A. Septic cardiomyopathy. *Ann Intens Care* 2011;1(6):1–7.

Vincent JL, De Backer D. Circulatory shock. *N Engl J Med* 2013;369:1726–1734.

15. ANSWER: A

This patient is experiencing a postoperative type II MI after major vascular surgery (the image shown demonstrates T-wave inversions in the V lead). The definition of MI is based on a rise in cardiac biomarkers (preferably troponin) in the setting of myocardial ischemia defined by symptoms, ECG changes, or imaging finding. Most perioperative MIs (PMIs) occur within 24 to 48 hours of surgery.

Two distinct mechanisms may lead to PMI. The first, designated a type 1 MI, is an acute coronary syndrome. The second, designated type 2 MI, is due to prolonged myocardial oxygen supply–demand imbalance in the presence of stable coronary artery disease. Therapeutic considerations depend on this distinction.

Type I PMI occurs when an unstable plaque undergoes spontaneous rupture, causing acute coronary thrombosis, ischemia, and infarction. Intraplaque inflammation plays a key role in this phenomenon, along with external stressors such as high sympathetic tone and increased cortisol levels postoperatively. Tachycardia and hypertension may exert shear stress on unstable coronary plaques. The postoperative procoagulant state may also contribute to acute coronary thrombosis.

HR-related ST-segment depression is common postoperatively and is associated with long-term morbidity and even mortality. Prolonged transient ST-segment depression leads to troponin release. ST depression myocardial ischemia represents the most common cause of PMI. Type 2 PMI runs the spectrum from silent, low-level troponin elevations to overt ischemia in multiple ECG leads with clinically obvious PMI. Tachycardia represents the most common cause of postoperative oxygen supply–demand imbalance. HR higher than 80 to 90 bpm in patients with significant coronary artery disease and low resting HR can lead to prolonged ischemia and PMI. Postoperative hypotension, hypertension, anemia, hypoxemia, and hypercarbia may all aggravate ischemia. Stress-induced and ischemia-induced coronary vasoconstriction may further inhibit coronary perfusion.

Early mortality from PMI ranges from 3.5 to 25%, increasing with elevation of troponin levels. However, even low-level troponin elevation predicts increased long-term mortality.

Beta-blockade may be used to reduce HR and myocardial oxygen demand. The landmark POISE trial demonstrated increased mortality and stroke when beta-blockers were administered prophylactically during the perioperative period. However, there was a reduction in nonfatal MI by 26%. The increase in mortality was due to hypotension and failure to maintain adequate cardiac output. In the setting of clinically overt ischemia due to myocardial oxygen demand mismatch, decreasing myocardial oxygen demand through the judicious use of beta-blockers may prove life-saving provided that adequate systemic BP and cardiac output are maintained. A reasonable goal is to target HR less than 80 bpm. There is little role for cardiac catheterization in this setting. ST-elevation MI would imply a type I mechanism and would mandate coronary intervention.

Furosemide's role would be to relieve pulmonary congestion and decrease preload in the setting of clinically overt congestive heart failure but would not treat the underlying myocardial ischemia. Aspirin and IV heparin would be more useful in the setting of a type I PMI due to coronary plaque rupture by inhibiting the subsequent coronary thrombus.

Keywords: ECG; Coronary artery disease; Myocardial ischemia/infarction; Nuclear imaging

REFERENCES

Devereaux PJ. Effects of extended release metoprolol succinate in patients undergoing non-cardiac surgery (POISE trial): a randomized controlled trial. Lancet 2008;371:1839–1847.

Landesberg MD, Beattie S, Mosseri M, et al. Perioperative myocardial infarction. *Circulation* 2009;119:2936–2944.

Priebe HJ. Perioperative myocardial infarction-aetiology and prevention. Br J Anaesth 2005;95(1):3–19.

16. ANSWER: D

This patient is most likely having a type I MI due to in-stent thrombosis of his DES and needs to go immediately to the catheterization lab to have his stent opened up if he has any chance of survival. There is no role for thoracotomy in this setting. Inotropes will not help break the arrhythmia, and procainamide will not help in the setting of ongoing ischemia due to an occluded stent. Of note, along with electrical cardioversion, procainamide and amiodarone are drugs of choice in WPW syndrome–induced tachyarrhythmias.

Timing of noncardiac surgery and the management of antiplatelet drugs in the perioperative period have become a critical topic for the anesthesiologist. The 2016 American College of Cardiology/American Heart Association (ACC/AHA) guideline and the European Society of Cardiology guideline both recommend use of dual antiplatelet therapy (DAPT) after PCI with DES implantation with both low-dose aspirin and a thienopyridine (P2Y12-receptor antagonist) such as clopidogrel for a minimum of 6 months after DES implantation. Both societies also recommend lifelong aspirin monotherapy after completion of DAPT. This is a change from the 2011 ACC/AHA guideline for minimum of 12 months of DAPT after DES implantation. Recent data have demonstrated that patients who undergo implantation of a second-generation DES may safely discontinue DAPT therapy after 3 to 6 months while remaining on lifelong aspirin monotherapy. The conundrum lies in the balance between a delay in surgical care and significant perioperative bleeding. Compared with bare metal stents, DES reduces the need for repeat coronary revascularization due to in-stent restenosis by inhibiting adverse neointimal proliferation. The downside is that without DAPT, they are prone to acute thrombosis in the early period after implantation.

Depending on what type of DES this patient has, DAPT should have been continued for a minimum of 3 to 6 months, and the patient should have remained on low-dose aspirin. A discussion should have occurred between the cardiologist, urologist, and anesthesiologist regarding the appropriate timing of this operation. If it was reasonable to delay this operation from an oncological standpoint, then it should have been delayed for the patient to complete DAPT. The patient should then have been left on aspirin monotherapy throughout the perioperative period. After abrupt cessation of DAPT, it is hypothesized that there is a period of "rebound hypercoagulability" lasting up to 90 days resulting from an inflammatory prothrombotic state, leading to increased platelet adhesion and aggregation, putting the patient at excessive risk for in-stent coronary thrombosis.

The most commonly used thienopyridine drugs include clopidogrel, prasugrel, and ticagrelor. Clopidogrel is a prodrug that requires metabolism by the hepatic CYP2-C19 isoenzyme to become clinically effective. A certain percentage of the population is deficient in this enzyme, and clinical genotyping may be used to test for platelet response to clopidogrel. Prasugrel is also a prodrug, but it is more efficiently converted into its active form during absorption by intestinal CYP3A and carboxylesterase-2 hydrolysis, resulting in more effective platelet inhibition. Ticagrelor binds reversibly and directly to the P2Y12 receptor without any biotransformation. It has a more rapid onset of action than clopidogrel and greater inhibition of platelet aggregation.

Keywords: Rhythm disturbances; Shock states; Anticoagulants and antithrombotics, antiplatelet agents; Coronary artery disease; Myocardial infarction; Ischemia

REFERENCES

Banerjee S, Angiolillo DJ, Boden WE et al. Use of antiplatelet therapy/DAPT for post-PCI patients undergoing noncardiac surgery. *J Am Coll Cardiol* 2017;69:1861–1870.

Darvish-Kazem S, Gandhi M, Marcucci M et al. Perioperative management of antiplatelet therapy in patients with a coronary stent who need noncardiac surgery: a systematic review of clinical practice guidelines. *Chest* 2013;144(6):1848–1856.

Essandoh MK, Dalia AA, George BS et al. Perioperative coronary thrombosis in a patient with multiple second-generation drug-eluting stents: is it time for a paradigm shift? *JCVA* 2016;30(6):1698–1708.

Vetter TR, Cheng D. Perioperative antiplatelet drugs with coronary stents and dancing with surgeons: can we ever agree about bleeding versus ischemic risk? IARS 2013 Review Course Lectures. Available at www.iars.org.

Vetter TR, Hunter JM, Boudreaux AM. Preoperative management of antiplatelet drugs for a coronary artery stent; how can we hit a moving target? *BMC Anesthesiol* 2014;14:73.

Vetter TR, Short RT, Hawn MT, Marques MB. Perioperative management of the patient with a coronary artery stent. *Anesthesiology* 2014;121:1093–1098.

17. ANSWER: C

This patient is experiencing an acute Stanford type A aortic dissection Figure 13.2). This is a life-threatening surgical emergency, and the patient needs to go directly to the operating room. The wall motion abnormalities and ST elevations are not due to an acute coronary syndrome but

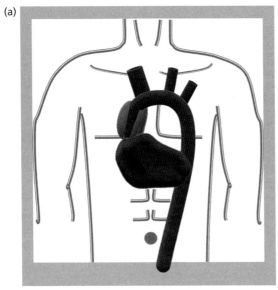

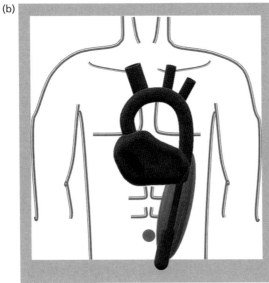

Figure 13.2 A: Stanford type A dissection. B: Stanford type B dissection.
(Courtesy of George Williams, MD, FASA, FCCP.)

to progression of the dissection flap into the right coronary ostium in the aortic root, causing acute ischemia in the RCA distribution. The pulmonary edema is secondary to acute aortic valve insufficiency as the dissection extends into the aortic valve annulus. The pericardial effusion is an ominous sign. Blood can rapidly collect in the pericardial space causing acute pericardial tamponade. Heparin would clearly not help this process. While CT scan would be helpful to delineate the extent of the dissection and perhaps help with the surgical planning, the patient will be dead by the time that can be done. Emergent surgery is critical if there is to be any hope of survival.

The most commonly used classification system for aortic dissections is the Stanford classification. Stanford type A involves the ascending aorta and may extend into the arch and descending aorta. Stanford type B involves only the descending aorta, distal to the left subclavian artery. Stanford type A dissections require immediate surgery, while Stanford type B dissections are best managed with conservative medical therapy under most circumstances.

Aortic dissections are most common in males with a peak incidence between 50 and 70 years of age. They result either from a tear in the intima with propagation of blood into the media or from intramural hemorrhage into the media with perforation into the intima. Hypertension and aortic dilation are known risk factors, along with integral wall abnormalities, such as with Marfan syndrome.

TTE can be used to make the diagnosis, as in this case, but TEE and CT are far more sensitive and allow examination of much more of the aorta.

This patient needs emergency surgery. While waiting to get the patient to the operating room, the intensivist should attempt to reduce the force of LV contraction and reduce cardiac shear forces that may propagate the dissection or lead to aortic rupture. Beta-blockers, along with short-acting IV antihypertensive agents, can be used. Beta-blockers should always be administered first to prevent any reflex catecholamine release from vasodilation. Intubation and mechanical ventilation should be considered to facilitate getting the patient to the operating room or if there is hemodynamic instability or neurological compromise. Adequate IV access and hemodynamic monitoring should be established immediately.

Keywords: Peripheral vascular disease; Dissections; Vasoactive or modulating drugs; antihypertensives, vasodilators; Coronary artery disease, myocardial ischemia

REFERENCES

Hebbali R, Swanevelder J. Diagnosis and management of aortic dissection. *Continuing Education in Anaesthesia, Critical Care & Pain* 2009;9(1):14–18.

Mussa FF, Horton JD, Moridzadeh R et al. Acute aortic dissection and intramural hematoma-a systematic review. *JAMA* 2016;316(7):754–763.

18. ANSWER: C

This patient is suffering secondary sequelae of his acute type A dissection. The dissection flap was seen to go below the diaphragm on TEE. In fact, the flap has compromised the ostium of the superior mesenteric artery, leading to mesenteric ischemia. This is responsible for the rising lactate and developing septic shock. Now that the acute type A dissection has been repaired (the entry site for initiation of the tear), the patient should essentially be treated as if he has a

Stanford type B dissection. Because there is compromise of a branch arterial territory, surgical or endovascular intervention is needed.

The incidence of organ malperfusion has been quoted as high as 20 to 40% after type A dissection and may involve cerebral, cardiac, limb, mesenteric, renal, and spinal perfusion zones. Preoperative CT scan may be able to identify areas of malperfusion, but malperfusion may not develop until intraoperatively after the initiation of cardiopulmonary bypass with a shift of the intimal flap. Visceral malperfusion is lethal, and its diagnosis constitutes yet another surgical emergency for this patient. Its presentation may occasionally by delayed. Emergent vascular surgical consultation should be obtained. A CT angiogram will most likely be needed to confirm involvement of the superior mesenteric artery. This patient may be amenable to endovascular treatment with fenestration, aortic stent grafting, or branch stenting of the visceral arterial supply. Resection of any necrotic intestine may also be necessary.

Acute kidney injury will certainly increase the morbidity and mortality of this patient, but it is not emergently life-threatening. Rhabdomyolysis is a possibility after type A dissection and circulatory arrest but can be medically managed. Acute cholecystitis is unlikely to present in isolation as an ischemic manifestation after aortic dissection.

Keywords: Peripheral vascular disease; Dissections; Shock states; Imaging, CT, interventional imaging

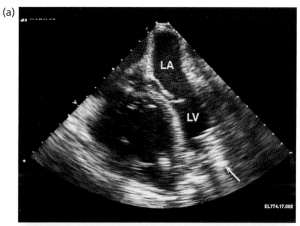

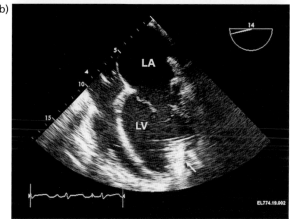

Figure 13.3 A: Left ventricular collapse along the route of the left ventricular assist device inflow. B: Left ventricular collapse resolved following volume administration.

REFERENCES

Morisaki A, Kato Y, Motoki M. delayed intestinal ischemia after surgery for type A acute aortic dissection. *Ann Vasc Dis* 2015;8(3):255–257.

Nauta JH, Trimarchi S, Kamman AV. Update in the management of type B aortic dissection. *Vasc Med* 2016;21(3):251–263.

Shimamoto T, Komiya T. Clinical dilemma in the surgical treatment of organ malperfusion caused by acute type A aortic dissection. *Gen Thorac Cardiovasc Surg* 2014;62:398–406.

19. ANSWER: A

This patient is experiencing an acute suction event (Figure 13.3). This is primarily caused by hypovolemia or catastrophic RV failure. The continuous flow device implanted at the LV apex generates negative pressure. If the LV is underfilled, the interventricular septum can get sucked into the LV, causing obstruction of the ventricular assist device inflow. The result is a power surge, a rise in RV filling pressures, and a drop in cardiac output and systemic pressure. Treatment is to acutely relieve the negative LV pressure by dialing the device RPM back, allowing the interventricular septum to pop back into its normal position. Intravascular volume can then be administered, and the RPM can then slowly be increased to restore cardiac output.

High-dose epinephrine will do nothing to relieve the LVAD inflow obstruction. Inhaled NO might be useful in the case of a struggling RV due to pulmonary hypertension if it is limiting LV fill. However, this is not the case here. Furosemide is the exact opposite of what is needed. The patient requires volume resuscitation.

Keywords: Myocardial function/dysfunction, left ventricular, right ventricular; Shock states, cardiogenic; Hemodynamic monitoring, arterial, CVP; Cardiac ultrasound, vasoactive or modulating drugs, inotropes; Circulatory support systems, left ventricular assist device

REFERENCES

Mauermann WJ, Rehfeldt KH, Park SJ. Transesophageal echocardiography in a patient in hemodynamic compromise after Jarvik 2000 implantation: the suckdown effect. *Anesth Analg* 2008;107(3):791–792.

Sen A, Larson JS, Kashani KB et al. Mechanical circulatory assist devices: a primer for critical care and emergency physicians. *Crit Care* 2016;20:153.

Slaughter MS, Pagani FD, Rogers JG, et al. Clinical Management of Continuous-Flow Left Ventricular Assist Devices in Advanced Heart Failure. J of Heart and Lung Transplantation 2010;29(4S): S1–S38.
Stainback RF, Estep JD, Agler DA et al. Echocardiography in the management of patients with left ventricular assist devices: recommendations from the American Society of Echocardiography. *JASE* 2015;28:853–909.

20. ANSWER: C

SAM can be a life-threatening condition. Instead of closing normally in systole, the anterior mitral leaflet is pulled into the LV outflow tract. It can result in severe LV outflow tract obstruction and severe mitral regurgitation due to the distortion of the mitral leaflet coaptation. It is associated with up to a 20% risk for sudden death. It is more commonly seen after mitral valve repairs when the posterior mitral annulus is brought closer to the LV outflow tract. Certain anatomical conditions such as hypertrophic cardiomyopathy also predispose patients to develop SAM.

Once identified, proper treatment is essential to avoid rapid hemodynamic collapse. Absolute hypovolemia, tachycardia, and afterload reduction all predispose to the development of SAM in those with the proper cardiac anatomical predisposition. Given that this patient did not demonstrate SAM postoperatively on the TEE in the operating room, there is every reason to think this patient will respond to conservative therapy. Medical treatment consists of beta-blockade, or at least cessation of beta-agonists, decreasing heart rate, increasing afterload, and giving intravascular volume. These maneuvers are generally done concomitantly in the face of hemodynamic instability from SAM.

Stopping epinephrine and rapid administration of IV fluids is an appropriate first step for this patient. Judicious administration of beta-blockers and phenylephrine may also help to relieve the SAM. If the patient proves refractory to medical therapy, then a discussion must be held with the surgeon. The patient may now be so anatomically predisposed to SAM that reoperation is occasionally necessary.

A Barlow valve is a synonym for mitral valve prolapse, as are click-murmur syndrome and floppy mitral valve.

Keywords: Diagnostic modalities, hemodynamic monitoring; Valvular heart disease; Shock states, cardiogenic, management strategies; Vasoactive or modulating drugs; cardiac ultrasound

REFERENCES

Alfieri O, Lapenna E. Systolic anterior motion after mitral valve repair: where do we stand in 2015? *Eur J Cardiothorac Surg* 2015;48:344–346.
Anyanwu AC, Adams DH. Etiologic classification of degenerative mitral valve disease: Barlow's disease and fibroelastic deficiency. *Semin Thorac Cardiovasc Surg* 2007;19:90–96.
Ibrahim M, Rao C, Ashrafian H et al. Modern management of systolic anterior motion of the mitral valve. *Eur J Cardiothorac Surg* 2012;41:1260–1270.

14.

RENAL ACID–BASE

Olakunle Idowu

QUESTIONS

1. A 59-year-old female with a history of gallstone pancreatitis, type 2 diabetes mellitus, hypertension, and chronic renal insufficiency is admitted to the intensive care unit (ICU) intubated following endoscopic retrograde cholangiopancreatography (ERCP). Her vital signs are as follows: blood pressure (BP) 88/50 mm Hg, heart rate (HR) 115 bpm, respiratory rate (RR) 16 breaths/minute, O_2 saturation 93% on a forced inspiratory oxygen (FiO_2) of 1. She is febrile with a temperature of 101.2° F. A fluid challenge is given, and her antibiotic regimen is broadened to meropenem and vancomycin. A Foley catheter is placed to closely monitor her urine output. Which of the following measures will MOST decrease this patient's risk for developing a catheter-associated urinary tract infection?

A. Keep the Foley catheter in place
B. Keep the urine collection bag level at the level of the bladder
C. Intermittent bladder irrigation with antimicrobials
D. Routine screening for asymptomatic bacteriuria

2. A 79-year-old African American male presents to the emergency department (ED) with new-onset tonic-clonic seizures that are treated with intravenous (IV) lorazepam and levetiracetam (Keppra). His seizures subside, and he appears slightly somnolent but easily arousable. He is protecting his airway, and his vital signs are temperature 98.2° F, BP 85/45 mm Hg, HR 101 bpm, RR 14 breaths/minute, O_2 saturation 98% on 2-L/minute nasal cannula. His labs in the ED are within normal limits except for a lactate of 4 mmol/L, serum sodium of 109 mEq/L, and chloride of 93 mEq/L. He has a past medical history significant for prostate cancer, type 2 diabetes mellitus, and hypertension. His diabetes is controlled with lifestyle modification, but he takes hydrochlorothiazide and lisinopril for hypertension.

What is the MOST appropriate next step in the management of this patient?

A. Emergently intubate the patient for airway protection
B. Send the patient for emergent imaging
C. Initiate hypertonic saline therapy
D. Administer a dose of Lasix

3. A 54-year female with chronic myeloid leukemia is admitted to the ICU with neutropenic fevers and worsening respiratory failure due to *Stenotrophomonas* pneumonia. She is intubated and placed on mechanical ventilation. Her antibiotic regimen is meropenem, Sulfamethoxazole/ Trimethoprim (Bactrim), caspofungin, and linezolid. Her serum creatinine (Cr) is 1.2 mg/dL, and her urine output is 0.6 mL/kg per hour. She has a serum potassium of 5.5 mEq/L, which remains elevated despite giving calcium, dextrose, insulin, and kayexalate. Arterial blood gas (ABG) analysis shows pH 7.40, $PaCO_2$ 35 mm Hg, PaO_2 187 mm Hg, HCO_3 20 mmol/L, base excess (BE) – 4 mmol/L, O_2 saturation 98%. An electrocardiogram (ECG) is obtained that shows normal sinus rhythm.
What is the MOST appropriate next step to treat her hyperkalemia?

A. Continuous albuterol nebulizer treatments
B. Renal consult to initiate emergent dialysis
C. Continue to observe
D. Discontinue Bactrim, switch to ceftazidime

4. A 29-year-old male presents to the ED with new-onset right-sided flank pain. He reports that his pain is intermittent and occasionally associated with fevers, chills, nausea, and vomiting. His vital signs are temperature 101.3° F, BP 80/45 mm Hg, HR 128 bpm, RR 24 breaths/ minute, O_2 saturation 98% on room air. An ECG is obtained that reveals sinus tachycardia. His labs are significant for a white blood cell (WBC) count of 22.4

K/µL, potassium 4.6 mEq/L, HCO$_3$ 19 mEq/L, blood urea nitrogen (BUN) 32 mmol/L, and Cr 1.63 mmol/L. He is started on empiric antibiotics with ciprofloxacin, given morphine for pain, and administered a 2-L bolus of normal saline. His repeat BP is 90/52 mm Hg. The ED physician initiates a norepinephrine infusion to stabilize his BP and transfers the patient to the ICU for further management.

Which of the following is the MOST sensitive and specific diagnostic test for the workup of this patient?

A. Renal ultrasound
B. Plain radiography—kidney, ureters, bladder (KUB)
C. Noncontrast helical computed tomography (CT)
D. Intravenous pyelography (IVP)

5. A 55-year-old female with a history of newly diagnosed ovarian cancer is admitted with a 3-day history of persistent nausea and vomiting due to a small bowel obstruction seen on abdominal CT. A nasogastric tube has been placed to low intermittent suction. She reports chronic constipation, decreased appetite, and 7 pounds weight loss over the last week. Her blood work is significant for Na 128 mEq/L, K 3.3 mEq/L, Cl 91 mEq/L, CO$_2$ 26 mEq/L, BUN 33 mg/dL, Cr 1.6 mg/dL. Urinalysis shows a pH of 7.32.

Which of the following supports a diagnosis of prerenal acute kidney injury?

A. Urinalysis with epithelial cell casts and a specific gravity of 1.010
B. Urinary Na >40 mmol/L
C. Left hydronephrosis
D. Fractional excretion of urea <35%

6. A 23-year-old male is admitted to the neurosurgical ICU following a traumatic brain injury from a motor vehicle collision. His CT shows a large intracranial hemorrhage with mass effect and midline shift. He was intubated in the field and has a Glasgow Coma Scale (GCS) score of 6. His pupils are 2 mm, equal, and sluggish. In the ICU, he is placed on mechanical ventilation. His labs are unremarkable. Vital signs are BP 162/89 mm Hg, HR 64 bpm, RR 14 breaths/minute, O$_2$ saturation 100% on 40% FiO$_2$. The neurosurgery service plans to place an external ventricular drain at bedside. What is the MOST appropriate fluid therapy for this patient?

A. Dextrose 5 g in normal saline
B. Dextrose 10 g in 0.45% normal saline
C. 0.9% Normal saline
D. Dextrose 5 g in sterile water

7. A 78-year-old female with a history of type 2 diabetes mellitus, hypertension, and chronic obstructive pulmonary disease (COPD) has been transferred to the ICU for a trial of noninvasive ventilation (biphasic positive airway pressure [BiPAP]) due to a COPD exacerbation. Vital signs are BP 146/85 mm Hg, HR 89 bpm, RR 16 breaths/minute, O$_2$ saturation 100%. Her work of breathing appears normal, and her initial ABG shows pH 7.24, PaCO$_2$ 60 mm Hg, PaO$_2$ 98 mm Hg, HCO$_3$ 26 mmol/L, BE 4 mmol/L, O$_2$ saturation 100% on 28% FiO$_2$. After 1 hour on BiPAP, her ABG shows pH 7.30, PaCO$_2$ 51 mm Hg, PaO$_2$ 65 mm Hg, HCO$_3$ 24 mmol/L, BE 3 mmol/L, O$_2$ saturation 94%. BiPAP settings are inspiratory positive airway pressure (IPAP) 10 cm H$_2$O, expiratory positive airway pressure (EPAP) 5 cm H$_2$O, rate 8, FiO$_2$ 21%, minute ventilation (MV) 3.7 L/minute.

What is the MOST appropriate next step in the management of this patient?

A. Emergent endotracheal intubation
B. Initiate a sodium bicarbonate infusion
C. Increase the IPAP and reassess in 1 hour
D. Increase FiO$_2$

8. An 18-year-old African American male with a history of insulin-dependent diabetes mellitus is admitted to the ICU for management of diabetic ketoacidosis (DKA). He reports that he hasn't had an appetite for the last 4 days and stopped taking his insulin 2 days ago. In the emergency center, he was treated with IV fluids and started on an insulin drip. His labs are as follow: WBC 14.3 K/µL, hemoglobin (Hgb) 12.5 g/dL, platelets 303 K/µL, Na 130 mEq/L, K 3.3 mEq/L, Cl 91 mEq/L, CO$_2$ 18 mEq/L, BUN 21 mg/dL, Cr 1.2 mg/dL, glucose 354 mg/dL, ABG shows pH 7.24, PaCO$_2$ 33 mm Hg, PaO$_2$ 95 mm Hg, bicarbonates 18 mEq/L, BE –5 mmol/L, O$_2$ saturation 98% on room air.

Which acid–base disorder is present in this patient?

A. Metabolic alkalosis
B. Non–anion gap metabolic acidosis, anion gap metabolic acidosis, acute respiratory alkalosis
C. Non–anion gap metabolic acidosis and a concurrent acute respiratory acidosis
D. Anion gap metabolic acidosis

9. A 17-year male is brought to the ED by emergency medical services (EMS) immediately following a motor vehicle collision. He was a restrained driver in a head-on collision. His vitals in the ED are BP 105/60 mm Hg, HR 105 bpm, RR 22 breaths/minute, temperature 96.7°F, O$_2$ saturation 98% on 4-L nasal cannula. The

patient is alert and responsive. His primary survey is unremarkable, and his focused assessment with sonography for trauma (FAST) exam is negative. He is sent for imaging, which reveals grade 2 left kidney injury. Repeat vital signs are BP 95/62 mm Hg, HR 103 bpm, RR 18 breaths/minute, temperature 96.7°F O_2 saturation 98% on 4-L nasal cannula. His Hgb 11.2 g/dL. What is the BEST next step in the management of this patient?

A. Emergent left nephrectomy
B. Supportive management and monitoring
C. Angiography
D. Repeat imaging within 72 hours

10. A 78-year-old male with hypertension, COPD, and type 2 diabetes mellitus lives alone at home, and his family is concerned that he has had a progressive decline in his functional status. He has lost 10 pounds over the past month due to poor nutritional intake. He also has a productive cough for the past 2 weeks. His daughter brings him to the ED, and he is emergently intubated due to a COPD exacerbation from community-acquired pneumonia. He is started empirically on levofloxacin and transferred to the ICU for close monitoring. Seven days into his ICU course, the patient remains on the ventilator due to generalized weakness. Enteral nutrition was started 3 days earlier, and he is unable to pass his spontaneous breathing trial because of tachypnea. His ABG analysis shows pH 7.56, $PaCO_2$ 20 mm Hg, PaO_2 105 mm Hg, bicarbonate 23 mEq/L, O_2 saturation 100%. What is the next step in the management of this patient?

A. Extubate to noninvasive ventilation
B. Initiate extracorporeal membrane oxygenation (ECMO)
C. Tracheostomy
D. Phosphate repletion

11. Peritoneal dialysis would be appropriate for which of the following patients?

A. A 50-year-old female with a history of type 2 diabetes, hypertension, and stage 5 chronic kidney disease who is admitted to the hospital for management of acute diverticulitis
B. A 22-year-old African American parturient with lupus in her third trimester who has a lupus flare and develops acute renal failure
C. A 76-year-old male with a history of colon cancer admitted to the hospital after undergoing an emergent hemicolectomy due to bowel obstruction who developed acute renal failure on postoperative day 5

D. A 67-year-old female with a history of hypertension, diastolic heart failure, and stage 5 chronic renal failure with chronic fluid retention and overload

12. Which of the following risk factors has the GREATEST impact on the development of contrast induced nephropathy in the perioperative setting.

A. Diabetes mellitus
B. Chronic kidney disease
C. Hypovolemia
D. Liver cirrhosis

13. A 55-year-old white woman with a history of hypertension and newly diagnosed squamous cell carcinoma of the lung is intubated in the ED because of seizures and altered mental status. She was treated with lorazepam and loaded with phosphenytoin. She also received a 2-L bolus of normal saline due to hypotension and started on a hypertonic saline infusion. Her husband reports that her internist started her on furosemide because of fluid retention. Her labs in the emergency center are significant for a serum sodium of 114 mEq/L; renal function is normal. Urine osmolality is 600 mOsm/kg of water.
What is the MOST likely cause of her hyponatremia?

A. Syndrome of inappropriate secretion of antidiuretic hormone (SIADH)
B. Diuretics
C. Diabetes insipidus
D. Polydipsia

14. A 66-year-old male with lung cancer presents to the emergency center with generalized weakness, shortness of breath, and refractory hypotension. While receiving IV fluids, he has a grand mal seizure that is treated with 2 mg of IV lorazepam. His labs are significant for Na 136 mEq/L, K 3.4 mEq/L, Cl 106 mEq/L, CO_2 21 mEq/L, BUN 35 mg/dL, Cr 1.5 mg/dL, Mg 2.3 mg/dL, ionized calcium 0.6 mmol/L, and phosphorus 7.6 mg/dL. He is intubated because of severe weakness and has been started on a norepinephrine infusion.
What is the MOST appropriate next step in management of this patient?

A. Furosemide infusion
B. IV calcium
C. Emergent hemodialysis
D. Steroids

15. A 35-year-old woman is brought to the ED by EMS following a cardiac arrest. Cardiopulmonary resuscitation (CPR) was performed in the field, and she was intubated. In the ED, she appears lethargic but is

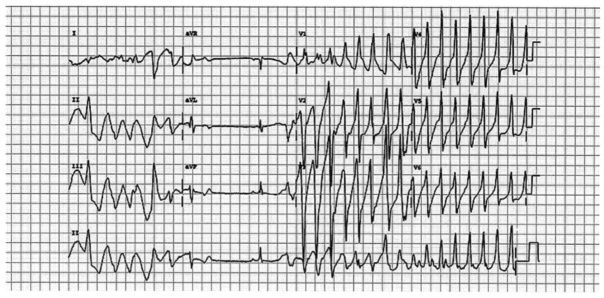

Figure Q15.1

arousable and has nonpurposeful movements. She is accompanied by her sister, who reports that she was recently started on ciprofloxacin for a urinary tract infection. Her labs are significant for WBC 4.6 K/μL, Hgb 12.3 g/dL, platelets 245 k/μL, Na 138 mEq/L, K 3.2 mEq/L, Cl 108 mEq/L, CO_2 23 mEq/L, BUN 10 mg/dL, Cr 0.65 mg/dL, Mg 1.2mg/dL, ionized calcium 0.9 mmol/L, and phosphorus 2.6 mg/dL. The patient is transferred to the ICU for further management, and on arrival she is pulseless. CPR is initiated, and her ECG is depicted here (image courtesy of https://upload.wikimedia.org/wikipedia/commons/2/22/112_%28CardioNetworks_ECGpedia%29.jpg).

What is the next appropriate step in management of this patient?

A. IV calcium
B. IV magnesium
C. Hypothermia to 36° C
D. Synchronized cardioversion

16. Which of the following would be MOST indicated in the management of chloride-sensitive metabolic alkalosis?

A. Furosemide
B. Acetazolamide
C. Hydrochlorothiazide
D. Sodium bicarbonate

17. A 68-year-old African American male with a history of hypertension and benign prostatic hypertrophy is admitted to the ICU from the emergency center with acute renal failure. He reported shortness of breath, abdominal distention, decreased urination, and fluid retention for the past 2 weeks. The ED physician ordered a CT of the abdomen and pelvis that showed a large pelvic mass with bilateral hydroureter and hydronephrosis. His labs are significant for WBC 13.4 K/μL, Hgb 11.8 g/dL, platelets 334 K/μL, Na 128 mEq/L, K 5.4 mEq/L, Cl 98 mEq/L, CO_2 16 mEq/L, BUN 76 mg/dL, Cr 5.63 mg/dL, phosphorus 6.5 mg/dL. ABG shows pH 7.30, $PaCO_2$ 29 mm Hg, PaO_2 89 mm Hg, bicarbonate 17 mEq/L, BE −8 mmol/L. Vital signs are BP 188/102 mm Hg, HR 115 bpm, RR 26 breaths/minute, O_2 saturation 99% on room air. What is the MOST appropriate next step in management?

A. Emergent hemodialysis
B. Continuous renal replacement therapy (CRRT)
C. Continue to monitor closely
D. Bilateral nephrostomy placement

18. A 28-year-old African American woman with lupus is intubated in the emergency center and transferred to the ICU for management of acute respiratory failure. Her chest radiograph is significant for multilobar pneumonia. She has had a progressive decline in her overall functional status over the past month, and she complains of a productive cough and dyspnea on exertion for the past week. She takes prednisone 5 mg daily and hydroxychloroquine but ran out of her medication a few days ago. In the ICU, she is empirically started on levofloxacin for pneumonia and placed on pressure-control ventilation. Her labs are significant for WBC 18.4 K/μL, Hgb 11.7 g/dL, platelets 334 K/μL, Na 143 mEq/L, Cl 117 mEq/L, CO_2 16 mEq/L, BUN

35 mg/dL, Cr 1.75 mg/dL. ABG shows pH 7.28, $PaCO_2$ 36 mm Hg, PaO_2 63 mm Hg, bicarbonate 17 mmol/L, BE −5 mmol/L. Vital signs are BP 168/86 mm Hg, HR 133 bpm, RR 26 breaths/minute, O_2 saturation 95% on 4-L nasal cannula. What is the next appropriate step in management of this patient's renal dysfunction?

A. Renal biopsy
B. Urinalysis
C. Emergent hemodialysis
D. 24-Hour protein

19. Which of the following features is MOST common to type II renal tubular acidosis (RTA)?

A. Chronic hyperkalemia
B. Association with autoimmune disease
C. Impairment in proximal bicarbonate reabsorption
D. Urine pH <5.5

20. A 52-year-old male with hypertension and end-stage renal disease (ESRD) due to polycystic kidney disease is transported to the ICU intubated following a cadaveric renal transplantation. Intraoperative course was uneventful, but he remained intubated because of difficulty with oxygenation at the end of the case. His vital signs are BP 187/102 mm Hg, HR 101 bpm, RR 16 breaths/minute, O_2 saturation 92% on 100% FiO_2. Within 2 hours of arriving in the ICU, he develops anuria, and his O_2 saturation drops to 87%. His skin is mottled and cyanotic, and expiratory wheezes are audible on exam. What is the MOST appropriate next step in management?

A. Emergent nephrectomy
B. Initiation of ECMO
C. Increased doses of tacrolimus and steroids
D. Emergent hemodialysis

21. A 78-year-old male with ESRD, hypertension, and congestive heart failure presents to the ED with shortness of breath after missing his last two dialysis sessions. He is auric, and his vital signs are BP 187/102 mm Hg, HR 101 bpm, RR 24 breaths/minute, O_2 saturation 92% on 3-L/minute nasal cannula. Which of the following is the MOST appropriate next stage of management?

A. Sodium bicarbonate
B. Peritoneal dialysis
C. CRRT
D. Intermittent hemodialysis

22. An 18-year-old morbidly obese African American male with a history of insulin-dependent diabetes mellitus is admitted to the ICU for management of DKA. He reports that he hasn't had an appetite for the past 4 days

and stopped taking his insulin 2 days ago. In the emergency center, he was treated with IV fluids and started on an insulin drip. His labs are as follows: WBC 14.3 K/μL, Hgb 12.5 g/dL, platelets 303 K/μL, Na 130 mEq/L, K 3.3 mEq/L, Cl 91 mEq/L, CO_2 19 mEq/L, BUN 21 mg/dL, Cr 1.2 mg/dL, glucose 354 mg/dL, aspartate transaminase (AST) 34 U/L, alanine aminotransferase (ALT) 45 U/L, total bilirubin 0.4 mg/dL, total protein 5.6 g/dL, albumin 3.4 g/dL. Urinalysis shows ketones positive, leukocyte esterase positive. ABG shows pH 7.19, $PaCO_2$ 45 mm Hg, PaO_2 95 mm Hg, bicarbonate 19 mmol/L, BE −10 mmol/L, O_2 saturation 95% on room air. Which acid–base disorder is present in this patient?

A. Metabolic alkalosis
B. Non–anion gap metabolic acidosis, anion gap metabolic acidosis, acute respiratory alkalosis
C. Anion gap metabolic acidosis and a concurrent acute respiratory acidosis
D. Anion gap metabolic acidosis

23. A 16-year-old male is brought to the emergency center following a gunshot wound to the abdomen. He is emergently taken to the operating room for an exploratory laparotomy, splenectomy with diaphragmatic repair, and chest tube placement. In the operating room, he received 10 units of packed red blood cells and 2 units of fresh frozen plasma (FFP). Postoperatively, he is transferred to the ICU intubated. His vital signs are BP 88/49 mm Hg, HR 123 bpm, RR 18 breaths/minute, O_2 saturation 92% on 100% FiO_2, temperature 97° F. His last Hgb in the operating room was 6.5 g/dL, and his postop labs are pending. His nurse reports that 200 mL of blood has drained from his chest tube in the last hour and he has no urine output. What is the BEST next step of action to improve his urine output?

A. Normal saline bolus
B. Transfuse FFP only
C. Transfuse blood, platelets, and FFP
D. Transfuse platelets only

24. A 54-year-old female presents to the emergency center with complaints of severe fatigue and easy bruising. Her WBC count is 400,000 cells/μL, and a bone marrow biopsy is performed that confirms acute myeloid leukemia. She is started on induction chemotherapy with daunorubicin and cytarabine. Her uric acid level is 10 mg/dL. Which of the following measures will minimize the progression of tumor lysis syndrome and acute kidney injury?

A. Volume restriction
B. Rasburicase

C. Allopurinol

D. Close observation

25. A 78-year-old female with a history of type 2 diabetes mellitus, hypertension, and COPD has been transferred to the ICU for a trial of noninvasive ventilation (BiPAP) due to a COPD exacerbation. Vital signs are BP 146/85 mm Hg, HR 89 bpm, RR 16 breaths/min, O_2 saturation 100%. Her work of breathing appears normal, and her initial ABG shows pH 7.24, $PaCO_2$ 60 mm Hg, PaO_2 98 mm Hg, HCO_3 26 mmol/L, BE 4 mmol/L, O_2 saturation 100% on 28% FiO_2. After 2 hours on BiPAP, her ABG reveals pH 7.23, $PaCO_2$ 63 mm Hg, PaO_2 58 mm Hg, bicarbonate 24 mmol/L, BE 3 mmol/L, O_2 saturation 89%. BiPAP settings are IPAP16 cm H_2O, EPAP 8 cm H_2O, rate 8 FiO_2 60%, MV 3.7 L/minute.

What is the MOST appropriate next step in the management of this patient?

A. Emergent endotracheal intubation

B. Sodium bicarbonate infusion

C. Increase the IPAP and reassess in 1 hour

D. Increase FiO_2

ANSWERS

1. ANSWER: A

Catheter-associated urinary tract infections (CAUTIs) are one of the most common causes of infection in the ICU and the second leading cause of nosocomial bloodstream infections. Foley catheterization should be reserved for patients with critical illness, perioperative monitoring during surgical procedures, prolonged immobilization from injuries related to trauma, incontinence, and comfort associated with end-of-life measures. Foley catheters should be promptly removed when they are no longer needed. The urine collection bag should drain with gravity at a level below the bladder at all times. Intermittent irrigation of the bladder and collection bag with antimicrobials and routine screening for asymptomatic bacteriuria are not recommended. Of note, per Medicare guidelines, a Foley needs to be in place 2 midnights (not 48 hours) for a positive urinary tract infection to qualify for designation as a CAUTI.

Keywords: Renal; infection

REFERENCE

Parrillo JE, Dellinger RP. *Critical care medicine principles of diagnosis and management in the adult,* 4th edition. Philadelphia: Elsevier/Saunders; 2014, pp. 859–861.

2. ANSWER: C

This patient's hypovolemic hyponatremia is likely due to renal sodium losses from hydrochlorothiazide, a thiazide diuretic, which impairs renal diluting ability. Cerebral salt wasting is another cause of hypovolemic hyponatremia. Symptomatic hyponatremia requires hypertonic saline therapy for rapid correction. Hypertonic saline also serves as a volume expander. Serum sodium should not be corrected faster than 10 to 12 mEq/L over 24 hours or faster than 4 to 6 mEq/L over the 2 hours owing to the risk for osmotic demyelinating syndrome. Hypertonic saline therapy is typically not needed when serum sodium is greater than 120 mEq/L.

Emergent intubation would be appropriate if this patient had signs of airway obstruction or if there were a need for airway protection based on a poor clinical exam. CT imaging and further diagnostic studies would be appropriate after initiating hypertonic saline therapy and providing volume expansion. Lasix is not indicated because this patient is hypotensive due to hypovolemia.

Keywords: Acid–base abnormalities; Hyponatremia

REFERENCE

Marino PL. *Marino's the ICU book,* 4th edition. Philadelphia: Wolters Kluwer Health/Lippincott Williams & Wilkins; 2014, pp. 665–670.

3. ANSWER: D

High doses of Bactrim can cause hyperkalemia by acting like a potassium-sparing diuretic and causing inhibition of distal epithelial sodium channels. Hyperkalemia typically manifests 7 to 10 days after initiation of treatment and is usually associated with higher doses. Ceftazidime can provide adequate coverage for *Stenotrophomonas*. Emergent dialysis is not indicated based on the clinical picture. The patient has adequate urine output, no significant ECG abnormalities, and a normal acid–base status. Life-threatening hyperkalemia may worsen if Bactrim is not discontinued. Because this patient did not respond to medical management, the next best step would be to remove the offending agent based on the clinical picture.

Keywords: Acid–base abnormalities; Electrolyte abnormalities; Potassium

REFERENCES

Perazella MA. Hyperkalemia and trimethoprim-sulfamethoxazole: a new problem emerges 25 years later. *Conn Med* 1997;61(8):451–458.

Perazella MA. Trimethoprim-induced hyperkalaemia. *Drug Saf* 2000;22(3):227–236.

Velazquez H, Perazella MA, Wright FS, Ellison DH. Renal mechanism of trimethoprim-induced hyperkalemia. *Ann Intern Med* 1993;119(4):296–301.

4. ANSWER: C

Urolithiasis should be considered for patients who present with episodic unilateral flank or groin pain, which may be associated with nausea and vomiting. Diagnosis is based on patient history, physical examination, urinalysis, and diagnostic imaging. Urolithiasis can lead to urinary tract infections, hydronephrosis, acute renal failure, sepsis, and pyelonephritis. Nonhelical CT is the most sensitive and specific modality for diagnosing urolithiasis and ruling out other pathology. Ultrasonography has limited use for detecting ureteral calculi but is helpful for diagnosing hydronephrosis and assessing the renal parenchyma. Radiography is most helpful for radiopaque calculi such as calcium oxalate and calcium phosphate stones. Calculi seen on radiography can easily be obscured by stool or bowel gas. IVP is more sensitive than ultrasonography and KUB in

Table 14.1 IMAGING MODALITIES FOR DIAGNOSIS OF URETERAL CALCULI

TEST	SENSITIVITY (%)	SPECIFICITY (%)
Ultrasonography	19	97
Plain radiography— kidney, ureters, bladder	45–59	71–77
Intravenous pyelography	64–87	92–94
Noncontrast helical computer tomography	95–100	94–96

detecting renal calculi (Table 14.1). One major limitation of IVP is the risk for worsening renal function.

Keywords: Renal; Diagnostic Modalities; Imaging; CT, Radiography; Ultrasound

REFERENCE

Portis AJ, Sundaram CP. Diagnosis and initial management of kidney stones. *Am Fam Physician* 2001;63(7):1329–1340.

5. ANSWER: D

Urinary Na <20 mmol/L, fractional excretion of urea <35%, and fractional excretion of Na <1% support the diagnosis of prerenal acute kidney injury. Urine sediment may also show hyaline casts. This patient was likely dehydrated from nausea, vomiting, and decreased fluid intake. In renal causes of acute kidney injury, the kidneys are not able to reabsorb sodium appropriately, which leads to higher urine sodium values. Elevated urine sodium can also occur as a result of diuretics; therefore, the fractional excretion of urea can be used as a surrogate marker. Epithelial cell casts or muddy-brown casts and a urinary Na >40 mmol/L are found in patients with acute tubular necrosis. Hydronephrosis is an example of obstructive acute kidney injury.

Keywords: Renal; Diagnosis; Renal failure, intrinsic renal, prerenal

REFERENCE

Parrillo JE, Dellinger RP. *Critical care medicine principles of diagnosis and management in the adult*, 4th edition. Philadelphia: Elsevier/Saunders; 2014, pp. 965–983.

6. ANSWER: C

Hypo-osmolar fluids should be avoided in patients with traumatic brain injury. The goal is to use iso-osmolar

Table 14.2 FLUID OSMOLALITY

FLUID	OSMOLALITY (MOSM/L)
Plasma	290
0.9% NaCl	309
Ringer's lactate	273
Normosol/PlasmaLyte	295

solutions when resuscitating patients with cerebral edema and elevated intracranial pressure. Normal saline, Normosol, and PlasmaLyte are ideal solutions (Table 14.2). Dextrose solutions can lead to hyperglycemia, which promotes ischemic neurological injury. Normal saline is slightly hyperosmolar in relation to extracellular fluid, which makes it an effective extracellular volume expander.

Keywords: Renal; Fluid and electrolyte management

REFERENCES

Marino PL. *Marino's the ICU book,* 4th edition. Philadelphia: Wolters Kluwer Health/Lippincott Williams & Wilkins; 2014, pp. 218–224.

Murray MJ, Rose SH, Wedel DJ et al. *Faust's anesthesiology review e-book: expert consult*. St. Louis: Elsevier Health Sciences; 2014, pp. 309–310.

7. ANSWER: C

This patient has a respiratory acidosis due to her COPD exacerbation. Noninvasive ventilation decreases mortality, invasive ventilation, and nosocomial infections in patients with COPD exacerbations. The next appropriate step would be to increase the IPAP to improve her minute ventilation and reassess the patient for further interventions. Emergent intubation is not indicated because her ABG is improving and her work of breathing appears normal. A sodium bicarbonate infusion is not the appropriate therapy in a patient with hypercapnic respiratory failure because it can cause worsening acidosis.

Keywords: Acid–base and electrolyte abnormalities; Respiratory

REFERENCES

Deutschman CS, Neligan PJ. *Evidence-based practice of critical care e-book*. St. Louis: Elsevier Health Sciences; 2015, pp. 176–178.

Scala R, Nava S, Conti G et al. Noninvasive versus conventional ventilation to treat hypercapnic encephalopathy in chronic obstructive pulmonary disease. *Intensive Care Med* 2007;33(12):2101–2108.

Soler N, Torres A, Ewig S et al. Bronchial microbial patterns in severe exacerbations of chronic obstructive pulmonary disease (COPD) requiring mechanical ventilation. *Am J Respir Crit Care Med* 1998;157(5 Pt 1):1498–1505.

8. ANSWER: D

DKA typically causes an anion gap metabolic acidosis with decreased serum bicarbonate and the presence of ketones in blood or urine. Serum glucose levels are moderately elevated to at least 250 mg/dL, and pH is typically less than 7.30. The mainstay of treatment of DKA includes insulin therapy, judicious fluid administration, and electrolyte management. This patient has an anion gap metabolic acidosis with the appropriate respiratory compensation. Winters formula 1.5 $(HCO_3) + 8 \pm 2$; $1.5 (18) + 8 \pm 2 = (33$ to $37)$. Of note, recall that the HCO_3 on an ABG is not measured, it is estimated; conversely, the HCO_3 on a serum chemistry is measured.

Keywords: Acid–base and electrolyte abnormalities; Acid–base abnormalities, metabolic

REFERENCE

Marino PL. *Marino's the ICU book,* 4th edition. Philadelphia: Wolters Kluwer Health/Lippincott Williams & Wilkins; 2014, pp. 587–592.

9. ANSWER: B

Grade 2 liver injury correlates with a nonexpanding perirenal hematoma or less than 1 cm laceration of the kidney without urinary extravasation. In a patient with stable hemodynamics, emergent nephrectomy is not indicated. Patients with grades 1 through 4 kidney injuries can undergo conservative management. Repeat imaging within 72 hours is based on changes in the patient's clinical status and may not be needed unless the patient has a grade 3 injury or higher. In patients who are unstable, have grade 5 injury, or have active extravasation of IV contrast on imaging, exploratory laparotomy or angiography is indicated (Table 14.3).

Keywords: Renal; Diagnosis; Renal trauma

REFERENCE

Shoobridge JJ, Corcoran NM, Martin KA et al. Contemporary management of renal trauma. *Rev Urol* 2011;13(2):65.

Table 14.3 AMERICAN ASSOCIATION FOR THE SURGERY OF TRAUMA RENAL INJURY SCALE

GRADE	TYPE	DESCRIPTION
I	Contusion	Microscopic or gross hematuria, urologic studies normal
	Hematoma	Subcapsular, nonexpanding without parenchymal laceration
II	Hematoma	Nonexpanding perirenal hematoma confined to renal retroperitoneum
	Laceration	<1-cm parenchymal depth of renal cortex with no urinary extravasation
III	Laceration	>1-cm parenchymal depth of renal cortex without collecting system rupture or urinary extravasation
IV	Laceration	Parenchymal laceration extending through renal cortex, medulla, and collecting system
	Vascular	Main renal artery or vein injury with contained hemorrhage
V	Laceration	Completely shattered kidney
	Vascular	Avulsion of renal hilum that devascularizes kidney

10. ANSWER: D

Hypophosphatemia has been associated with impaired contractility of the diaphragm, decreased maximal inspiratory force, and a failure to wean from mechanical ventilation. This patient has refeeding syndrome due to his history of poor nutritional intake, and electrolyte repletion is the mainstay of management. Patients with refeeding syndrome have hypophosphatemia, which results from increased production of adenosine triphosphate (ATP) and the intracellular shift of phosphorus. Respiratory alkalosis can also cause hypophosphatemia due to the intracellular shift of phosphorus but typically does not require repletion. Extubation to noninvasive ventilation would be an option if his electrolytes were repleted and he passed his spontaneous breathing trial. ECMO is not indicated, and tracheostomy should be considered after electrolyte correction.

Keywords: Acid–base and electrolyte abnormalities; Electrolyte abnormalities, phosphorus

REFERENCES

Amanzadeh J, Reilly RF. Hypophosphatemia: an evidence-based approach to its clinical consequences and management. *Nature Clin Pract Nephrol* 2006;2(3):136–148.

Aubier M, Murciano D, Lecocguic Y et al. Effect of hypophosphatemia on diaphragmatic contractility in patients with acute respiratory failure. *N Engl J Med* 1985;313(7):420–424.

Gravelyn TR, Brophy N, Siegert C, Peters-Golden M. Hypophosphatemia-associated respiratory muscle weakness in a general inpatient population. *Am J Med* 1988;84(5):870–876.

Hoppe A, Metler M, Berndt TJ et al. Effect of respiratory alkalosis on renal phosphate excretion. *Am J Physiol Renal Physiol* 1982;243(5):F471–F475.

Mostellar ME, Tuttle Jr EP. Effects of alkalosis on plasma concentration and urinary excretion of inorganic phosphate in man. *J Clin Invest* 1964;43(1):138.

11. ANSWER: D

Peritoneal dialysis is an alternative to hemodialysis and typically preferred in the pediatric population. Patients who are highly active with vascular access failure, intolerance to hemodialysis, congestive heart failure, and limited access to a dialysis center are ideal candidates of peritoneal dialysis. Patient preference is also a factor. Peritoneal dialysis is typically contraindicated for patients with active intraabdominal infections, persons with cognitive impairment and limited support, and parturients in the third trimester of pregnancy.

Peritoneal dialysis catheters care required and can be placed by open surgical technique, laparoscopically, or by percutaneous approach. Dialysate is infused into the peritoneal space at prescribed intervals, allowing waste products to pass from the blood to the dialysate, which is eventually drained. The cycle is repeated multiple times and can be performed manually or in an automated fashion. Dialysate typically contains a high amount of dextrose, which can cause weight gain and lead to hyperglycemia; insulin can be added to the dialysate fluid. Peritoneal dialysis can be helpful in patients with ESRD and heart failure by allowing consistent fluid management and service as an alternative of hemodialysis.

Patients receiving peritoneal dialysis are at high risk for developing peritonitis.

Keywords: Renal; Management strategies; Renal replacement therapies, peritoneal dialysis

REFERENCES

Ansari N. Peritoneal dialysis in renal replacement therapy for patients with acute kidney injury. *Int J Nephrol* 2011;2011:739794.

Blagg CR. The early history of dialysis for chronic renal failure in the United States: a view from Seattle. *Am J Kidney Dis* 2007;49(3):482–496.

Teitelbaum I, Burkart J. Peritoneal dialysis. *Am J Kidney Dis* 2003;42(5):1082–1096.

12. ANSWER: B

The most important risk factor for developing contrast-induced nephropathy (CIN) is preexisting renal disease. CIN typically manifests within 72 hours after a contrast load. Diabetes mellitus, hypovolemia, and liver cirrhosis are also risk factors. Administration of isotonic fluid and euvolemia up to 12 hours before a contrast load and 24 hours after the procedure minimize the risk for renal impairment. Data on *N*-acetylcysteine and sodium bicarbonate are conflicting; however, they are commonly used before procedures. Furosemide, fenoldopam, dopamine, calcium channel blockers, and mannitol have not proved to be efficacious in the prevention of CIN.

Keywords: Renal failure; Contrast-induced nephropathy

REFERENCE

Parrillo JE, Dellinger RP. *Critical care medicine principles of diagnosis and management in the adult*, 4th edition. Philadelphia: Elsevier/ Saunders; 2014, pp. 965–983.

13. ANSWER: B

SIADH is associated with euvolemia and not hypotension. Paraneoplastic syndromes can manifest with SIADH, especially in patients with lung cancer. Diabetes insipidus would be expected if the patient were hypernatremic and hypotensive and had a low urine osmolarity. Polydipsia is inconsistent with the patient's history, and patients with polydipsia are euvolemic.

Symptomatic hyponatremia requires hypertonic saline therapy for rapid correction. Hypertonic saline also serves as a volume expander. Serum sodium should not be corrected faster than 10 to 12 mEq/L over 24 hours or faster than 4 to 6 mEq/ L over the 2 hours owing to the risk for osmotic demyelinating syndrome. Hypertonic saline therapy is typically not needed when serum sodium is greater than 120 mEq/L.

Keywords: Renal; Management strategies; Pharmacologic therapies; Diuretic therapy; Osmolarity

REFERENCE

Marino PL. *Marino's the ICU book*, 4th edition. Philadelphia: Wolters Kluwer Health/Lippincott Williams & Wilkins; 2014, pp. 666–670.

14. ANSWER: B

Hypocalcemia can occur as a result of hypoparathyroidism, diuretic use, sepsis, pancreatitis, renal failure, and alkalosis. Patients can present with seizures, weakness, bronchospasm, paresthesias, tetany, hypotension, heart block, and arrhythmias. Severe hypocalcemia should be immediately treated with IV calcium, which can be administered as calcium chloride or calcium gluconate. IVs calcium is short-acting, so the initial calcium bolus should be followed by an infusion. Emergent dialysis should be considered in the presence of acute kidney injury and hyperphosphatemia. Lasix and steroids are not indicated in the management of hypocalcemia.

Keywords: Acid–base and electrolyte abnormalities; Electrolyte abnormities; Calcium

REFERENCES

Marino PL. *Marino's the ICU book,* 4th edition. Philadelphia: Wolters Kluwer Health/Lippincott Williams & Wilkins; 2014, pp. 701–706.

Parrillo JE, Dellinger RP. *Critical care medicine principles of diagnosis and management in the adult*, 4th edition. Philadelphia: Elsevier/Saunders; 2014, pp. 1029–1046.

15. ANSWER: B

Hypomagnesemia and aminoglycosides increase the risk for torsade de pointes, which is a polymorphic form of ventricular tachycardia caused by an acquired long QT syndrome. All drugs that produce long QT syndrome can increase the risk for developing torsade de pointes. Mainstay of treatment is to stop the precipitating cause and give IV magnesium. Nonsynchronized electrical cardioversion, temporary pacing, and administration of isoproterenol are also effective therapies for acute management. By accelerating the HR >100 bpm with isoproterenol or by pacing, the QT interval is shortened in acquired long QT syndrome.

Keywords: Acid–base and electrolyte abnormalities; Electrolyte abnormities, magnesium

REFERENCES

Khan IA. Long QT syndrome: diagnosis and management. *Am Heart J* 2002;143(1):7–14.

Passman R, Kadish A. Polymorphic ventricular tachycardia, long QT syndrome, and torsades de pointes. *Med Clin North Am* 2001;85(2):321–341.

Table 14.4 URINE CHLORIDE IN METABOLIC ALKALOSIS

Chloride responsive	Urine chloride <15 mEq/L
Chloride resistant	Urine chloride >25 mEq/L

16. ANSWER: B

Metabolic alkalosis can be classified as chloride responsive and chloride resistant (Table 14.4). Chloride-responsive metabolic alkalosis can be caused by administration of diuretics such as thiazides or furosemide, laxative use, volume depletion, or vomiting. Chloride-resistant hypochloremia is typically caused by mineralocorticoid excess and severe hypokalemia. The mainstay of treatment for chloride-responsive metabolic alkalosis is to stop the precipitating cause along with the administration of normal saline, hydrochloric acid, acetazolamide, or potassium chloride.

Keywords: Acid–base and electrolyte abnormalities; electrolyte abnormities, chloride

REFERENCE

Marino PL. *Marino's the ICU book*, 4th edition. Philadelphia: Wolters Kluwer Health/Lippincott Williams & Wilkins; 2014, pp. 625–628.

17. ANSWER: D

Postrenal failure is typically caused by ureteral strictures, retroperitoneal and pelvic tumors, hematomas, prostate hypertrophy, prostate tumors, and bladder tumors. The mainstay of management is to treat the underlying cause. Often, emergent nephrostomy tube placement is needed to return kidney function to normal. Less severe obstruction can be managed with placement of a Foley catheter. Emergent dialysis is indicated for severe acid–base and electrolyte abnormalities. There is no difference in survival outcomes between CRRT and intermittent hemodialysis. CRRT is usually reserved for hemodynamically unstable patients.

Keywords: Renal; Diagnosis; Postrenal; Hemodialysis; Continuous Renal Replacement Therapy

REFERENCE

Parrillo JE, Dellinger RP. *Critical care medicine principles of diagnosis and management in the adult*, 4th edition. Philadelphia: Elsevier/Saunders; 2014, pp. 965–983.

Class I	Minimal mesangial lupus nephritis
Class II	Mesangial proliferative lupus nephritis
Class III	Focal lupus nephritis
Class IV	Diffuse lupus nephritis
Class V	Membranous lupus nephritis
Class VI	Advancers sclerosis lupus nephritis

18. ANSWER: B

Along with obtaining serum BUN and creatinine levels, a urinalysis can help to quickly assess for protein, red blood cells, and cellular casts. A spot urine and 24-hour urine test for creatinine clearance and protein excretion can also be obtained to evaluate for urinary protein-to-creatinine ratio, which is normally less than 0.2. Renal biopsy is helpful to determine the histologic pattern and the stage of renal disease. Biopsy can be helpful in guiding prognosis and treatment. Lupus nephritis has varying severities, from asymptomatic to rapidly progressive as well as acute or chronic (Table 14.5).

Keywords: Renal failure; Diagnostic modalities, renal biopsy

REFERENCE

Dooley MA. Clinical and epidemiologic features of lupus nephritis. In: Wallace DJ, Hahn BH, eds. *Dubois' lupus erythematosus and related syndromes*. Philadelphia: Elsevier Saunders; 2013, pp. 438–454.

19. ANSWER: B

RTA should be suspected in a patient with hyperchloremic non–anion gap metabolic acidosis. Type I RTA is associated with an impairment in distal acidification of urine and can be associated with autoimmune diseases. Patients will have a urine pH >5.5 and elevated urine ammonium excretion in type I RTA because of the inability to excrete excess hydrogen ions. Type II RTA occurs as a result of impaired proximal bicarbonate reabsorption or acetazolamide or topiramate administration and can be treated by administering sodium bicarbonate and thiazide diuretics. Type 4 RTA is due to hypoaldosteronism either from decreased aldosterone secretion or aldosterone resistance and can be treated with fludrocortisone.

Keywords: Diagnosis; Renal failure; Renal tubular acidosis

REFERENCES

Burton D, Theodore W. Metabolic acidosis. In: Rose B, Post T, eds., *Clinical physiology of acid-base and electrolyte disorders*, 5th edition. New York: McGraw-Hill, 2001, pp. 578–635; 612.
Soriano JR. Renal tubular acidosis: the clinical entity. *J Am Soc Nephrol* 2002;13(8):2160–2170.

20. ANSWER: A

Hyperacute renal transplant rejection occurs immediately to within hours after transplantation as a result of ABO incompatibility, and the treatment is emergent nephrectomy. Before transplantation, patients are screened for ABO compatibility, HLA typing, serum antibodies, and crossmatching. Renal transplant donors can be living or cadaveric, and rejection is typically T-cell or antibody mediated. Cyclosporine, tacrolimus, and antilymphocyte antibodies are the mainstay of treatment, but other therapies such as IV immune globulin, plasmapheresis, and complement pathway inhibitors are used.

Keywords: Renal; Diagnosis; Renal transplantation

REFERENCES

Heptinstall RH. *Pathology of the kidney*, vol. 3. Boston: Little Brown; 1992.
Patel R, Terasaki PI. Significance of the positive crossmatch test in kidney transplantation. *N Engl J Med* 1969;280(14):735–739.
Trpkov K, Campbell P, Pazderka F et al. Pathologic features of acute renal allograft rejection associated with donor-specific antibody: analysis using the Banff grading schema. *Transplantation* 1996;61(11):1586–1592.

21. ANSWER: D

Urgent indications for emergent dialysis include fluid overload, severe electrolyte abnormalities, metabolic acidosis, or drug overdose. There are no data to support superiority or survival benefit for intermittent hemodialysis over CRRT. Hemodialysis, in general, is not administered to hypotensive or hemodynamically unstable patients because of rapid fluid and solute removal that can exacerbate hypotension. CRRT is as effective at solute removal as IHD but can take up to 24 to 48 hours to achieve the same clearance. In this case, a patient previously stabilized on hemodialysis is presenting after missing two sessions, so changing the method of dialysis to peritoneal dialysis would not be practical. Sodium bicarbonate is a buffer administered in the setting of acidosis but would not resolve the presenting symptoms of this patient.

Keywords: Renal; Management strategies, renal replacement therapies, intermittent hemodialysis, continuous renal replacement therapies

REFERENCES

Cole L, Bellomo R, Silvester W, Reeves JH; Victorian Severe Acute Renal Failure Study Group. A prospective, multicenter study of the epidemiology, management, and outcome of severe acute renal failure in a "closed" ICU system. *Am J Respir Crit Care Med* 2000;162(1):191–196.

Golper TA. Indications, technical considerations, and strategies for renal replacement therapy in the intensive care unit. *J Intensive Care Med* 1992;7(6):310–317.

22. ANSWER: C

DKA typically causes an anion gap metabolic acidosis with decreased serum bicarbonate and the presence of ketones in blood or urine. Serum glucose levels are moderately elevated greater than or equal to 250 mg/dL, and serum pH is typically less than 7.30. The mainstay of treatment of DKA includes insulin therapy, judicious fluid administration, and electrolyte management. This patient has an anion gap metabolic acidosis with a concurrent appropriate respiratory acidosis. Winters formula 1.5 (HCO_3) + 8 ± 2; 1.5 (19) + 8 ± 2 = (34 to 38) indicates inappropriate compensation because $PaCO_2$ is 45. Gap-to-gap ratio = (AG excess/bicarbonate deficit) = (20 – 12)/(24 –19) = 1.6; therefore, no concurrent non–anion gap metabolic acidosis exists because the gap-to-gap ratio is more than 1.

Keywords: Acid–base and electrolyte abnormalities; Acid–base abnormalities, mixed

REFERENCE

Marino PL. *Marino's the ICU book*, 4th edition. Philadelphia: Wolters Kluwer Health/Lippincott Williams & Wilkins; 2014, pp. 587–592.

23. ANSWER: C

This patient has developed a coagulopathy and possibly disseminated intravascular coagulation related to his trauma and from acute blood loss. He is hypotensive and tachycardic and has high output from his chest tube. His chest tube should be monitored closely over the next hour because there may be a missed thoracic injury. Low urine output is a result of hypovolemia, and transfusing platelets, blood, and FFP would be the appropriate course of action. He received 10 units of blood and only 2 units of FFP, which could also cause a dilutional coagulopathy. Recommended transfusion practice in trauma is 1:1:1 or 1:1:2 for blood, FFP, and platelets. These transfusion practices have been associated with decreased mortality.

Keywords: Renal; Management strategies; Fluid and electrolyte management

REFERENCE

Holcomb JB, Tilley BC, Baraniuk S et al. Transfusion of plasma, platelets, and red blood cells in a 1: 1: 1 vs a 1: 1: 2 ratio and mortality in patients with severe trauma: the PROPPR randomized clinical trial. *JAMA* 2015;313(5):471–482.

24. ANSWER: B

Tumor lysis syndrome describes metabolic derangements that occur as a result of rapid lysis of malignant cells that release intracellular components into the bloodstream. Typical manifestations include hyperkalemia, hypocalcemia, hyperphosphatemia, and hyperuricemia. Uric acid and calcium phosphate can precipitate in the renal tubules and lead to renal failure, which is associated with worse outcomes. The mainstays of therapy are IV hydration, medical management of hyperkalemia, and rasburicase. Allopurinol is reserved for prevention because it cannot reduce preexisting high levels of uric acid. Owing to calcium phosphate precipitation, calcium supplementation is only recommended when patients have symptoms. The approved dosing for rasburicase is 0.2 mg/kg per day for up to 5 days. Rasburicase is contraindicated in patients with glucose-6-phosphate deficiency.

Keywords: Renal; Management strategies, fluid and electrolyte management; Tumor lysis syndrome

REFERENCE

Roberts PR, Todd SR. *Comprehensive critical care: adult*. Mount Prospect, IL: Society of Critical Care Medicine; 2012, pp. 603–604.

25. ANSWER: A

This patient has a respiratory acidosis due to her COPD exacerbation. Noninvasive ventilation decreases mortality, invasive ventilation, and nosocomial infections in patients with COPD exacerbations; however, after 2 hours of noninvasive therapy without improvement, endotracheal intubation is recommended. Other adjuncts to consider in the management of an acute COPD exacerbation are steroids, optimization of bronchodilators, and antibiotics. A sodium bicarbonate infusion is not the appropriate therapy in a patient with hypercapnic respiratory failure because it can cause worsening acidosis.

Keywords: Acid–base and electrolyte abnormalities; Respiratory

REFERENCES

Deutschman CS, Neligan PJ. *Evidence-based practice of critical care e-book*. Philadelphia: Elsevier Health Sciences; 2015, pp. 176–178.

Scala R, Nava S, Conti G et al. Noninvasive versus conventional ventilation to treat hypercapnic encephalopathy in chronic obstructive pulmonary disease. *Intensive Care Med* 2007;33(12):2101–2108.

Soler N, Torres A, Ewig S et al. Bronchial microbial patterns in severe exacerbations of chronic obstructive pulmonary disease (COPD) requiring mechanical ventilation. *Am J Respir Crit Care Med* 1998;157(5 Pt 1):1498–1505.

15.

PROCEDURES

Navneet Kaur Grewal

1. A 62-year-old male from a nursing home is admitted to intensive care unit (ICU) with right middle lobe recurrent aspiration pneumonia. After 10 days in the unit with unsuccessful weaning from ventilator secondary to poor neurological status, the MOST appropriate next step in management is:

A. Percutaneous tracheostomy
B. Slow PS weaning
C. Continue assist control/volume control (AC/VC) mode
D. Change to inverse ratio ventilation

2. A 55-year-old male with a history of heart failure has an arterial blood gas (ABG) analysis that reveals pH 7.35, PaO$_2$ 67 mm Hg, PaCO$_2$ 52 mm Hg, HCO$_3$ 21 mmol/L. His ventilator settings are assist control 450 mL, respiratory rate (RR) 20 breaths/minute, positive end-expiratory pressure (PEEP) 5 cm H$_2$O on 100% FiO$_2$. The patient's chest radiograph is shown here.

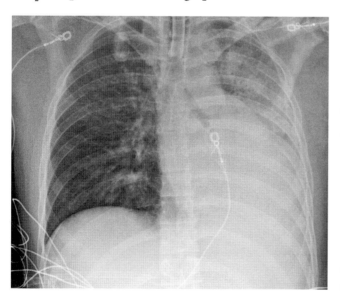

Which of the following is the MOST appropriate next step in the management of this patient?

A. Increase PEEP to 10 cm H$_2$O
B. Thoracentesis
C. Bronchoscopy
D. Chest computed tomography (CT) angiogram

3. A 45-year-old female is admitted for management of severe seasonal flu. The patient's course in the ICU is complicated by acute respiratory distress syndrome (ARDS), and current ventilator settings are assist control with volume settings of 400 mL, RR of 22 breaths/minute, PEEP of 18 cm H$_2$O, and 100% FiO$_2$. Bronchoscopy is performed to obtain specimen for bronchoalveolar lavage (BAL) and bronchial washings. After bronchoscopy is performed, the patient is noted to have acute desaturation and elevated peak pressures. The MOST likely cause of deterioration of the patient's condition is:

A. Pneumothorax
B. Worsening of ARDS
C. Pulmonary embolism
D. Pulmonary edema

4. The patient in question 3 continues to deteriorate, with drop in blood pressure (BP), elevated peak pressures on the ventilator, and decrease in O$_2$ saturation. As part of the workup, a chest radiograph is done, which is shown here. The MOST appropriate next step in the management of this patient is:

A. Placement of chest tube
B. Decrease PEEP to 5 cm H$_2$O
C. Pressure support mode
D. Observation

5. You are called to a code on a patient on the hemodialysis floor. The patient suddenly became asystolic

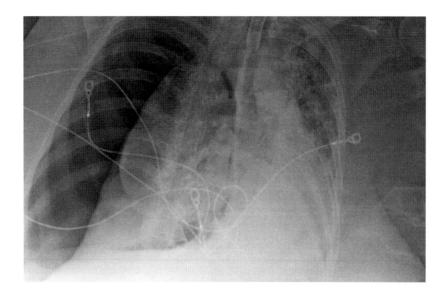

Figure Q4.1

during hemodialysis by an arteriovenous (AV) fistula. Attempts to obtain peripheral or femoral central venous access are unsuccessful. A bedside ultrasound reveals a thrombus in the right internal jugular vein. The MOST appropriate next step in management of this patient is:

A. Internal jugular cannulation
B. Subclavian cannulation
C. Intraosseous access placement
D. Reattempt femoral access by a different provider

6. A patient with maxillary fractures has a tracheostomy placed with difficulty in the operating room. Postoperatively, the patient is noted to have a temperature of 100.7° F, heart rate (HR) of 118 bpm, and BP of 97/58 mm Hg. Percutaneous tracheostomy has been associated with increased risk of:

A. Infection
B. Bleeding
C. Mortality
D. Posterior tracheal wall perforations

7. The intensivist is called to the bedside of a patient in a code. The code is conducted as per advanced cardiac life support (ACLS) guidelines, and return of spontaneous circulation (ROSC) is achieved. A bedside ultrasound with a transthoracic echocardiogram is performed, and a diagnosis of tamponade is suspected. Which of the following echocardiographic finding is MOST sensitive for diagnosis of cardiac tamponade?

A. Right atrial collapse
B. Right ventricular collapse
C. Left ventricular collapse
D. Increased ventricular dependence

8. After a difficult central line placement, the patient is noted to be markedly tachypneic and tachycardic with increased work of breathing. A bedside ultrasound is performed. Ultrasound findings diagnostic of pneumothorax on lung ultrasonography include:

A. Absence of lung sliding, absence of B lines
B. Presence of lung sliding, presence of A lines
C. Absence of B lines, presence of A lines
D. Absence of lung point

9. The patient after trauma is brought to the emergency department (ED) with extensive bleeding from the face. The patient is unresponsive, and the airway is noted to be bloody. Three attempts by the ED physician to secure the airway are unsuccessful, and at this time mask ventilation is possible but is becoming difficult. The patient's O₂ saturation is 90%. The MOST appropriate next step in the management of this airway is:

A. Direct laryngoscopy by a different provider
B. Placement of supraglottic device
C. Fiberoptic bronchoscopy
D. Video laryngoscopy

10. Regarding the patient in question 9, laryngeal mask airway (LMA) placement is attempted and unsuccessful. The patient cannot be mask-ventilated and has an O₂ saturation of 84%. The MOST appropriate next step in management of this airway is:

A. Cricothyroidotomy
B. Bronchoscopy
C. Video laryngoscopy
D. Direct laryngoscopy

11. A 75-year-old male patient is admitted to the ICU for 2 weeks with persistent hypotension requiring vasopressors. He is noted to have digital ischemia and necrosis. Flushing the catheter with which of the following would MOST likely have prevented thrombosis of the arterial line catheter and embolization?

A. Heparin
B. Normal saline
C. Sodium citrate
D. Papaverine

12. A 42-year-old male patient is transported to the trauma bay after a serious motor vehicle collision. A focused assessment with sonography for trauma (FAST) exam is negative, and the patient is hemodynamically stable at this time. The NEXT most appropriate step in the management of this patient is:

A. CT scan
B. Exploratory laparotomy
C. Monitor in the ICU
D. No further intervention needed.

13. A 75-year-old male is weaned from the ventilator after 2 weeks of respiratory failure secondary to pneumonia. The patient passed a spontaneous breathing trial and is extubated. Soon after extubation, the patient develops inspiratory stridor, increased work of breathing, and drop in O_2 saturation to 85%. Bronchoscopy is performed that shows the following image:

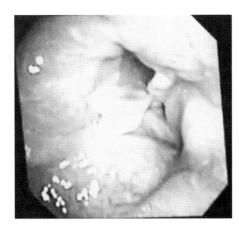

The MOST likely etiology of the above presentation is:

A. Bronchospasm
B. Aspiration event

C. Glottic edema
D. Critical illness myopathy

14. A 65-year-old male is admitted to the critical care unit with altered mental status, fever, and headaches. As part of the workup, lumbar puncture is planned. It is noted in the past medical history that the patient has been treated with enoxaparin for treatment of deep vein thrombosis (DVT) in the lower extremities. Which of the following is the MOST appropriate next step in the management of this patient?

A. Delay lumbar puncture until 24 hours after enoxaparin
B. Proceed with lumbar puncture
C. CT imaging of the head
D. Transfuse platelets before lumbar puncture

15. A 64-year-old male patient is admitted to the ICU for management of ventilator-dependent respiratory failure. The patient's ICU course has been complicated by sepsis, acute renal failure, and thrombocytopenia. He had a tracheostomy placed 14 days ago. You are called to the bedside for evaluation of bleeding around the tracheostomy site. On exam, the patient is noted to have a brisk bright-red bleeding at the tracheostomy site. The bedside nurse also notes that the patient did have a similar short episode a few days ago that resolved with application of a hemostatic dressing. A CT scan of the neck is obtained and shown here.

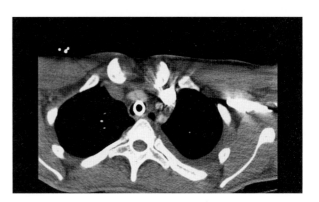

The next MOST appropriate step in the management of this patient is:

A. Transfuse platelets
B. Stat operating room intervention
C. Repack with Surgicel
D. No intervention

ANSWERS

1. ANSWER: A

This patient is debilitated with recurrent aspiration pneumonia; hence, prolonged ventilator support is anticipated. Despite all weaning measures, the patient is not extubated and needs ventilator support for the near future. Therefore, the appropriate measure at this time is to proceed with percutaneous tracheostomy. Slow pressure support weaning versus AC/VC and inverse ratio ventilation (e.g., airway pressure release ventilation [APRV], bilevel) modes are not appropriate at this time. The most relevant issue is an obvious need for long-term ventilator support; however, whether to provide early (7–10 days) versus late (>15 days) support is still controversial, and data so far have been inconclusive, but there are obvious benefits to early tracheostomy. Tracheostomy has its benefits of ease of liberation from ventilator and patient comfort. Studies have evaluated "early" versus "late" tracheostomy in the past decade. In 2005, a meta-analysis of five randomized trials was conducted between 1990 and 2004 involving a total of 406 patients with diverse conditions, including trauma, head injury, medical, surgical, and burn patients. It was limited by the relatively small number of patients, small number of trials included, and significant degree of heterogeneity, which existed across included studies with regard to definitions of "early" versus "late" tracheostomy. Overall, however, no difference was observed in mortality or rate of ventilator-associated pneumonia. However, a significant decrease in the duration of mechanical ventilation and ICU length of stay was observed for early tracheostomy (defined as <7 days).

Keywords: Specialized areas; Procedures, airway, tracheostomy

REFERENCES

Griffiths J, Barber VS, Morgan L, Young JD. Systematic review and meta-analysis of studies of the timing of tracheostomy in adult patients undergoing artificial ventilation. *BMJ* 2005;330(7502):1243.

Rumbak MJ, Newton M, Truncale T et al. A prospective, randomized study comparing early percutaneous dilational tracheotomy to prolonged translaryngeal intubation (delayed tracheotomy) in critically ill medical patients. *Crit Care Med* 2004;32(8):1689–1694.

Scales DC, Ferguson ND. Early vs late tracheotomy in ICU patients. *JAMA* 2010;303(15):1537–1538.

Terragni PP, Antonelli M, Fumagalli R et al. Early vs late tracheotomy for prevention of pneumonia in mechanically ventilated adult ICU patients: a randomized controlled trial. *JAMA* 2010; 303(15):1483–1489.

2. ANSWER: C

The patient is noted to have extensive thick mucus secretions in the setting of pneumonia; hence, the likelihood of mucus plugging as a cause of the radiographic findings is highly likely. Bronchoscopy is the most indicated procedure at this time because it could be diagnostic and also therapeutic when the mucous plug is aspirated through bronchoscope. Repeat chest radiograph must be done to confirm improvement in aeration of the lung fields. Thoracentesis is not immediately indicated because we do not have anything to suggest a diagnosis of pleural effusion as of yet. Flexible bronchoscopy is a very often used tool in the diagnosis and management of many pulmonary diseases. Bronchoscopy is indicated for assessment of the airway, diagnosis, and staging of bronchogenic carcinoma, evaluation of hemoptysis, and diagnosis of pulmonary infections. It can be used for transbronchial lung biopsy, endobronchial biopsy, BAL, and removal of retained secretions and foreign bodies from the airway. The procedure is contraindicated in severe bronchospasm or a bleeding disorder. Complications, although rare (< 1%), include hemorrhage and transient hypoxemia.

Keywords: Specialized areas; Procedures; Monitoring techniques and troubleshooting (e.g., cardiac, neurological)

REFERENCES

Aziz M. Advances in laryngoscopy. *F1000Res* 2015;4:pii: F1000 Faculty Rev-1410.

Bauer TL, Berkheim DB. Bronchoscopy: diagnostic and therapeutic for non-small cell lung cancer. *Surg Oncol Clin N Am* 2016;25(3):481–491.

Collins SR. Direct and indirect laryngoscopy: equipment and techniques. *Respir Care* 2014;59(6):850–864.

3. ANSWER: A

Pneumothorax is the most feared complication after bronchoscopy. This patient is particularly at risk. High ventilator setting of PEEP and FiO_2 increase the risk, and procedures involving bronchial washings and biopsies also put pneumothorax high on the differential. Known complications of bronchoscopy include:

1. Risk for anesthesia and sedation. Risks are higher in elderly patients and those with preexisting hepatic and renal dysfunction. There is potential for respiratory depression and systemic absorption of topical anesthetics (e.g., methemoglobinemia from lidocaine/benzocaine use).
2. Pneumothorax. This is most common after transbronchial and endobronchial biopsies. Pneumothorax following TBB occurs in 4 to 5% of cases and in approximately 1% after routine bronchoscopies. The risk is increased in patients with immunocompromised status, mechanical ventilation, and bullous lung disease.

3. Hemorrhage. Bleeding is more common in patients with thrombocytopenia, uremia, liver disease, pulmonary hypertension, and concurrent anticoagulation.

Keywords: Specialized areas; Procedures; Monitoring techniques and troubleshooting (e.g., cardiac, neurological)

REFERENCES

Cordasco EM Jr, Mehta AC, Ahmad M. Bronchoscopically induced bleeding: a summary of nine years' Cleveland clinic experience and review of the literature. *Chest* 1991;100(4):1141–1147.

Facciolongo N, Patelli M, Gasparini S et al. Incidence of complications in bronchoscopy: multicentre prospective study of 20,986 bronchoscopies. *Monaldi Arch Chest Dis* 2009;71(1):8–14.

Izbicki G, Shitrit D, Yarmolovsky A et al. Is routine chest radiography after transbronchial biopsy necessary? A prospective study of 350 cases. *Chest* 2006;129(6):1561–1564.

O'Brien JD, Ettinger NA, Shevlin D, Kollef MH. Safety and yield of transbronchial biopsy in mechanically ventilated patients. *Crit Care Med* 1997;25(3):440–446.

4. ANSWER: A

Management of pneumothorax in this patient includes placement of chest tube because the patient is symptomatic and the pneumothorax is greater than 20%. Since the patient is on full positive pressure mode of ventilation, the size of the pneumothorax is likely to increase and cause tension a pneumothorax. Decreasing PEEP and placing the patient on pressure support mode may theoretically reduce the rate of pneumothorax expansion but should not be considered an intervention. Additionally, worsening hemodynamics should be expected up to and including cardiac arrest if this pneumothorax is resolved.

Keywords: Specialized areas; Procedures; Chest tube placement

REFERENCES

Ball CG, Lord J, Laupland KB et al. Chest tube complications: how well are we training our residents? *Can J Surg* 2007;50(6):450.

Jones PW, Moyers JP, Rogers JT et al. Ultrasound-guided thoracentesis: is it a safer method? *Chest* 2003;123(2):418.

Lim KE, Tai SC, Chan CY et al. Diagnosis of malpositioned chest tubes after emergency tube thoracostomy: is computed tomography more accurate than chest radiograph? *Clin Imaging* 2005;29(6):401.

5. ANSWER: C

This patient most likely is a difficult central line placement candidate because he presents with a history of multiple central vein cannulation and possible thrombosis versus stenosis of central veins. The patient is also in cardiac arrest; hence, line placement is urgent. The best and quickest approach at this time is intraosseous line placement.

Keywords: Specialized areas; Procedures; Vascular access; Intraosseous

REFERENCES

Horton MA, Beamer C. Powered intraosseous insertion provides safe and effective vascular access for pediatric emergency patients. *Pediatr Emerg Care* 2008;24(6):347.

Luck RP, Haines C, Mull CC. Intraosseous access. *J Emerg Med* 2010;39(4):468.

Ngo AS, Oh JJ, Chen Y et al. Intraosseous vascular access in adults using the EZ-IO in an emergency department. *Int J Emerg Med* 2009;2(3):155.

Reades R, Studnek JR, Garrett JS et al. Comparison of first-attempt success between tibial and humeral intraosseous insertions during out-of-hospital cardiac arrest. *Prehosp Emerg Care* 2011;15(2):278.

6. ANSWER: D

Percutaneous tracheostomy has many advantages, including that it can be performed quickly and with lower cost at the bedside. It is best performed by surgeons and trained critical care physicians under bronchoscopic guidance. Two meta-analyses have shown a decreased risk for infection with percutaneous dilational tracheostomy compared with surgical tracheostomies. There is also evidence that, compared with surgical tracheostomies, the bleeding risk and mortality are lower with percutaneous tracheostomies. One meta-analysis showed no difference in terms of mortality, and another showed no difference in terms of bleeding risk or risk for tracheal stenosis. Hence, it can be said that percutaneous tracheostomies do not carry increased risk and possibly carry decreased risk for infection, bleeding, and mortality. There have been cases documenting increased risk for anterior and posterior tracheal wall injury with percutaneous tracheostomy, and physicians must be watchful for these complications. Another life-threatening complication of tracheostomies (surgical and percutaneous) is trachea-arterial fistula and subsequent massive hemorrhage. This mostly occurs from erosion of the tip or cuff of the tracheostomy into the innominate artery at the anterior aspect of the trachea. Outcomes in these cases are dependent on having a high index of suspicion after a sentinel bleed and immediate surgical action to stop the bleeding.

Keywords: Specialized areas; Procedures; Airway; Tracheostomy

REFERENCES

Brass P, Hellmich M, Ladra A et al. Percutaneous techniques versus surgical techniques for tracheostomy. *Cochrane Database Syst Rev* 2016;(7):CD008045.

Delaney A, Bagshaw SM, Nalos M. Percutaneous dilatational tracheostomy versus surgical tracheostomy in critically ill patients: a systematic review and meta-analysis. *Crit Care* 2006;10(2):R55.

Dempsey GA, Morton B, Hammell C et al. Long-term outcome following tracheostomy in critical care: a systematic review. *Crit Care Med* 2016;44(3):617–628.

Friedman Y, Fildes J, Mizock B et al. Comparison of percutaneous and surgical tracheostomies. *Chest* 1996;110(2):480.

Silvester W, Goldsmith D, Uchino S et al. Percutaneous versus surgical tracheostomy: a randomized controlled study with long-term follow-up. *Crit Care Med* 2006;34(8):2145.

Trottier SJ, Hazard PB, Sakabu SA et al. Posterior tracheal wall perforation during percutaneous dilational tracheostomy: an investigation into its mechanism and prevention. *Chest* 1999;115(5):1383.

7. ANSWER: A

Echocardiography has been used extensively in the diagnosis of pericardial diseases and recommended by American College of Cardiology, American Heart Association, and American Society of Echocardiography. The European Society of Cardiology Guidelines in 2015 recommend its use as the first step in evaluating cardiac tamponade and its subsequent use to perform pericardiocentesis.

The initial evaluation by ultrasound shows a moderate to large pleural effusion and the presence of a "swinging heart." Chamber collapse is the next most significant finding and can be diagnostic of impending hemodynamic collapse. Diastolic collapse of the right atrium is the most sensitive finding, especially when present for more than one third of the cardiac cycle. Right ventricular collapse also occurs but is less sensitive and more specific for cardiac tamponade. The left ventricle is a more muscular structure and its collapse is seen less often and is not always diagnostic early in the course of tamponade

Keywords: Specialized areas; Procedures; Ultrasound; Interpretation

REFERENCES

Adler Y, Charron P, Imazio M, et al. 2015 ESC guidelines for the diagnosis and management of pericardial diseases: The Task Force for the Diagnosis and Management of Pericardial Diseases of the European Society of Cardiology (ESC) Endorsed by: The European Association for Cardio-Thoracic Surgery (EACTS). *Eur Heart J* 2015;36(42):2921.

Gillam LD, Guyer DE, Gibson TC et al. Hydrodynamic compression of the right atrium: a new echocardiographic sign of cardiac tamponade. *Circulation* 1983;68(2):294.

Kerber RE, Gascho JA, Litchfield R et al. Hemodynamic effects of volume expansion and nitroprusside compared with pericardiocentesis in patients with acute cardiac tamponade. *N Engl J Med* 1982;307(15):929.

Reydel B, Spodick DH. Frequency and significance of chamber collapses during cardiac tamponade. *Am Heart J* 1990;=119(5):1160.

8. ANSWER: A

Lung ultrasound is low-risk portable bedside imaging that can be done to diagnose and treat various pleural abnormalities, including pleural effusions and pneumothorax. Ultrasound guidance has been shown to reduce the risk for pneumothorax when used during thoracentesis. Ultrasound can be very easily used for bedside detection of pneumothorax after procedures with this associated risk. The two US findings essential for the diagnosis of pneumothorax are:

1. Absence of lung sliding. Lung sliding represents the horizontal movement of the lung relative to the pleural surface.
2. Absence of B lines. B lines are vertical multiple comet-tail lines extending from the pleural lines to the lower edge of the screen. These lines move with the movement of the lung, and the presence of B lines rules out pneumothorax.

Additional findings include absence of lung pulse and presence of lung point. Lung point is defined as the part of the lung where the lung is adherent to the parietal pleura in a part of the lung and not so in the part with pneumothorax. However, lung point is not always present and is not as accurate as the absence of B lines and absence of lung sliding.

Keywords: Specialized areas; Procedures; Ultrasound; Interpretation

REFERENCES

Lichtenstein DA, Menu Y. A bedside ultrasound sign ruling out pneumothorax in the critically ill: lung sliding. *Chest* 1995;108(5):1345.

Lichtenstein D, Mezière G, Biderman P, Gepner A. The "lung point": an ultrasound sign specific to pneumothorax. *Intensive Care Med* 2000;26(10):1434.

Mercaldi CJ, Lanes SF. Ultrasound guidance decreases complications and improves the cost of care among patients undergoing thoracentesis and paracentesis. *Chest* 2013;143(2):532.

Volpicelli G. Sonographic diagnosis of pneumothorax. *Intensive Care Med* 2011;37(2):224.

9. ANSWER: B

Supraglottic devices are used to provide oxygenation and ventilation in emergency situations when direct laryngoscopy has been unsuccessful. In a patient with bleeding making visualization of the larynx difficult, supraglottic devices like LMA can be placed blindly and can provide much-needed ventilation and oxygenation and thus are an essential part of the Failed Airway Algorithm. More than three attempts at direct laryngoscopy even by another provider are not recommended because risk for further airway trauma and injury are markedly increased. Also, given the ongoing bleeding, fiberoptic bronchoscopy and video laryngoscopy are not recommended according to the Failed Airway Algorithm. Because this patient is very close to a "can't ventilate" situation, the supraglottic device is a better recommendation and more likely to be successful until a more definite airway can be secured.

Keywords: Specialized areas; Procedures; Airway, LMA, others

REFERENCES

Bair AE, Filbin MR, Kulkarni RG, Walls RM. The failed intubation attempt in the emergency department: analysis of prevalence, rescue techniques, and personnel. *J Emerg Med* 2002;23(2):131.

Brown CA 3rd, Bair AE, Pallin DJ, Walls RM; NEAR III Investigators. Techniques, success, and adverse events of emergency department adult intubations. *Ann Emerg Med.* 2015;65(4):363–370.

Walls RM. The emergency airway algorithms. In: Walls RM, Murphy MF, eds. *Manual of emergency airway management*, 3rd edition. Philadelphia: Lippincott Williams & Wilkins; 2008, p. 8.

10. ANSWER: A

This patient's care has reached a very critical point, with a "can't ventilate, can't intubate" situation. The patient is at high risk for having hypoxic sequelae if the airway is not secured in a timely fashion. Cricothyroidotomy is a very realistic option at this time. Other alternate airway devices may be able to secure the airway, but time is of critical importance here, which usually means that a surgical airway is warranted.

Keywords: Specialized areas; Procedures; Airway; Transtracheal tubes

REFERENCES

Bair AE, Panacek EA, Wisner DH et al. Cricothyrotomy: a 5-year experience at one institution. *J Emerg Med* 2003;24(2):151.

Eisenburger P, Laczika K, List M et al. Comparison of conventional surgical versus Seldinger technique emergency cricothyrotomy performed by inexperienced clinicians. *Anesthesiology* 2000;92(3):687.

Sagarin MJ, Barton ED, Chng YM, Walls RM; National Emergency Airway Registry Investigators. Airway management by US and Canadian emergency medicine residents: a multicenter analysis of

more than 6,000 endotracheal intubation attempts. *Ann Emerg Med* 2005;46(4):328.

11. ANSWER: A

Presence of arterial catheters has been associated with thrombosis in up to 25% of patients, although subsequent clinically significant embolism has been noted in only 1%. Risk factors associated with arterial catheter thrombosis include duration of catheterization (>72 hours associated with increased risk), presence of peripheral vascular disease, longer catheters, and presence of vasospastic disorders. Heparin flushes have been associated with lower risk for thrombosis compared with normal saline. Sodium citrate is another agent that can be used in patients when heparin is contraindicated. It has similar patency rates to heparin; however, there are not a enough studies comparing them. Papaverine can be injected in patients with vasospasm, but it is not indicated in patients with thrombosis.

Keywords: Specialized areas; Procedures; Vascular access, arterial

REFERENCES

Clifton GD, Branson P, Kelly HJ, Dotson LR, Record KE, Phillips BA, Thompson JR: Comparison of normal saline and heparin solutions for maintenance of arterial catheter patency. Heart Lung.1991;20(2):115.

Evaluation of the effects of heparinized and nonheparinized flush solutions on the patency of arterial pressure monitoring lines: the AACN Thunder Project. By the American Association of Critical-Care Nurses. *Am J Crit Care*1993; 2(1):3.

Kulkarni M, Elsner C, Ouellet D, Zeldin R: Heparinized saline versus normal saline in maintaining patency of the radial artery catheter. Can J Surg. 1994;37(1):37.

Zevola DR, Dioso J, Moggio R: Comparison of heparinized and nonheparinized solutions for maintaining patency of arterial and pulmonary artery catheters. Am J Crit Care. 1997;6(1):52.

12. ANSWER: A

FAST exam has various limitations that prevent its use as a definitive test to rule out intra-abdominal injuries. Some studies have shown sensitivities as low as 42%, but mostly its sensitivity is considered to be in the 63 to 100% range. If a patient is suspected to have significant injuries, even though the FAST is negative and the patient is stable, further imaging such as CT scan should be done to rule out injuries that may need surgical interventions. Many injuries are not detected by ultrasound. FAST cannot rule out bowel perforations, mesenteric injuries, and diaphragmatic tears. Also, the ability of ultrasound to detect free fluid in amounts less than 200 mL or retroperitoneal and pelvic injuries is very limited. The sensitivity and accuracy of FAST can be improved by doing serial FAST exams. One observational study in trauma patients showed that sensitivity improved to 94% when a repeat FAST was done within 24 hours of a negative FAST exam.

Keywords: Specialized areas; Procedures; Ultrasound, indications, application

REFERENCES

Blackbourne LH, Soffer D, McKenney M et al. Secondary ultrasound examination increases the sensitivity of the FAST exam in blunt trauma. *J Trauma* 2004;57(5):934.

Dolich MO, McKenney MG, Varela JE et al. 2,576 Ultrasounds for blunt abdominal trauma. *J Trauma* 2001;50(1):108.

Hoffman L, Pierce D, Puumala S. Clinical predictors of injuries not identified by focused abdominal sonogram for trauma (FAST) examinations. *J Emerg Med* 2009;36(3):271.

Lingawi SS, Buckley A. Focused abdominal US in patients with trauma. *Radiology* 2000;217(2):426.

Natarajan B, Gupta PK, Cemaj S et al. FAST scan: is it worth doing in hemodynamically stable blunt trauma patients? *Surgery* 2010;148(4):695.

Tayal VS, Nielsen A, Jones AE et al. Accuracy of trauma ultrasound in major pelvic injury. *J Trauma* 2006;61(6):1453.

13. ANSWER: C

Laryngeal injuries are common after intubation and most often present as dysphonia and hoarseness after extubation. Severe injuries (bilateral vocal cord paralysis and laryngotracheal stenosis) can present as acute stridor and extubation failure, requiring reintubation. The cause is most likely secondary to inflammation and direct pressure from the presence of the endotracheal tube (ETT). Various risk factors have been described. The most common are prolonged intubation (>36 hour), traumatic intubation, larger size of the ETT, aspiration, and unplanned extubation. Laryngeal edema must be suspected in cases with absence of cuff leak. Diagnosis in most cases involves assessment of the airway by laryngoscopy or bronchoscopy. Most cases of laryngeal edema resolve in 24 to 48 hours with supportive management, including racemic epinephrine, glucocorticoid therapy, Heliox, or reintubation in cases with severe symptoms.

Keywords: Specialized areas; Procedures; Airway, LMA/others

REFERENCES

Colice GL, Stukel TA, Dain B. Laryngeal complications of prolonged intubation. *Chest* 1989;96(4):877.

Darmon JY, Rauss A, Dreyfuss D et al. Evaluation of risk factors for laryngeal edema after tracheal extubation in adults and its prevention by dexamethasone: a placebo-controlled double blind, multicenter study. *Anesthesiology* 1992;77(2):245.

Santos PM, Afrassiabi A, Weymuller EA Jr. Risk factors associated with prolonged intubation and laryngeal injury. *Otolaryngol Head Neck Surg* 1994;111(4):453.

Shadmehr MB, Abbasidezfouli A, Farzanegan R et al. The role of systemic steroids in postintubation tracheal stenosis: a randomized clinical trial. *Ann Thorac Surg* 2017;103(1):246.

Whited RE. A prospective study of laryngotracheal sequelae in long-term intubation. *Laryngoscope* 1984;94(3):367–377.

14. ANSWER: A

All patients with suspected meningitis should have cerebrospinal fluid obtained by lumbar puncture unless contraindicated. Therapeutic anticoagulation is a relative contraindication because the patient is definitely at risk for bleeding and developing spinal hematoma. Delaying the lumbar puncture for 24 hours seems to be a prudent course of action to take in this situation while empiric antibiotics can be started for the treatment of meningitis. CT scan of the head is sometimes done in patients with suspected meningitis to rule out mass lesion or if elevated intracranial pressure or cerebral herniation is suspected, but it is not helpful in diagnosing or ruling out meningitis, which is the most likely diagnosis in this patient. Transfusing platelets before lumbar puncture is unlikely to be helpful in decreasing the risk for bleeding in this patient.

Keywords: Specialized areas; Procedures; Monitoring techniques and troubleshooting (e.g., cardiac, neurological)

REFERENCES

Horlocker TT. Low molecular weight heparin and neuraxial anesthesia. *Thromb Res* 2001;101(1):V141.

Pitkänen MT, Aromaa U, Cozanitis DA, Förster JG. Serious complications associated with spinal and epidural anaesthesia in Finland from 2000 to 2009. *Acta Anaesthesiol Scand* 2013;57(5):553–564.

Ruff RL, Dougherty JH Jr. Complications of lumbar puncture followed by anticoagulation. *Stroke* 1981;12(6):879.

Sinclair AJ, Carroll C, Davies B. Cauda equina syndrome following a lumbar puncture. *J Clin Neurosci* 2009;16(5):714.

15. ANSWER: B

Fistulas can form between the innominate artery and tracheobronchial tree after a tracheostomy placement, more likely in a tracheostomy placed too low. The tracheostomy tube can erode into the innominate artery as it crosses the

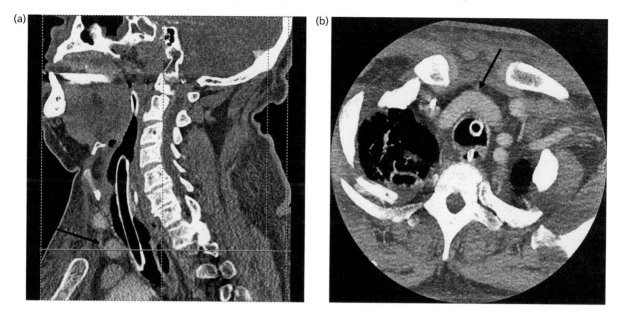

Figure 15.1 High-riding innominate artery (*black arrow*) in both sagittal (A) and axial (B) views in a patient scheduled for a tracheostomy. (Courtesy of George Williams, MD, FASA, FCCP.)

anterolateral surface of the trachea at the level of the upper sternum. Tracheal–innominate artery fistulas can cause rare but life-threatening hemorrhage, usually preceded by a sentinel bleed before massive hemorrhage. When that happens, it involves a stat trip to the operating room with cardiovascular surgery. About 2 weeks after tracheostomy placement is the timeframe for this complication to happen, and the critical care team must be vigilant for it. All the other options in the question are not likely to resolve the acute massive hemorrhage that occurs in these patients. Figure 15.1 demonstrates a high-riding innominate artery in a patient who was scheduled for a tracheostomy; this was discovered before the procedure was completed by a diligent surgical team.

REFERENCES

Dixit MD, Gan M, Narendra NG et al. Aortopulmonary fistula: a rare complication of an aortic aneurysm. *Tex Heart Inst J* 2009;36(5):483.

Hung JJ, Hsu HS, Huang CS, Yang KY. Tracheoesophageal fistula and tracheo-subclavian artery fistula after tracheostomy. *Eur J Cardiothorac Surg* 2007;32(4):676–678.

Komatsu T, Sowa T, Fujinaga T et al. Tracheo-innominate artery fistula: two case reports and a clinical review. *Ann Thorac Cardiovasc Surg* 2013;19(1):60–62.

16.

NUTRITION

George W. Williams

QUESTIONS

1. A 42-year-old 70-kg male is admitted to the intensive care unit (ICU) with postoperative sepsis after emergent abdominal surgery. Following 8 days of admission to the ICU, he remains on low-dose vasopressors to maintain a normal blood pressure (BP). The computed tomography (CT) scan shown here is obtained:

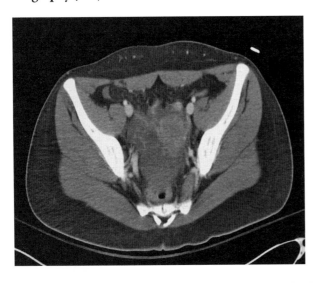

The patient is tolerating 1 kcal/mL tube feeds, which have been infusing at 100 mL/hour. Which of the following is the MOST appropriate next step?

   A. Decrease tube feeds
   B. Repeat CT in 72 hours
   C. Indirect calorimetry
   D. Stool ova and parasites

2. While performing your morning assessments, the unit dietitian informs you that a patient who was admitted to the hospital 3 days ago is receiving 1 g/kg per day of protein intake. You determine that the patient's wounds are healing slowly and that further intervention may be warranted. Which of the following is the MOST useful next study to perform?

   A. Prealbumin
   B. Nitrogen balance
   C. Transferrin
   D. Paracetamol absorption

3. A patient is diagnosed with severe protein-calorie malnutrition and admitted from the emergency department (ED) in order to monitor for refeeding syndrome. A colonoscopy is performed with no noted intestinal lesions, and nutrition is initiated. Which of the following provides the MOST energy per gram?

   A. Lipids
   B. Protein
   C. Glucose
   D. Arginine

4. A peripherally inserted central catheter (PICC) line is placed in a patient with deep vein thrombosis and type 2 diabetes mellitus who requires intravenous (IV) antibiotics for osteomyelitis and total parenteral nutrition (TPN). Two days after placement, the patient is noted to be hypothermic, hypotensive, and delirious. He is transferred to the ICU for further management. Which of the following is the MOST likely cause of his presentation?

   A. Thrombophlebitis
   B. Peripheral vascular disease
   C. Hypothermia
   D. TPN

5. A 28-year-old male is admitted following a motor vehicle collision. He has persistently altered mental status without obvious signs of trauma. His family states that he was once treated for cocaine abuse. Toxicology does not reveal illicit substances or alcohol intoxication. The

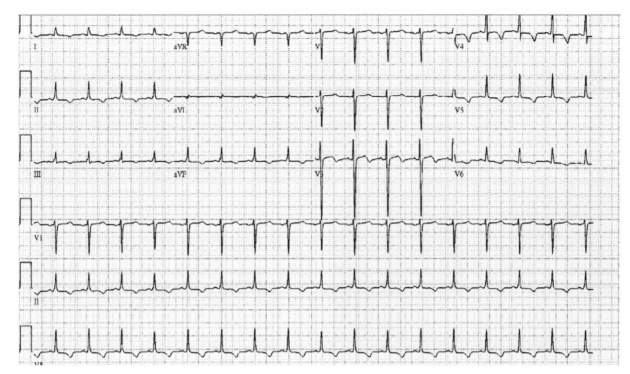

Figure Q6.1

level of which of the following is MOST likely to be deficient in this patient?

A. Thiamine
B. Vitamin E
C. Selenium
D. Linoleic acid

6. A patient from the general medical floor is transferred to your ICU for workup of protracted diarrhea. *Clostridium difficile* polymerase chain reaction (PCR) has been sent, and results are pending; labs reveal a white blood cell (WBC) count of 13.5×10^9. Although vital signs are within normal limits, the patient complains of weakness. The electrocardiogram (ECG) is shown here.

Which of the following is the MOST appropriate to administer?

A. Packed red blood cells
B. Potassium
C. D_5 water
D. Antibiotics

7. An 81-year-old male who on postoperative day 2 after a transurethral resection of the prostate presents with fever, elevated WBC count, abdominal distention, and altered mental status. A kidney-ureter-bladder radiograph (KUB) is obtained and is shown here:

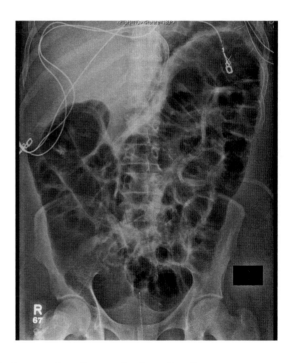

He is noted to be producing cloudy nonconcentrated urine. Which of the following would be the MOST appropriate next step?

A. TPN
B. IV fluid bolus
C. Antibiotics
D. Endoscopy

8. A 70-kg, 175-cm female with past medical history significant for dyslipidemia is in the ICU following an ST-elevation myocardial infarction. She is intubated, sedated with midazolam, and fed with 1 kcal/mL tube feeds at a rate of 70 mL/hour. Additionally, she is afebrile and on scheduled acetaminophen for pain and a multivitamin elixir. The nurse reports diarrhea and that the stool "does not smell like C Diff." Her KUB is shown here:

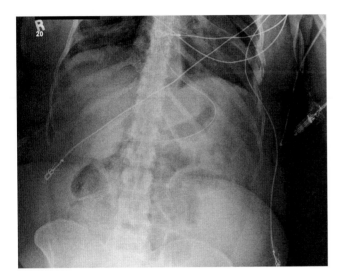

Which of the following is the MOST appropriate to resolve the patient's diarrhea?

A. Oral cimetidine
B. Oral vancomycin
C. Discontinuation of oral medications
D. Reduction of tube feeds

9. A 96 -year-old female with a past medical history significant for Brugada syndrome is found unconscious in her home by her family after she did not respond to phone calls for 4 days. After interrogation, her pacemaker indicates frequent premature ventricular contractions with no shocks delivered. Laboratory findings include:

Sodium: 130 mEq/L
Potassium: 2.7 mEq/L
Chloride: 110 mEq/L
Bicarbonate: 31 mEq/L
Urea: 62 mg/dL
Creatinine: 2.1 mg/dL

Following initiation of tube feeds, the patient appears clinically weaker and remains lethargic. Which of the following is the MOST appropriate next step in management?

A. Reduce tube feeds
B. Hemodialysis
C. Replete potassium
D. Administer hypertonic saline

10. A 100-kg patient on postoperative day 8 after an emergent colectomy is now status post tracheostomy insertion, and all abdominal drains have been removed. The patient is currently not on tube feeds, is receiving 50 mcg/kg per minute of propofol, 100 mcg/hour of fentanyl, and routine gastrointestinal prophylaxis and thromboprophylaxis. You are called to the bedside while she us undergoing indirect calorimetry assessment, with results on the screen shown here (image courtesy of George Williams).

After considering the patient's resting energy expenditure (REE) as her clinical status, which rate BEST approximates the patient's tube feed requirement?

A. 700 kcal/day
B. 1400 kcal/day
C. 2100 kcal/day
D. 2800 kcal/day

11. A patient is transferred from the floor with altered mental status and marginally responsive to stimulus. The hospitalist service reports that the patient has a history of polysubstance abuse. You decide to place a feeding tube. Which of the following is the BEST indication for placement of a postpyloric feeding tube?

A. Reduced aspiration risk
B. Ease of placement
C. More physiological digestion
D. Acute pancreatitis

12. A patient has failed trials of enteric feeding for 8 days following a complex nephrectomy due to renal cell carcinoma. The team dietitian suggests initiating TPN with lipids. Which of the following is NOT a risk of TPN administration?

A. Inflammation
B. Acalculous cholecystitis
C. Hyperkalemia
D. Hypercapnia

13. Four days after a small bowel resection, a patient with a body mass index of 16 kg/m² has gastric output of 1200 mL/shift, abdominal distention, and no bowel movements. During the morning assessment, the

Time	VCO2	VO2	RQ	REE	REE_Covar	FIO2	Vt BTPS
7:46	241	304	0.79	2110	10	38.39	449
7:49	241	304	0.79	2110	10	38.39	449
7:53	239	300	0.79	2086	10	38.39	446
7:56	241	304	0.79	2110	10	38.39	449

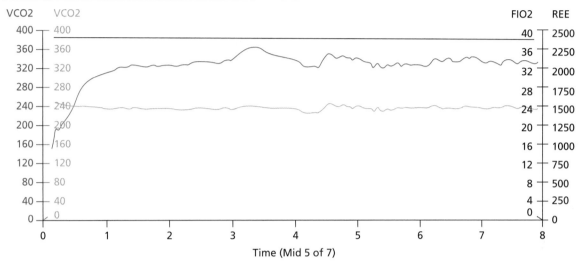

Figure Q10.1

patient apparently has had flatus but no other examination changes. There is no central line present, and the family is concerned about the patient's nutritional status. Which of the following is the MOST appropriate next step?

A. Insert duodenal feeding tube
B. Initiate TPN
C. Indirect calorimetry
D. Resume gastric feeding

14. A patient with a large left lower extremity wound is scheduled for daily plastic surgery procedures over the next two weeks. Although he is conscious and communicating, he cannot swallow and has a duodenal feeding tube placed in order to provide nutrition while not in the operating room. Which of the following would be the MOST effective means of gastric ulcer prophylaxis?

A. Administer tube feeds
B. Antacids
C. Sucralfate
D. Cimetidine

15. A 56-year-old female becomes acutely hypotensive and is requiring vasopressors. She is intubated because of hypoxia that was refractory to high-flow nasal cannula oxygen. Blood cultures are negative, but bronchial alveolar lavage cultures reveal 10,000 CFU of methicillin-resistant *Staphylococcus aureus*. Which of the following would be the MOST appropriate nutritional approach to this patient's care?

A. Arginine supplementation
B. Underfeeding
C. Early TPN
D. Trace elements

ANSWERS

1. ANSWER: C

This patient is receiving 35 kcal/kg per day at his current rate, which can be reasonably calculated in the testing environment. While the range of caloric demand for a critically ill patient is 25 to 35 kcal/kg per day, this requirement tends to change as the admission progresses. After 7 days, most patients enter a recovery phase, which results in a 35- to 50-kcal/kg per day caloric requirement. While the amount of calories that the patient is currently receiving is within this range, it is prudent and most appropriate to measure indirect calorimetry so as to avoid overfeeding and its related complications. Similarly, reducing tube feeds would likely be counterproductive because more clinical data regarding the patient's actual metabolism are needed.

Overfeeding of fats or glucose can stress the patient physiologically and compound insulin resistance. Additionally, when substrate excess is administered, metabolically induced increased oxidative processes and reactive oxygen molecules are promoted. The CT scan demonstrates free abdominal fluid, a clinical finding consistent with the abdominal sepsis that the patient presents with here. As such, repeating the CT scan would likely serve no clinical benefit. While the patient is critically ill, a stool ova and parasites would not be most appropriate.

Keywords: Metabolic assessment (basal and stress energy requirements); Indirect calorimetry

REFERENCES

Cynober L, Moore FA. Nutrition and critical care. In Nitenberg G, ed. Nutritional support in sepsis and multiple organ failure. Nestlé Nutrition Workshop Series Clinical and Performance Program, volume. 8. Basel: Nestec Ltd. Vevey/S. Karger AG; 2003, pp. 223–244.

Griffiths RD. Too much of a good thing: the curse of overfeeding. *Crit Care* 2007;11(6):176.

Rattanachaiwong S, Singer P. Should we calculate or measure energy expenditure? Practical aspects in the ICU. *Nutrition* 2018;55–56:71–75.

2. ANSWER: B

Nitrogen balance is an important tool to determine adequacy of nutrition. Nitrogen balance can be effectively calculated by determining the amount of protein administered (in this case given in the question stem), and the amount of protein lost. Of note, 16% of the weight of protein given is actually nitrogen; therefore, the total amount of protein administered can be divided by 6.25 to obtain the nitrogen administered. With regard to losses, because protein is primarily lost in the urine (~67% of all protein relating to metabolism) and the feces (~4–6 g/day), measuring the urinary urea nitrogen (UUN) and adding 4 to 6 g can provide the total amount of nitrogen lost. Therefore, nitrogen balance = protein administered (g)/6.25 – [UUN + ~4 g].

Prealbumin can be used to measure overall nutrition status because it has a relatively short half-life (2 days) compared with transferrin (7 days). While these tests may be useful, they do not provide an immediate assessment of the patient's hospital nutrition status. Paracetamol absorption is a method of determining absorption in the small intestine and is not affected by absorption in the stomach. This effectively makes paracetamol a measure of the gastric emptying rate. While this may be useful in certain clinical situations, a test of gastric emptying is not related to overall nutritional status.

Keyword: Nitrogen balance, other

3. ANSWER: A

The energy provided by a nutrient type is equal to the heat produced by the nutrient following oxidation; this is normally expressed as kcal/g. Lipids provide the highest amount of energy per gram (9.1 kcal/g), followed by protein (4 kcal/g) and glucose (3.7 kcal/g). When the metabolic oxidation of all provided nutrients are added together, this can be used to determine the REE. The REE should be used to determine the amount of nutrition to provide to a patient owing to the tremendous changes in metabolism that can be seen during critical illness.

Arginine is a precursor to nitric oxide and is used to help rebuild muscle because it is a substrate in that process; it is particularly prone to depletion following trauma. The exact amount of arginine needed to meet metabolic needs is not known, although it is an additive in several types of nutrition formulas.

Keywords: Metabolic assessment (basal and stress energy requirements); Nitrogen balance, other

REFERENCES

Cynober L, Moore FA. Nutrition and critical care. In Nitenberg G, ed. Nutritional support in sepsis and multiple organ failure. Nestlé Nutrition Workshop Series Clinical and Performance Program, volume. 8. Basel: Nestec Ltd. Vevey/S. Karger AG; 2003, pp. 223–244.

Marino P. *The ICU book*. Philadelphia: Wolters Kluwer Health/ Lippincott Williams & Wilkins; 2014, pp. 847–848.

4. ANSWER: D

This patient is presenting with clinical signs of sepsis and is on TPN. It is surmised that the possible immunosuppressive effect of lipids in the septic patient occurs because long-chain fatty acids reduce the functionality of the reticulo-endothelial system, neutrophils, and the relative presence of helper and suppressor T cells. While oxidization of fatty acids is not shown to be impaired, sepsis appears to reduce the metabolism of fatty acids, leading to higher lipid concentrations in the blood and further exacerbating the potential for worsening of the sepsis.

While peripheral vascular disease is possible given the presence of diabetes, the stem does not provide any information making this selection more likely. Although hypothermia may result in metabolic dysfunction, this presentation is more likely the result of overwhelming sepsis and not the cause of infection or immunosuppression. Deep vein thrombosis may result in fever, but it is not characteristically associated with fever and hypotension.

Keyword: Nutritional support (enteral, parenteral)

REFERENCES

Marino P. *The ICU book*. Philadelphia: Wolters Kluwer Health/Lippincott Williams & Wilkins; 2014, pp. 847–848.
Vincent J, Abraham E, Moore F et al. *Textbook of critical care*, 6th edition. Philadelphia: Elsevier Saunders; 2011, p. 724.

5. ANSWER: A

Thiamine (vitamin B_1) is key in carbohydrate metabolism because it functions as a coenzyme for pyruvate dehydrogenase (which allows pyruvate to enter mitochondria). Because of this, thiamine deficiency affects the brain, which is sensitive to disruptions in availability of adenosine triphosphate. Overall, it is likely that vitamin requirements are higher for septic patients than for normal patients because reports of deficiency have been written in the absence of supplementation.

Vitamin E is helpful in reducing reperfusion injury following aortic cross-clamping, and serum levels may be useful to monitor if deficiency is suspected; it does not appear to be pertinent in this presentation. Selenium deficiency has been shown to be associated with sepsis, and supplementation of selenium may be helpful in reducing mortality in sepsis, although no effect on length of stay or pneumonia was found. As such, more data are needed to confirm the role of selenium in sepsis. Linoleic acid is the only fatty acid that must be ingested or provided in the diet. A scaly rash, susceptibility to infection, and cardiac dysfunction are seen with this deficiency. Linoleic acid is provided automatically in most nutritional regimens, and safflower oil should be the additive in order to provide this essential item.

Keyword: Nutritional deficiencies

REFERENCES

Alhazzani W, Jacobi J, Sindi A et al. The effect of selenium therapy on mortality in patients with sepsis syndrome: a systematic review and meta-analysis of randomized controlled trials. *Crit Care Med* 2013;41(6):1555–1564.
Marino P. *The ICU book*. Philadelphia: Wolters Kluwer Health/Lippincott Williams & Wilkins; 2014, pp. 851–853.

6. ANSWER: B

The patient presents following protracted diarrhea with likely associated volume loss and hypokalemia. The ECG shown demonstrates T-wave inversion with mild tachycardia, which would be consistent with both hypokalemia and hypovolemia. While muscle weakness may be seen in hypokalemia, most patients do not have symptoms. Approximately 50% of patients present with ECG changes. None of the provided answers would result in fluid resuscitation appropriate for this presentation because only 7% of D_5 water administered would remain intravascular after administration, and it could also lead to hypovolemic hyponatremia in this case. There is no indication of anemia based on the clinical data provided. Because being afebrile is implied (normal vital signs), with a marginally elevated WBC count, the need for antibiotics is questionable and therefore not the BEST answer based on the information provided.

Keywords: Diarrhea, nausea, vomiting

REFERENCE

Marino P. *The ICU book*. Philadelphia: Wolters Kluwer Health/Lippincott Williams & Wilkins; 2014, p. 677.

7. ANSWER: C

The KUB and presentation described are consistent with an ileus. While less common, urinary tract infections may lead to an ileus or a small bowel obstruction picture. Although an ileus may prevent administration of tube feeds, TPN should not be given immediately because it is associated with disruption of gut mucosa and infectious complications. IV fluids may be helpful and commonly needed in the setting of ileus, but a bolus does not appear to be needed under these circumstances because the patient is urinating well. IV fluids are certainly useful while providing bowel rest for patients with an ileus (e.g., Ogilvie syndrome or pseudo-obstruction).

Endoscopy may eventually be part of the patient's workup, but at this junction in his care, allowing the ileus to resolve would be more appropriate. If further workup is required, oral contrast with Gastrografin may aid both in diagnosis of the degree of obstruction and in resolving an obstruction owing to its osmotic effect. Antibiotics to treat the urinary tract infection would be the most helpful option out of the choices given for this specific presentation.

Keyword: Ileus

REFERENCE

Miraflor E, Green A. Small bowel obstruction. In: Harken A, Moore E, eds. *Abernathy's surgical secrets*, 7th edition. Philadelphia: Elsevier; 2018.

8. ANSWER: C

Diarrhea is a common presentation in the ICU and has many potential causes. Overfeeding is a common cause of diarrhea and occurs in 33% of ICU patients. In this case, a 70-kg patient is being fed slightly less than 25 kcal/kg per day; it is important to note that this is following a calculation of her ideal body weight, which is 70 kg based on a height of 175 cm [ideal body weight = height (cm) – 100 (in males)…*or* = height (cm) – 105 (in females). Therefore, this diarrhea is not resulting from overfeeding, and reduction in tube feeding amount is unlikely to be helpful. Undigested proteins can lead to diarrhea, especially when postpyloric tubes are being used; in this case, the KUB demonstrates a tube that is in the stomach. High fructose may lead to this as well (no indication of this based on the question), and gastrointestinal tract atrophy may cause diarrhea as well. Although the patient is on acetaminophen, an antipyretic would not likely suppress a *C. difficile* mega colonic fever, and therefore vancomycin would not be appropriate (although it remains the preferred first-line therapy).

Given the previous discussion, sorbitol-containing drugs are the most likely way to resolve or reduce this patient's diarrhea and related malabsorption. Sorbitol is considered inert by the US Food and Drug Administration and is frequently added to medications to provide sweetness and texture. However, just 10 to 20 grams of sorbitol can cause diarrhea; this amount can be contained in just two to three doses of medication. Oral cimetidine contains sorbitol and would therefore likely worsen the patient's presentation.

Keyword: Malabsorption

REFERENCES

Btaiche IF, Chan LN, Pleva M, Kraft MD. Critical illness, gastrointestinal complications, and medication therapy during enteral feeding in critically ill adult patients. *Nutr Clin Pract* 2010;25(1):32–49.

Vincent J, Abraham E, Moore F et al. *Textbook of critical care*, 7th edition. Philadelphia: Elsevier; 2017, pp. 103–104.

9. ANSWER: A

This patient is demonstrating the overall electrolyte derangements consistent with refeeding syndrome. Refeeding syndrome is manifested by acute reduction in many of the electrolytes, which are principally intracellular, including potassium, sodium, magnesium, and phosphorus. Additionally, water balance may be altered, and thiamine deficiency can occur. The patient appears to have a hypovolemic hyponatremia, and her weakness suggests hypophosphatemia. Hypertonic saline may improve the lab results but is not indicated given her volume status and does not address the underlying problem. Reducing tube feedings to less than 500 kcal/day is indicated when signs of refeeding syndrome are noted. Hemodialysis does not have a role in managing a patient with refeeding syndrome.

Keyword: Refeeding syndrome

REFERENCE

Vincent J, Abraham E, Moore F et al. *Textbook of critical care*, 7th edition. Philadelphia: Elsevier; 2017, p. 207.

10. ANSWER: B

Propofol contains 1.1 kcal/mL of lipid-based calories. Given the frequency of propofol's use as a sedation agent in the ICU, understanding and being able to calculate the degree to which propofol may affect nutrition is important and frequently germane to the content of daily rounds. The calculation of propofol's calories is manifested by:

[(Propofol mcg/kg/min) × (patient weight in kg) × (60 min)] × (1 mg/1000 mcg) = hourly mg of propofol

So, by entering the information from the question stem:

[(50 mcg/kg/min) × (100 kg) × (60 min)/1000] = (50 × 100 × 60)/1000 = (300,000)/1000 = 300 mg

Since propofol is only available in a concentration of 10 mg/mL, one can immediately determine that the actual pump rate of propofol for this patient is 30 mL/hour, which effectively means that the patient is receiving 30 kcal/hour of propofol, or 720 kcal/day. After knowing this information, and then knowing from the indirect calorimetry report shown that the patient has an REE of about 2110 kcal/day, the patient only *needs* the remaining calories not provided by propofol [2110 kcal (REE) – 720 kcal (propofol)], which is 1390 kcal. Anything more that this would, by definition, be overfeeding.

Keyword: Enteral and parenteral nutrition (formula, caloric intake)

11. ANSWER: D

Because a postpyloric tube bypasses the stomach and potentially the duodenum, there is less stimulation of the exocrine function of the pancreas while still maintaining the intestinal barrier. In either case, guidelines still recommend feeding in acute pancreatitis because several meta-analyses demonstrate a reduction in length of stay and complications. While a nasojejunal tube may be smaller, placement is not easier compared with placement of a gastric tube because a gastric tube may be placed at the bedside by most hospital personnel with a minor amount of training. It should be noted that 1% of feeding tube insertions go into the trachea and that a chest radiograph is required before use of a feeding tube (auscultating for bowel sounds with a push of air can be misleading).

Feeding into the stomach is more physiological and allows the intrinsic digestive process to regulate gastric emptying and to introduce food into the small bowel. Valentine et al. demonstrated that gastric feeding is also thought to reduce gastric pH compared with postpyloric feeding. Unless the presentation is consistent with gastric ileus, there is no difference in the rate of aspiration between gastric and duodenal feeding.

Keyword: Enteral tubes

REFERENCES

Marik PE, Zaloga GP. Gastric versus post-pyloric feeding: a systematic review. *Crit Care* 2003;7:R46–R51.
Tenner S, Baillie J, DeWitt J, Vege SS; American College of Gastroenterology. American College of Gastroenterology guideline: management of acute pancreatitis. *Am J Gastroenterol* 2013;108(9):1400–1416.
Valentine RJ, Turner WW Jr, Borman KR, Weigelt JA. Does nasoenteral feeding afford adequate gastroduodenal stress prophylaxis? *Crit Care Med* 1986;14(7):599–601.

12. ANSWER: C

With TPN administration, glucose is expected to move intracellularly with an accompanied movement of potassium;
therefore, potassium levels will decrease, not increase. Similarly, because phosphate also follows glucose in order to participate in glucose metabolism, hypophosphatemia may occur when TPN is initiated. Hypercapnia may be produced with excess carbohydrate retention associated with overfeeding in general, which is seen in patients on TPN.

The lipids (including oleic acid) that are administered with TPN are thought to promote inflammation; in fact, when acute respiratory distress syndrome must be instigated in animal models in order to achieve basic science research, administration of oleic acids is a means to achieve this goal. In general, since lipid emulsions used in TPN have an abundance of oxidizable lipids, an inflammatory response should be expected. Because TPN is associated with discontinuation of fat content in the gut, the gallbladder is no longer required to contract. This process leads to sludge buildup in the gallbladder, which in time leads to acalculous cholecystitis.

Keyword: Acalculous cholecystitis

REFERENCE

Marino P. *The ICU book*. Philadelphia: Wolters Kluwer Health/Lippincott Williams & Wilkins; 2014, pp. 881.

13. ANSWER: A

The patient has symptoms consistent with a gastric ileus, which is common and even expected following abdominal surgery. Placement of a duodenal feeding tube could be helpful in bypassing the region of the ileus, although this would need to be done slowly to ensure that the patient tolerates feeding appropriately. TPN *could* be used in this patient, although given a high rate of complications, infection, intestinal barrier breakdown, and so forth (see earlier question), TPN is not normally started until after 5 to 7 days of no nutrition (unless it is expected that the lack of nutrition would be prolonged). Additionally, the patient would have to have central access in order to receive TPN. This is because the final concentration of TPN is commonly about 35% dextrose, which has a relative osmolality of 1800 mOsm/kg water; this concentration is poorly tolerated in the veins, necessitating a central line for administration. Once infused centrally, TPN is immediately diluted in the higher flow blood of the vena cava or femoral vein.

Indirect calorimetry could be useful in determining caloric needs of the patient but would not be helpful in achieving nutrition, making this choice not an ideal next step. Resuming gastric feeding may be possible eventually, but with high gastric residual and output being reported, this is not the appropriate time to initiate gastric feeding.

Keyword: Enteral nutrition

REFERENCE

Morgan S, Weinsier R, eds. *Fundamentals of clinical nutrition*, 2nd edition. St. Louis: Mosby; 1998, p. 201.

14. ANSWER: D

Cimetidine is a histamine-2 receptor antagonist, a commonly used class of medications to achieve ulcer prophylaxis, and has been demonstrated to be more effective than sucralfate alone. Additionally, sucralfate is a cytoprotective agent, which works by forming a protective layer physically in the stomach. Because of this mechanism, no change in gastric pH is expected, which can be helpful in maintaining normal flora. Sucralfate is not the best choice for a second reason: it does not work unless administered in the stomach or orally, and it does not have an effect if given in a postpyloric tube.

Antacids have not been demonstrated to be an adequate prophylactic agent and therefore should not be used. Enteral nutrition is considered by some as an option to reduce the risk for gastric bleeding; however, this has not been demonstrated consistently in the literature, possibly because it is challenging to consistently provide nutrition in the critical care setting. In this case, the question stem indicated frequent trips to the operating room; this patient would not realistically be able to benefit from the tube feedings that he eventually receives because of the intermittent nature of his feeding schedule.

Keywords: Gastrointestinal motility dysfunction; Malabsorption

REFERENCE

Deutschman C, Neligan P. *Evidence-based practice of critical care.* Philadelphia: Saunders; 2010, p. 487.

15. ANSWER: D

Trace elements such as selenium and zinc are commonly deficient in critically ill patients, and their repletion has minimal risks when dosed properly. Repletion should be based on levels assessed, and parenteral nutrition solution is not the ideal source for the entirety of the trace elements administered (the volumes would be too high); therefore, many of these supplements are given separately intravenously and cannot be given by nasogastric tube. Selenium and zinc levels are best checked between 7 and 10 days if the level is not known at baseline. Multiple observational studies have evaluated underfeeding as a mechanism of caring for critically ill patients. It generally appears that there may be a role in underfeeding around 80% or slightly less in many critically ill patients, but this has not been evaluated with a randomized control trial; current trials link increased length of stay with exceeding 80% of calorie goals. Currently, it appears that there is no mortality benefit, but there is a benefit in reducing infectious complication when enteral nutrition is chosen over parenteral nutrition; therefore, early TPN would not be the best choice.

Arginine supplementation has been demonstrated to improve wound healing immune function in humans and animals. The mechanisms of this benefit include effects mimicking growth hormone, stimulation of T cells, availability of collagen molecules, and substrate for the generation of nitric oxide. The problem is that arginine in sepsis is contraindicated because of worsening of septic shock in canine studies. Currently, arginine is not recommended in the setting of septic shock, as is the case in this patient.

Keyword: Enteral and parenteral nutrition (formula, caloric intake)

REFERENCES

Deutschman C, Neligan P. *Evidence-based practice of critical care.* Philadelphia: Saunders; 2010, pp. 461–477.

Hise ME, Halterman K, Gajewski BJ et al. Feeding practices of severely ill intensive care unit patients: an evaluation of energy sources and clinical outcomes. *J Am Diet Assoc* 2007;107:458–465.

INDEX